Clinical Anatomy
of the Eye

SECOND EDITION

Clinical Anatomy

of the Eye

SECOND EDITION

Richard S. Snell, M.D., Ph.D.

Emeritus Professor of Anatomy, The George Washington School of Medicine and Health Sciences, Washington, D.C.

Michael A. Lemp, M.D.

Clinical Professor of Ophthalmology, Georgetown University Medical Center, President, University of Ophthalmic Consultants of Washington, Washington, D.C.

Illustrations by Ira Grunther, B.S., A.M.I.

Blackwell
Science

© 1998 by Blackwell Science, Inc.
Blackwell Science Ltd, a Blackwell Publishing company

Editorial offices:
Blackwell Science Ltd, 9600 Garsington Road, Oxford OX4 2DQ, UK
    Tel: +44 (0) 1865 776868
Blackwell Publishing Inc., 350 Main Street, Malden, MA 02148-5020, USA
    Tel: +1 781 388 8250
Blackwell Science Asia Pty, 550 Swanston Street, Carlton, Victoria 3053, Australia
    Tel: +61 (0)3 8359 1011

First edition published 1989 (ISBN 978-0-865-42053-3)
Second edition first published 1998
12   2012

ISBN 978-0-6320-4344-6

Library of Congress Cataloging-in-Publication Data

Snell, Richard S.
    Clinical anatomy of the eye / Richard S. Snell, Michael A. Lemp.—2nd ed.
        p.   cm.
    Includes bibliographical references and index.
    ISBN 978-0-6320-4344-6
    1. Eye—Anatomy 2. Eye-sockets—Anatomy. I. Lemp, Michael A. II. Title.
    [DNLM: 1. Eye—anatomy & histology. 2. Orbit—anatomy & histology. 3. Cranial
Nerves—anatomy & histology. 4. Eye Diseases—diagnosis. WW 101 671c 1997]
    QM511.S64   1997
    611'.84—dc21
    DNLM/DLC
    for Library of Congress   97-39908
                                                                         CIP

A catalogue record for this title is available from the British Library

Typeset by Publication Services, WG, Inc
Printed and bound in Malaysia by Vivar Printing Sdn Bhd

For further information on Blackwell Publishing, visit our website:
www.blackwellpublishing.com

Contents

Preface

Clinical Anatomy of the Eye has proved to be a very popular textbook for ophthalmologists and optometrists in training both in the United States and in many other parts of the world. We wish to thank the many colleagues and students who have provided us with suggestions to improve the second edition.

The objective of the book remains unchanged: to provide the reader with the basic knowledge of anatomy necessary to practice ophthalmology. It is recognized that this medical specialty requires a detailed knowledge of the anatomy of the eyeball and the surrounding structures. The specialist's knowledge should include not only gross anatomic features and their development, but also the microscopic anatomy of the eyeball and the ocular appendages. The nerve and blood supply to the orbit, the autonomic innervation of the orbital structures, the visual pathway, and associated visual reflexes should receive great emphasis.

The practical application of anatomic facts to ophthalmology is emphasized throughout this book in the form of Clinical Notes in each chapter. Clinical Problems requiring anatomic knowledge for their solution are presented at the end of each chapter.

Most of the illustrations have been kept simple, and many are in color. Overview drawings of the distribution of the cranial and autonomic nerves have been included.

In this edition, a new chapter on the cranial nerves other than those present within the orbit has been added for completeness. Many new tables have been included to aid the learning process. The clinical material has been brought up-to-date and the anatomy involved with new clinical techniques has been introduced. The radiographs, CT scans, and MRIs have been updated and a PET scan has been added. Again, the surface anatomy and surface landmarks have been emphasized, with photographs of living subjects added to assist this study.

We extend grateful thanks to Drs. Geva E. Mannor, Douglas E. Gaasterland, and John F. O'Neill who carefully read chapters of the manuscript and made valuable suggestions, many of which have been incorporated into the final text.

We are greatly indebted to Dr. David O. Davis of the Department of Radiology at the George Washington University School of Medicine for the loan of radiographs and CT scans that have been reproduced in different sections of this book. We are also grateful to Dr. Gordon Sze of the Department of Radiology at Yale University Medical Center for examples of CT scans and MRIs of the brain.

We once again give our sincere thanks to Ira Alan Grunther for the very fine art.

To the staff of Blackwell Science, we express our appreciation for guiding this book through every phase of its production.

Richard S. Snell
Michael A. Lemp
1997

Development of the Eye and the Ocular Appendages

CHAPTER OUTLINE

Introduction

The eye is formed from both ectoderm and mesenchyme. The ectoderm that is derived from the neural tube gives rise to the retina, the nerve fibers of the optic nerve, and the smooth muscle of the iris. The surface ectoderm on the side of the head forms the corneal and conjunctival epithelium, the lens, and the lacrimal and tarsal glands. The mesenchyme forms the corneal stroma, the sclera, the choroid, the iris, the ciliary musculature, part of the vitreous body, and the cells lining the anterior chamber. The endothelium of the cornea is believed to be of neural crest origin.

The reader should note the importance of the induction of one ocular tissue by another during development. The lens, for example, is induced to develop by the presence of the optic vesicle. The presence of the developing lens induces the formation of the cornea and stimulates the development of the vitreous body. The presence of the developing lens is also important for the normal growth of the pigment layer of the retina, which in turn influences the differentiation of the mesenchyme into the choroid and the sclera. How this induction process is brought about remains to be determined.

The Eyeball

The rudimentary eyeball develops as an ectodermal diverticulum from the lateral aspect of the forebrain (Fig. 1-1). The diverticulum grows out laterally toward the side of the head, and the end becomes slightly dilated to form the *optic vesicle,* while the proximal portion becomes constricted to form the *optic stalk* (Fig. 1-1). At the same time, a small area of surface ectoderm overlying the optic vesicle thickens to form the *lens placode.* The lens placode invaginates and sinks below the surface ectoderm to become the *lens vesicle.* Meanwhile, the optic vesicle becomes invaginated to form the double-layered *optic cup.* The inferior edge of the optic cup is deficient, and this notch is continuous with a groove on the inferior aspect of the optic stalk called the *optic or choroidal fissure* (Fig. 1-1). Vascular mesenchyme now grows into the optic fissure and takes with it the *hyaloid artery.* Later, this fissure becomes narrowed by growth of its margins around the artery, and by the seventh week of embryonic development the fissure closes, forming a narrow tube, the *optic canal,* inside the optic stalk (Fig. 1-2). Failure of the fissure to close completely results in coloboma formation (see p. 18), which may include the pupil, ciliary body, and choroid or optic nerve. By the fifth week, the lens vesicle loses contact with the surface ectoderm and lies within the mouth of the optic cup, the edges of which form the future *pupil* (Fig. 1-3).

The Retina

The retina develops from the optic cup. For purposes of description, the retina may be divided into two developmental layers, the pigment layer and the neural layer.

The *pigment layer* is formed from the outer thinner layer of the optic cup (Fig. 1-3). It is a single layer of cells that become columnar in shape and develop pigment granules (melanosomes) within their cytoplasm.

● **Figure 1-1**

(A) Dorsal view, showing the formation of the optic vesicle, which grows out
as a diverticulum from the lateral aspect of the forebrain. (B) Coronal section of
diencephalon, showing a thickening of the surface ectoderm overlying the optic
vesicle to form the lens placode. (C) Coronal section of diencephalon, showing the
lens placode invaginating and sinking below the surface ectoderm. Note that the
optic vesicle is also becoming invaginated. (D) The formation of the lens vesicle,
the optic cup, and the choroidal fissure.

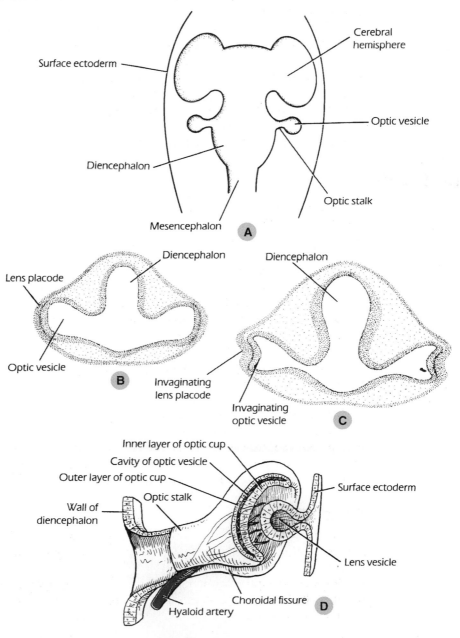

Figure 1-2

(A–E) A series of diagrams illustrating the formation of the optic cup from the optic vesicle. Note that the inferior edge of the optic cup is deficient, and that this notch is continuous with the choroidal fissure. The lips of the choroidal fissure fuse around the hyaloid artery and vein.

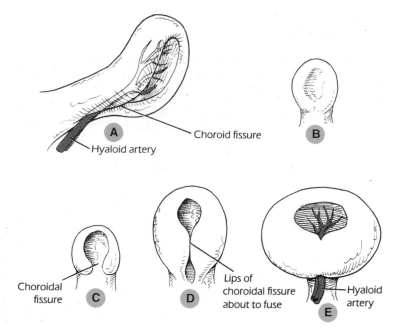

The *neural layer* is formed from the inner layer of the optic cup. However, in the region of the cup that overlaps the lens, the inner layer is not differentiated into nervous tissue. This anterior one-fifth of the inner layer persists as a layer of columnar cells, which, together with the pigmented epithelium of the outer layer, extend forward onto the posterior surface of the developing ciliary body and iris (Fig. 1-4).

The posterior four-fifths of the inner layer of the optic cup undergoes cellular proliferation, forming an outer *nuclear zone* and an inner *marginal zone*, devoid of nuclei (Fig. 1-3). Later, the cells of the nuclear zone invade the marginal zone so that the neural part of the retina is made up of an *inner and an outer neuroblastic layer*. The inner neuroblastic layer forms the ganglion cells, the amacrine cells, and the bodies of the sustentacular fibers of Müller. The outer neuroblastic layer gives rise to the horizontal and rod and cone bipolar nerve cells and the rod and cone cells. By the eighth month of fetal life all the layers of the retina can be recognized. It should be noted that the retinal photoreceptor cells continue to form after birth so that the retina develops the ability for increasing resolution and sensitivity.

Thus, the inner layer of the optic cup may be divided into a small nonnervous portion near the edge of the cup and a large photosensitive portion, the two being separated by a wavy line, the *ora serrata* (Fig. 1-4).

It is interesting to remember that the cavity of the optic vesicle is continuous through the optic canal with the cavity of the diencephalon (i.e., that part which will form the third ventricle). Early in development, the outermost layer of cells of the nuclear zone have cilia, which are continuous with the ciliated ependymal cells of the third ventricle. Later, during the seventh week of development, the cilia of the cells of the nuclear zone disappear and are believed to be replaced by the outer segments of the rods and cones during the fourth month.

Figure 1-3

The eye at different stages of development. (A) The formation of the lens from the lens vesicle and its nourishment by the hyaloid artery. Note the further development of the inner and outer layers of the optic cup and the continued presence of the cavity of the optic vesicle. (B) The development of the cornea, the anterior chamber, and the pupillary membrane. The cavity of the lens vesicle is still present. The eyelids have fused and remain so until the seventh month before birth.

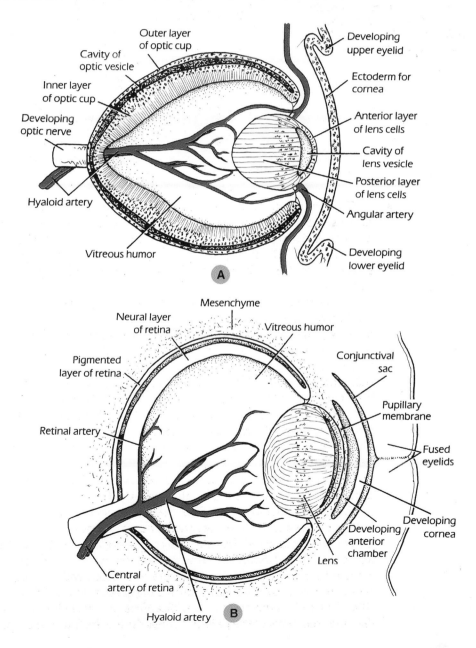

Figure 1-4

(A, B) The eye in advanced stages of development. Note the degeneration of the hyaloid vessels and the persistence of the hyaloid canal in the vitreous body. The remains of the hyaloid vessels become the central artery and vein of the retina. The lacrimal gland has developed as an outgrowth of the conjunctival sac.

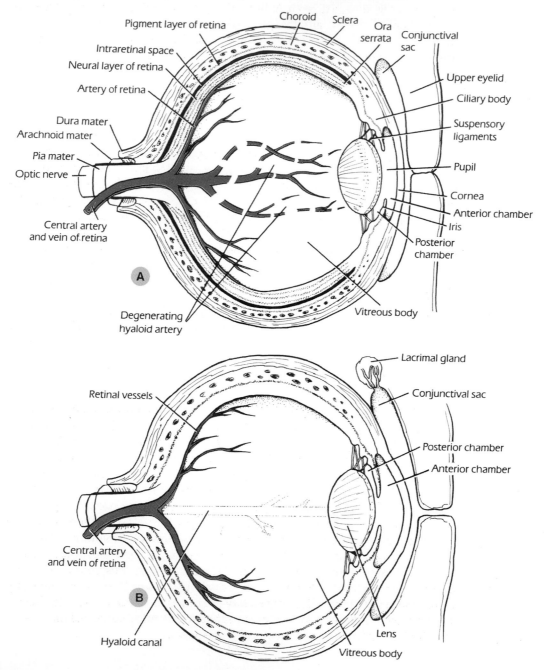

Macular Area and Fovea Centralis

The macular area first develops as a localized increase of superimposed nuclei in the ganglion cell layer, lateral to the optic disc, just after midterm. During the seventh month there is a peripheral displacement of the ganglion cells, leaving a central shallow depression, the *fovea centralis*. The inner segments of the foveal cones decrease in width, but the outer segments are elongated. This permits an increase in foveal cone density. At birth, the ganglion cells have been reduced to a single layer in the fovea, and by 4 months of age the cone nuclei in the center of the fovea have no ganglion cells covering them. The reason for the newborn's imperfect central fixation is that the cones do not fully develop until several months after birth.

The Optic Nerve

The ganglion cells of the retina develop axons that converge to a point where the optic stalk leaves the posterior surface of the optic cup. This site will later become the *optic disc*. The axons now pass among the cells that form the inner layer of the stalk (Fig. 1-5). Gradually, the inner layer encroaches on the cavity of the stalk until the inner and outer layers fuse. The cells of the optic stalk form neuroglial supporting cells to the axons, and the cavity of the stalk disappears. The stalk, together with the optic axons, forms the optic nerve. The axons of the optic nerve begin to develop their myelin sheaths just before birth, but the process of myelination continues for some time after birth. The partial decussation of the axons of the two optic nerves forms the *optic chiasma*. The hyaloid artery and vein become the *central artery* and *vein of the retina*.

The optic nerve axons leave the optic chiasma and grow backward as the *optic tracts* and the majority pass to the lateral geniculate body and to the tectum of the midbrain.

The Lens

The rudimentary lens is first seen as a thickening of the surface ectoderm, the *lens placode*, at 22 days' gestation; it overlies the optic vesicle (Fig. 1-1). The lens placode invaginates and sinks below the surface ectoderm to form the *lens vesicle*, which consists of a single layer of cells covered by a basal lamina.

The cells forming the posterior wall of the lens now rapidly elongate and become filled with proteins called *crystallins*, which make them transparent (Figs. 1-3 and 1-4). These densely packed elongated cells are known as the *primary lens fibers*. The base of each elongating cell remains attached to the basal lamina posteriorly while their apices grow forward toward the anterior lens epithelium so that the cavity of the lens vesicle gradually becomes obliterated. The lengthening of the cells first occurs at the center of the posterior wall, which projects forward into the lens cavity. The nuclei of the lens fibers move anteriorly within the cells to form a line convex forward called the *nuclear bow* (Fig. 1-6). The primary lens fibers now become attached to the apical surface of the anterior lens epithelium and their nuclei disappear.

Figure 1-5

A series of diagrams showing the formation of the optic nerve from the optic stalk, as seen in cross-section. (A) The cavity of the optic stalk. (B) The choroidal fissure occupied by the hyaloid vessels, which become the central artery and vein of the retina. Note the presence of the optic nerve axons growing among the cells forming the inner layer of the optic stalk. The neuroglial cells (oligodendrocytes and astrocytes) are derived from the cells of the inner layer of the optic stalk. (C) The cavity of the optic stalk diminishing in size. (D, E) The surrounding mesenchyme condensing and later differentiating into the meninges, which form a sheath for the optic nerve.

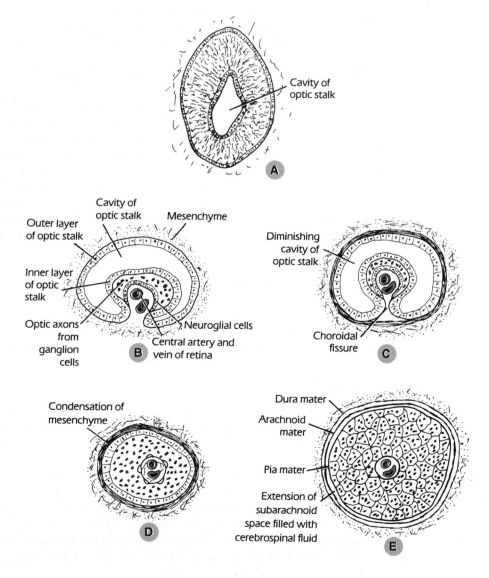

All additional lens fibers are formed by the mitotic division of the anterior epithelial cells at the equator (Fig. 1-7). These are known as the *secondary lens fibers*. New secondary lens fibers are formed throughout life and persist throughout life. The basal ends of the fibers remain attached to the basal lamina, while their apical ends extend around the primary fibers. Thus, each new set of lens fibers is added superficially to the previous layer at the equator and the lens enlarges and becomes more ellipsoid. Since the lens fibers are laid down concentrically, the lens on section has a laminated appearance (Fig. 1-6).

It is interesting to note that none of the lens fibers runs completely from the anterior to the posterior surface of the lens. The ends of the fibers come into apposition at sites referred to as *sutures*. The fibers run in a curved course from the sutures on the anterior surface to those on the posterior surface (Fig. 1-7). The anterior suture line is shaped like an upright Y, and the posterior suture line is like an inverted Y.

In the fetus the lens grows rapidly, because it is supplied by the hyaloid artery, which forms a plexus on the posterior surface of the lens. It is nearly spherical in shape, is soft, and has a reddish tint. By the time the infant is born, the anteroposterior diameter of the lens is nearly that of an adult; its equatorial diameter is about two-thirds of that reached in the adult. The increase in size of the equatorial diameter with age is due largely to the continued production of new secondary lens fibers. The lens increases in density during development as successive fibers become tightly apposed and the layers become interdigitated. Increased amounts of fibrillar material also appear within the fiber cytoplasm.

The structure of the lens is taken advantage of in certain phacoemulsification surgical techniques such as the "phaco chop" and the "phaco stop" and the "phaco stop and chop" techniques. See Chapter 6.

The Vascular Lens Capsule

The vascular capsule is formed from the mesenchyme that surrounds the lens. In the earliest stages of development, it receives an abundant arterial supply from the hyaloid artery. Later, this blood supply regresses, and the vascular capsule disappears before birth. For its nutrition, the lens now depends on diffusion from the aqueous and vitreous humors.

The Lens Capsule

The true lens capsule is a noncellular envelope that completely surrounds the lens. It is formed from the thickened basal lamina, which is developed from the lens epithelium.

The Ciliary Body and Suspensory Ligaments of the Lens

The mesenchyme, situated at the edge of the optic cup, differentiates into the connective tissue of the ciliary body, the smooth muscle fibers of the ciliary muscle, and the suspensory ligaments of the lens. The two layers of neuroectoderm forming the edge of the optic cup grow onto the posterior surface of the ciliary muscle, forming the two epithelial layers covering the ciliary body.

Figure 1-6

(A) Diagram of a section of a developing eye showing the invasion of the optic cup by surrounding mesenchyme. Note the great elongation of the cells forming the posterior wall of the lens vesicle and the forward movement of the nuclei to form the nuclear bow. The pigment layer and the neural layer of the retina can be easily recognized. (B) A much later stage in the development, showing the disappearance of the cavity of the lens vesicle and the arrangement of the primary lens fibers.

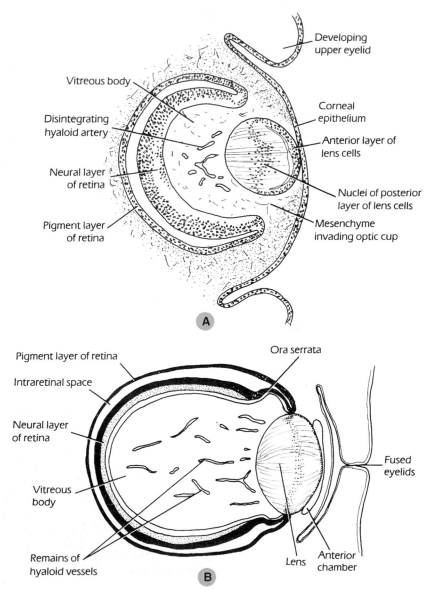

Figure 1-7

Diagrams showing the formation of the secondary lens fibers. (A, B) New secondary lens fibers are formed throughout life by the division of the anterior epithelial cells at the lens equator. The lens fibers (cells) elongate, the anterior end of each fiber extending forward and the posterior end extending backward. (C) The anterior and posterior ends of the fibers unite with each other at suture lines, which in the fetus have the form of an erect Y on the anterior surface and an inverted Y on the posterior surface. Succeeding generations of new fibers cover their predecessors and extend anteriorly and posteriorly, joining fellow fibers formed at about the same time all around the equator.

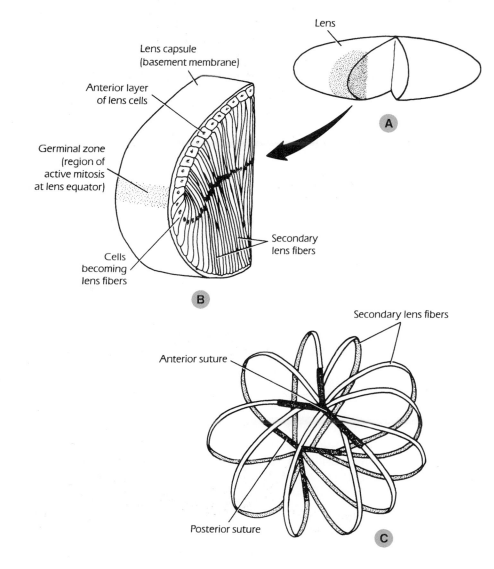

The Iris

The mesenchyme situated on the anterior surface of the lens condenses to form the *pupillary membrane* (Fig. 1-8). The two layers of neuroectoderm forming the edge of the optic cup, having covered the ciliary muscle, now extend onto the posterior surface of the pupillary membrane. These structures fuse to become the iris. The *sphincter* and *dilator muscles of the pupil* are derived from the pigment cells of the neuroectoderm. The mesenchyme forms the connective tissue and blood vessels of the iris. Pigment cells derived from the neuroectoderm penetrate the sphincter muscle and enter the connective tissue. The opening in the central part of the iris becomes the *pupil*. In its earliest development, the pupillary membrane to begin with is attached to the edge of the pupil. Later, as the result of a split in the mesenchyme, the pupillary membrane begins to separate from the iris but remains attached to the front of it. At about the eighth month the pupillary membrane starts to degenerate and eventually disappears. Fine fibrillary remnants often persist even after birth.

The Anterior and Posterior Chambers

The anterior chamber arises as a slit in the mesenchyme between the surface ectoderm and the developing iris. The posterior chamber develops as a split in the mesenchyme posterior to the developing iris and anterior to the developing lens (Fig. 1-4). The anterior and posterior chambers communicate when the pupillary membrane disappears and the pupil is formed. The aqueous humor now fills the anterior and posterior chambers of the eyeball.

The Vitreous Body

The vitreous body develops between the lens and the optic cup. The *primitive* or *primary vitreous* consists of a network of delicate cytoplasmic processes that are derived partly from the ectodermal cells of the developing lens and partly from the neuroectoderm of the retinal layer of the optic cup. The mesenchyme that enters the cup through the choroidal fissure contains many vascular elements, including the vasa hyaloidea propria, which join the primitive vitreous. At this stage the primitive vitreous is supplied by the hyaloid artery and its branches (Fig. 1-3).

The *definitive or secondary vitreous* arises between the primitive vitreous and the retina and develops from the retina. It is at first a homogeneous gel that rapidly increases in volume and pushes the primitive vitreous anteriorly to behind the lens. The secondary vitreous is basically an extracellular matrix consisting mainly of type II collagen.

Hyalocytes, derived from the mesenchyme around the hyaloid vessels and possibly from blood-derived monocytes, now migrate into the definitive vitreous. Later, the hyaloid vessels atrophy and disappear, leaving the acellular hyaloid canal.

The *tertiary vitreous* is the term applied to the phase of development in which large numbers of collagen fibers develop with formation of the zonular fibers, which extend between the ciliary processes and the lens capsule.

Figure 1-8

(A, B) Diagrams showing the development of the ciliary body and iris. The two layers of ectoderm forming the edge of the optic cup cover the ciliary muscle and then extend onto the posterior surface of the pupillary membrane.

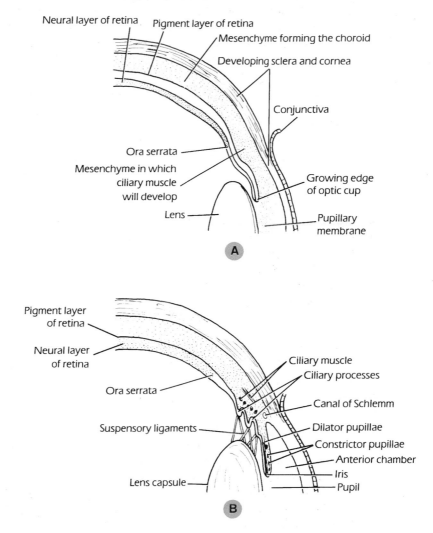

The Cornea

The formation of the cornea is induced by the lens and the optic cup (Fig. 1-3). The corneal epithelium forms from the surface ectoderm. The substantia propria is formed from mesenchyme. The endothelium covering its posterior surface is derived from the neural crest.

Bowman's membrane, which lies immediately beneath the basal lamina of the corneal epithelium, is formed from mesenchyme. *Descemet's membrane*, which is the basement membrane of the endothelial cells, is synthesized by the endothelial cells.

The Sclera

The sclera, the outer tough fibrous coat of the eyeball, is formed from a condensation of the mesenchyme outside the optic cup (Fig. 1-8). It first forms near the future insertion of the rectus muscles.

The Choroid

The choroid, the inner vascular coat of the eyeball, develops early and is formed from the mesenchyme surrounding the optic vesicle (Fig. 1-8).

The Extraocular Muscles

The four rectus muscles and the superior and inferior oblique muscles of the eyeball are formed from the mesenchyme in the region of the developing eyeball (prechordal mesenchyme). Originally represented as a single mass of mesenchyme, they later separate into distinct muscles, first at their insertions and later still at their origins. The levator palpebrae superioris is formed last, splitting off from the mesenchyme that forms the superior rectus muscle. During development the extraocular muscles become associated with the third, fourth, and sixth cranial nerves.

Accessory Eye Structures

The Eyelids

The *eyelids* develop as folds of surface ectoderm above and below the developing cornea (Fig. 1-3). As they grow, they become united with each other at about the third month of intrauterine life. The lids remain fused until about the fifth month, when they start to separate. Separation of the eyelids is complete by the seventh month. While the lids are fused, a closed space, the *conjunctival sac*, exists in front of the cornea. The mesenchymal core of the lids forms the connective tissue and *tarsal plates*. The *orbicularis oculi muscle* is formed from the mesenchyme of the second pharyngeal arch, which invades the eyelids and is supplied by the seventh cranial nerve.

The *eyelashes* develop as epithelial buds from the surface ectoderm. They arise first in the upper lid and are arranged in two or three rows, one behind the other. The ciliary *glands of Moll and Zeis* grow out from the ciliary follicles. The *tarsal glands* (meibomian glands) develop as columns of ectodermal cells from the lid margins.

The Lacrimal Gland

The *lacrimal gland* forms as a series of ectodermal buds that grow superolaterally from the superior fornix of the conjunctiva into the underlying mesenchyme. These buds later canalize, forming the secretory units and multiple ducts of the gland (Fig. 1-4). The gland becomes divided into orbital and palpebral parts with the development of the levator palpebrae superioris. Tears are not produced until the third month after birth.

The Lacrimal Sac and Nasolacrimal Duct

The lacrimal sac and nasolacrimal duct initially develop as a solid cord of ectodermal cells between the lateral nasal process and the maxillary process of the developing face. Later, the cord becomes canalized to form the *nasolacrimal duct*, and the superior end becomes dilated to form the *lacrimal sac*. Incomplete canalization, particularly in the lower end of the system is common, even in full-term infants (see p. 18). Further cellular proliferation results in the formation of *lacrimal ducts*, which enter each eyelid.

The Orbit

The orbital bones develop from the mesenchyme that encircles the optic vesicle. The medial wall forms from the lateral nasal process. The lateral wall and inferior wall develop from the maxillary process. The superior wall forms from the mesenchymal capsule of the forebrain. Posteriorly, the orbit is formed of the bones of the base of the skull. The bones of the orbit form in membrane except those belonging to the base of the skull, which develop in cartilage. Initially, the optic axes are directed laterally toward the side of the head; only later are they directed anteriorly. It is interesting to note that early in development the eyeball develops at a faster rate than the orbit, so that in the sixth month of fetal life the anterior half of the eyeball projects beyond the orbital opening.

Postnatal Growth

The eyeball increases rapidly in size during the first years of life. The rate of growth then slows but increases again at puberty. The cornea, which is relatively large at birth, reaches adult size by the time the child is 2 years old. Pigmentation of the iris stroma occurs during the first years after birth, so that usually the color of the iris changes by a deepening coloration. The lens grows rapidly after birth and continues to grow throughout life. At birth the eye is hypermetropic. Later, as the anteroposterior axis of the eye increases in length, this condition is corrected. Further increase in the anteroposterior axis could cause myopia but generally this is prevented by the simultaneous flattening of the lens as growth proceeds.

A newborn baby perceives light and closes the eyes whenever there is a bright light. Eye movements are uncoordinated at first, and transient deviation of the eyes may be present. This condition may last several months but should stabilize by the fourth month. Toward the end of the neonatal period, good fixation and following should be evident and accommodation (focusing) becomes better coordinated. The lacrimal glands do not function at birth; tears do not accompany crying until the third month.

Senile Changes in the Eye

Arcus senilis is a fatty infiltration of the cornea near its margin. This starts as two white crescents superiorly and inferiorly. Eventually the arcs fuse. The fatty degeneration occurs first in the superficial stroma and the Bowman's membrane.

Loss of accommodation results from hardening changes in the nucleus of the lens (see p. 202) and changes in the ciliary body.

Thickening of the sclera also occurs. The sclera becomes yellowish as the result of fatty infiltration.

Senile myosis or presbyopia occurs as the result of increasing rigidity of the ciliary body due to increasing deposits of connective tissue. This connective tissue interferes with the contraction of the ciliary muscle, preventing sufficient accommodation of the lens to focus objects.

Clinical Notes

Only the common congenital anomalies will be briefly discussed here.

Strabismus

Normal binocular vision begins to develop in very early infancy. If strabismus is present after the third month and is allowed to continue without treatment, amblyopia or diminished vision of the affected eye may result because of cortical suppression of the deviated image. There is a strong familial tendency to strabismus.

Cataract

In cases of congenital cataract, the lens becomes opaque (Fig. 1-9) during intrauterine life. The principal causes appear to be genetic, infection, and malnutrition. If the mother is exposed to the rubella virus before the seventh week of pregnancy—a time when the lens is actively developing—and before the development of the lens capsule, the child may have congenital cataract. If the mother contracts rubella after the seventh week, the lens is rarely affected. Many of the children with congenital cataract are of low birth weight and may have suffered from intrauterine malnutrition resulting from poor diet during the mother's pregnancy, maternal toxemia, or multiple pregnancy. Chromosomal abnormalities may be another factor; Down syndrome, for example, carries an increased incidence of congenital cataract.

Glaucoma

In congenital glaucoma, there is elevated intraocular pressure resulting from a developmental anomaly of the absorption mechanism of aqueous humor from

Figure 1-9

(A) Adhesion of the eyelids. The eyelids have failed to separate completely at the seventh month. (B) Congenital cataract. (C) Persistent pupillary membrane. (D) Coloboma of the iris. (All courtesy of Dr. D. Friendly.)

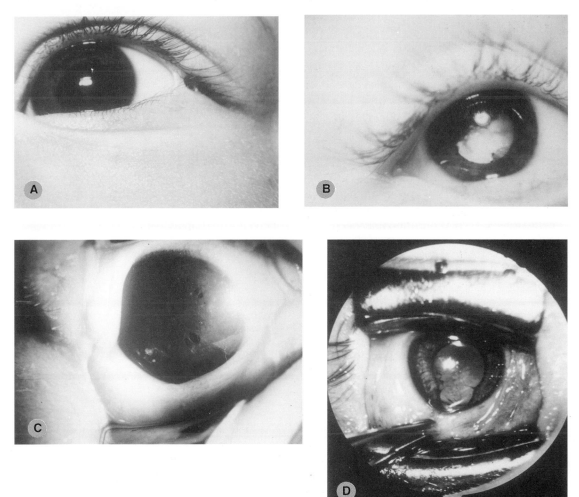

the anterior chamber of the eye. Eighty percent of cases are bilateral, and the condition is responsible for 5 to 10 percent of blindness in children. The eye may be enlarged.

Persistent Pupillary Membrane

Normally, the central part of the pupillary membrane disappears before birth. Very occasionally this part of the membrane persists as strands of connective tissue that stretch across the pupil (Figs. 1-9 and 1-10).

Figure 1-10

Some congenital anomalies of the eye. (A) Coloboma of the iris. (B) Cleft upper eye-lid. (C) Remnants of pupillary membrane stretching across the pupil.

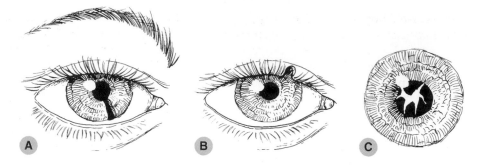

Coloboma

A coloboma—a notched defect of a sector of the iris, ciliary body, retina, or choroid—is caused by a failure of the optic fissure to close (Figs. 1-9 and 1-10). This condition may occur as an isolated lesion or in association with other mal-formations, especially cleft lip or palate.

Absence of Pigment in the Retina and Iris

This lack of retinal and iridic pigment is often part of the syndrome of albinism.

Cleft Eyelid

This defect usually occurs in the upper lid (Fig. 1-10). If the cornea is left exposed when the eyes are closed, the defect must be surgically closed at once.

Adhesion of Eyelid Margins

Rarely, the eyelid margins are connected by bands of tissue that reduce the palpebral fissure and impair the mobility of the eyelids (Fig. 1-9). Microscop-ically, the bands have a core of connective tissue and are covered on the outside with epithelium.

Atresia of the Nasolacrimal Duct

Atresia of the nasolacrimal duct causes watering from the affected eye and liabil-ity to infection of the lacrimal duct and sac. Failure of the developing duct to canalize causes this defect. It may occur at the upper end, but it usually occurs at the lower end, at the entrance into the nose.

Congenital Fistulas of the Lacrimal Sac

A lacrimal sac fistula is a relatively rare condition that can occur unilaterally or bilaterally. The orifice is usually found on the side of the nose a short distance below the inner canthus of the eye.

CHAPTER 1
Clinical Problems

Answers on Page 20

1 A 5-year-old boy was taken to an ophthalmologist because his right eye turned inward when he was tired or excited, and especially when he was looking at an object intently. On physical examination, it was noted that he had a convergent strabismus of the right eye. On questioning the child, the doctor ascertained that he did not have double vision. Examination of the fundus showed it to be normal in both the right and left eyes. Covering the nonstrabismic eye showed that the child had severe impairment of vision in the strabismic eye. Can strabismus be a congenital anomaly? Is this condition hereditary? Does this condition cure itself spontaneously?

2 A 2-month-old boy was taken to an ophthalmologist because the child's mother had noticed an opacity of his left eye since birth. The mother gave a history of rubella infection during the first trimester of the pregnancy. On physical examination, a pearly nuclear cataract of the left eye was found. The child also had impaired hearing in the right ear and evidence of a ventricular septal defect. Is there any connection between the rubella infection of the mother and the congenital defects noted in the child?

3 A 5-year-old boy undergoing routine examination by an ophthalmologist was found to have a small notch on the inferior nasal section of his left iris. The notch measured about 0.5 mm long and involved the pupillary margin. The boy's mother stated that he had had the notch since birth. What is your diagnosis? How would you explain this condition embryologically?

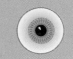

CHAPTER 1
Answers to Clinical Problems

1 This child has a congenital convergent strabismus of the right eye (esotropia), resulting from an imbalance of the extraocular muscles. Although abnormalities of the central nervous system can cause strabismus, in many cases the condition results from a simple congenital muscle imbalance, and about half the incidence is familial. The condition never cures itself spontaneously. In this case the deviating right eye, which was not being used for seeing, failed to develop good central vision, and the child actually suppressed the image. Covering the normal undeviated eye immediately revealed the impaired vision in the deviating eye.

2 Yes, there is a connection between rubella infection of the mother and the congenital defects in the child. The rubella virus is a potent teratogenic agent. The virus is transmitted to the fetus via the placenta, and the effects on the fetus usually are multiple. If the mother is infected with rubella before the seventh week of pregnancy, a time when the lens is actively developing, the child may have congenital cataract. In a similar manner, the organ of Corti of the ear may undergo viral destruction. The most common heart anomalies caused by rubella are pulmonary stenosis, patent ductus arteriosus, and ventricular septal defects. Remember that a child born of a mother infected by rubella will have the virus within his tissues for many months after birth.

3 This child has a small coloboma of the iris of the left eye. This condition results from a failure of closure of the optic fissure. The anomaly may be minimal, as in this instance, or it may extensively involve the uveal tissue, with defects in the ciliary body and retina.

An Overview of the Anatomy of the Skull

CHAPTER OUTLINE

Composition

The skull consists of a number of separate bones united at immobile joints called *sutures*. The connective tissue between the bones is called a *sutural ligament*. The mandible is an exception to this rule, for it is united to the skull by the mobile temporomandibular joint.

The bones of the skull may be divided into those of the *cranium* and those of the face. The *vault* is the upper part of the cranium, and the *base of the skull* is the lower part of the cranium (Figs. 2-1 and 2-2).

The skull bones are made up of *external* and *internal tables* of compact bone, separated by a layer of spongy bone called the *diploë*. The internal table is thinner and more brittle than the external table. The bones are covered on the outer and inner surfaces with periosteum; the outer layer is referred to as the *pericranium*; the inner covering, as the *endocranium*.

The *cranium* consists of the following bones, two of which are paired (Figs. 2-1 through 2-5):

Frontal bone	1	Temporal bones	2
Parietal bones	2	Sphenoid bone	1
Occipital bone	1	Ethmoid bone	1

Figure 2-1

Bones of the anterior aspect of the skull.

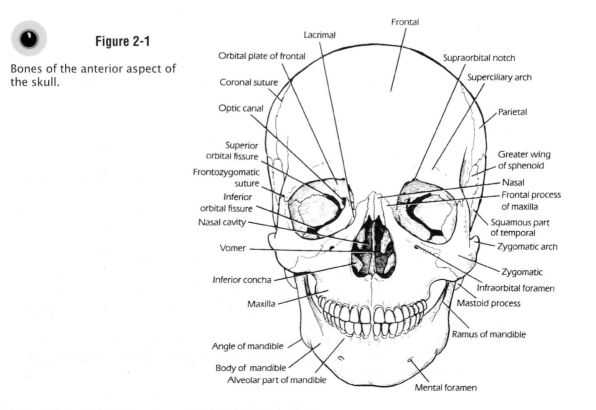

● **Figure 2-2**

Bones of the lateral aspect of the skull.

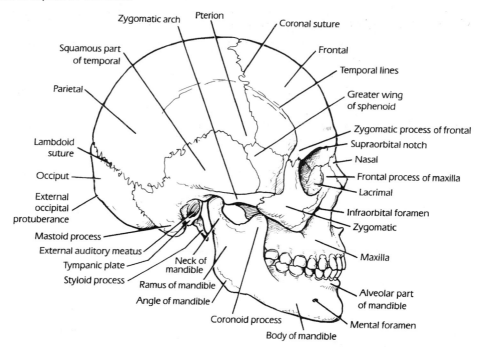

The *facial bones* consist of the following, two of which are single bones:

Zygomatic bones	2	Vomer	1
Maxillae	2	Palatine bones	2
Nasal bones	2	Inferior conchae	2
Lacrimal bones	2	Mandible	1

The reader will find it helpful to have a skull available for reference while reading the following description.

Anterior View ·

The *frontal bone* curves downward to form the upper margins of the orbits (Fig. 2-1). The *superciliary arches* can be seen on either side, as can the *supraorbital notch*, or *foramen*. Medially, the frontal bone articulates with the frontal processes of the maxillae and with the nasal bones. Laterally, the frontal bone articulates with the zygomatic bone.

The *orbital margins* are bounded by the frontal bone superiorly, the zygomatic bone laterally, the maxilla inferiorly, and the processes of the maxilla and frontal bone medially.

Figure 2-3

Bones of the skull viewed from
(A) the posterior aspect and
(B) the superior aspect.

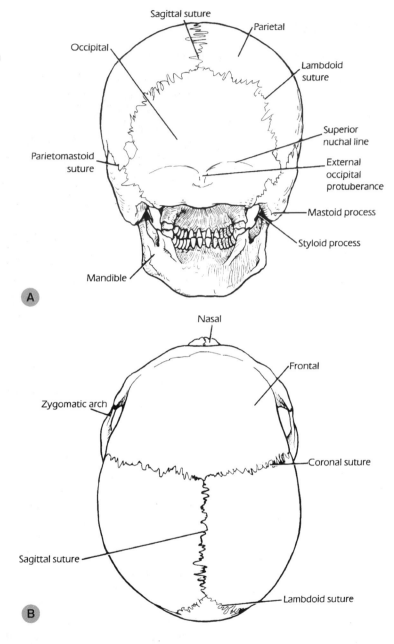

Within the *frontal bone,* just above the orbital margins, are two hollow spaces lined with mucous membrane, called the *frontal air sinuses.*

The two nasal bones form the bridge of the nose. Their lower borders, with the maxillae, make the *anterior nasal aperture.* The nasal cavity is divided into two parts by the bony nasal septum, which is largely formed by the vomer. The *superior* and *middle conchae* jut into the nasal cavity from the ethmoid on each side; the inferior conchae are separate bones.

Figure 2-4

The inferior surface of the base of the skull.

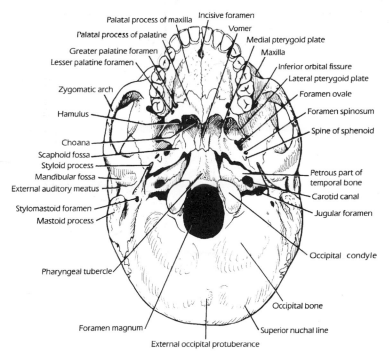

The two *maxillae* form the upper jaw, the anterior part of the hard palate, part of the lateral walls of the nasal cavities, and part of the floors of the orbital cavities. These two bones meet in the midline at the *intermaxillary suture* and form the lower margin of the nasal aperture. Below the orbit, the *infraorbital foramen* perforates the *maxilla*. The *alveolar process* projects downward and, together with the fellow of the opposite side, forms the *alveolar arch*, which carries the upper teeth. Within each maxilla is a large pyramid-shaped cavity lined with mucous membrane, the *maxillary sinus.*

The *zygomatic bone* forms the prominence of the cheek and part of the lateral wall and floor of the orbital cavity. Medially, it articulates with the zygomatic process of the temporal bone to form the *zygomatic arch*. The zygomatic bone is perforated by two foramina for the zygomaticofacial and zygomaticotemporal nerves.

The *mandible*, or lower jaw, consists of a horizontal *body* and two vertical *rami*; the body joins the ramus at the *angle of the mandible*. The *mental foramen* opens onto the anterior surface of the body of the mandible, below the second premolar tooth. The upper border of the mandible, the alveolar part, carries the lower teeth.

Figure 2-5

The internal surface of the base of the skull.

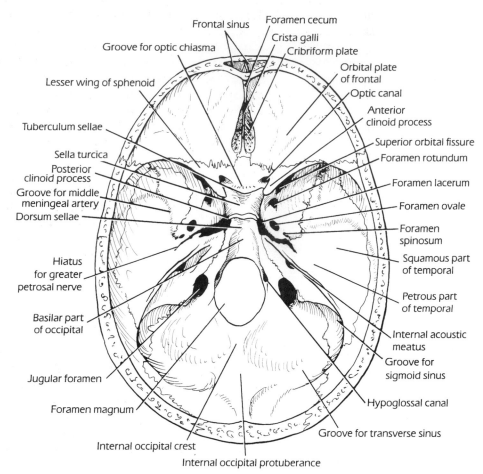

Lateral View

The *frontal bone* forms the anterior part of the side of the skull and articulates with the parietal bone at the *coronal suture* (Fig. 2-2).

The *parietal bones* form the sides and roof of the cranium and articulate with each other in the midline at the *sagittal suture*. They articulate with the occipital bone behind, at the *lambdoid suture*.

The skull is completed from the side by the squamous part of the *occipital bone*; parts of the *temporal bone*, namely, the *squamous, tympanic, mastoid process, styloid process,* and *zygomatic process*; and the *greater wing of the sphenoid*. The ramus and body of the mandible lie inferiorly.

Note that at the thinnest part of the lateral wall of the skull the anteroinferior corner of the parietal bone articulates with the greater wing of the sphenoid; this point is referred to as the *pterion*.

Clinically, the pterion is a very important area, because it overlies the anterior division of the *middle meningeal artery* and *vein*. On the outer surface of the skull, the pterion lies about 1 inch (2.5 cm) behind the frontal process of the zygomatic bone and about 1¹/₂ inches (4 cm) above the zygomatic arch.

The *temporal fossa* lies below the temporal lines (Fig. 2-2). The lower limit of the temporal fossa is the *infratemporal crest* of the greater wing of the sphenoid, which is level with the upper border of the zygomatic arch.

The *infratemporal fossa* lies below the infratemporal crest on the greater wing of the sphenoid. Th*e pterygomaxillary fissure* is a vertical fissure that lies within the fossa between the pterygoid process of the sphenoid bone and back of the maxilla. It leads medially into the *pterygopalatine fossa*.

The *inferior orbital fissure* is a horizontal fissure between the greater wing of the sphenoid bone and the maxilla (Fig. 2-1). It leads forward into the orbit.

The *pterygopalatine fossa* is a small space behind and below the orbital cavity. It communicates laterally with the infratemporal fossa through the pterygomaxillary fissure, medially with the nasal cavity through the *sphenopalatine foramen*, superiorly with the skull through the *foramen rotundum*, and anteriorly with the orbit through the *inferior orbital fissure*.

Posterior View

The posterior parts of the two parietal bones with the intervening *sagittal suture* are seen above (Fig. 2-3). Below, the parietal bones articulate with the squamous part of the occipital bone at the *lambdoid suture*. On each side the occipital bone articulates with the temporal bone. In the midline of the occipital bone is a roughened elevation called the *external occipital protuberance*, which gives attachment to muscles and to the ligamentum nuchae. On either side of the protuberance the *superior nuchal lines* extend laterally toward the temporal bone.

Superior View

Anteriorly, the frontal bone articulates with the two parietal bones at the *coronal suture* (Fig. 2-3). Occasionally, the two halves of the frontal bone fail to fuse, leaving a midline *metopic suture*. Behind, the two parietal bones articulate in the midline at the *sagittal suture*.

Inferior View

If the mandible is discarded, the anterior part of this aspect of the skull is seen to be formed by the *hard palate* (Fig. 2-4).

The *palatal processes of the maxillae* and the *horizontal plates of the palatine bones* can be identified. In the midline anteriorly are the *incisive fossa* and *foramen*. Posterolaterally are the *greater* and *lesser palatine foramina*.

Above the posterior edge of the hard palate are the *choanae* (posterior nasal apertures). These are separated from each other by the posterior margin of the vomer and are bounded laterally by the medial pterygoid plates of the sphenoid bone. The inferior end of the *medial pterygoid plate* is prolonged as a curved spike of bone, the *pterygoid hamulus*. The superior end widens to form the *scaphoid fossa*.

Posterolateral to the *lateral pterygoid plate*, the large *foramen ovale* and the small *foramen spinosum* pierce the greater wing of the sphenoid. Posterolateral to the foramen spinosum is the s*pine of the sphenoid*. Above the medial border of the scaphoid fossa, the *pterygoid canal* pierces the sphenoid bone.

Behind the spine of the sphenoid, in the interval between the greater wing of the sphenoid and the petrous part of the temporal bone, there is a groove for the cartilaginous part of the *auditory tube*. The opening of the bony part of the tube can be identified.

The *mandibular fossa* of the temporal bone and the *articular tubercle* form the upper articular surfaces for the temporomandibular joint. Separating the mandibular fossa from the tympanic plate posteriorly is the *squamotympanic fissure*, through the medial end of which (petrotympanic fissure) the chorda tympani exits from the tympanic cavity.

The *styloid process* of the temporal bone projects downward and forward from its inferior aspect. The opening of the *carotid canal* can be seen on the inferior surface of the petrous part of the temporal bone.

The medial end of the petrous part of the temporal bone is irregular and, together with the basilar part of the occipital bone and the greater wing of the sphenoid, forms the *foramen lacerum*. During life the foramen lacerum is closed with fibrous tissue, and only a few very small vessels pass through it from the cavity of the skull to the exterior.

The *tympanic plate*, which forms part of the temporal bone, is C-shaped on section and forms the bony part of the *external auditory meatus*.

In the interval between the styloid and mastoid processes, the *stylomastoid foramen* can be seen. Medial to the styloid process, the petrous part of the temporal bone has a deep notch, which, together with a shallower notch on the occipital bone, forms the *jugular foramen*.

Behind the posterior apertures of the nose and in front of the foramen magnum are the sphenoid bone and the basilar part of the occipital bone.

The *occipital condyles* should be identified; they articulate with the superior aspect of the lateral mass of the atlas. Superior to the summit of the occipital condyle is the *hypoglossal canal* containing the hypoglossal nerve.

Posterior to the foramen magnum is the *external occipital protuberance*.

The Cranial Cavity ·

The cranial cavity contains the brain and its surrounding meninges, portions of the cranial nerves, arteries, veins, and venous sinuses.

Vault of the Skull

The internal surface of the vault shows the coronal, sagittal, and lambdoid sutures. In the midline a shallow sagittal groove lodges the *superior sagittal sinus*. On each side of this groove are a number of small pits, called *granular pits*, which lodge the *lateral lacunae* and *arachnoid granulations* (see p. 41). A number of narrow grooves are present for the anterior and posterior divisions of the *middle meningeal vessels* as they pass up the side of the skull to the vault.

Base of the Skull

The interior of the base of the skull, for ease of description, is conveniently divided into three cranial fossae: anterior, middle, and posterior (Fig. 2-5).

Anterior Cranial Fossa

The anterior cranial fossa lodges the frontal lobes of the cerebral hemispheres. It is bounded anteriorly by the inner surface of the frontal bone; in the midline there is a crest for the attachment of the *falx cerebri*. Its posterior boundary is the sharp lesser wing of the sphenoid, which articulates laterally with the frontal bone and meets the anterior inferior angle of the parietal bone, or pterion. The medial end of the lesser wing of the sphenoid forms the *anterior clinoid process* on each side, to give attachment to the *tentorium cerebelli*. The median part of the anterior cranial fossa is limited posteriorly by the groove for the optic chiasma.

The floor of the fossa is formed by the ridged orbital plates of the frontal bone laterally and by the *cribriform plate* of the ethmoid medially (Fig. 2-5). The *crista galli* is a sharp upward projection of the ethmoid bone in the midline, for the attachment of the falx cerebri. Alongside the crista galli is a narrow slit in the cribriform plate for the passage of the *anterior ethmoidal nerve* into the nasal cavity. The upper surface of the cribriform plate supports the *olfactory bulbs*, and the small perforations in the cribriform plate are for the *olfactory nerves*.

Middle Cranial Fossa

The middle cranial fossa consists of a small median part and expanded lateral parts (Fig. 2-5). The body of the sphenoid forms the median raised part, and the expanded lateral parts form concavities on either side, lodging the *temporal lobes* of the *cerebral hemispheres*.

The middle cranial fossa is bounded anteriorly by the lesser wings of the sphenoid and posteriorly by the superior borders of the petrous parts of the temporal bones. Laterally lie the squamous parts of the temporal bones, the greater wings of the sphenoid, and the parietal bones.

The floor of each lateral part of the middle cranial fossa is formed by the greater wing of the sphenoid and the squamous and petrous parts of the temporal bone.

Anteriorly, the *optic canal* transmits the optic nerve and the ophthalmic artery, a branch of the internal carotid artery, to the orbit. The *superior orbital fissure*, which is a slitlike opening between the lesser and greater wings of the sphenoid, transmits the lacrimal, frontal, trochlear, oculomotor, nasociliary, and abducent nerves, together with the superior ophthalmic vein. The sphenoparietal venous sinus runs medially along the posterior border of the lesser wing of the sphenoid and drains into the cavernous sinus.

The *foramen rotundum*, which is situated behind the medial end of the superior orbital fissure, perforates the greater wing of the sphenoid and transmits the maxillary nerve from the trigeminal ganglion to the pterygopalatine fossa.

The *foramen ovale* lies posterolateral to the foramen rotundum (Fig. 2-5). It perforates the greater wing of the sphenoid and transmits the large sensory root and small motor root of the mandibular nerve to the infratemporal fossa; the lesser petrosal nerve also passes through it.

The small *foramen spinosum* lies posterolateral to the foramen ovale and also perforates the greater wing of the sphenoid. The foramen transmits the middle meningeal artery from the infratemporal fossa into the cranial cavity. The artery then runs forward and laterally in a groove on the upper surface of the squamous part of the temporal bone and the greater wing of the sphenoid (Fig. 2-5). After a short distance the artery divides into anterior and posterior branches. The anterior branch passes forward and upward to the anterior inferior angle of the parietal bone (Fig. 2-5). Here, the bone is deeply grooved or tunneled by the artery for a short distance before it runs backward and upward on the parietal bone (it is at this site that the artery may be damaged following a blow to the side of the head). The posterior branch passes backward and upward across the squamous part of the temporal bone to reach the parietal bone.

The large and irregularly shaped *foramen lacerum* lies between the apex of the petrous part of the temporal bone and the sphenoid bone (Fig. 2-5).

The *carotid canal* opens into the side of the foramen lacerum. The internal carotid artery enters the foramen through the carotid canal and immediately turns upward to reach the side of the body of the sphenoid bone. Here, the artery turns forward in the cavernous sinus to reach the region of the anterior clinoid process. At this point the internal carotid artery turns vertically upward, medial to the anterior clinoid process, and emerges from the cavernous sinus (Fig. 2-7).

Lateral to the foramen lacerum is an impression on the apex of the petrous part of the temporal bone for the *trigeminal ganglion*. The anterior surface of the petrous bone has two grooves for nerves; the larger, medial groove is for the *greater petrosal nerve*, a branch of the facial nerve; the smaller, lateral groove is for the *lesser petrosal nerve*, a branch of the tympanic plexus. The greater petrosal nerve enters the foramen lacerum deep to the trigeminal ganglion and joins the *deep petrosal nerve* (sympathetic fibers from around the internal carotid artery), to form the *nerve of the pterygoid canal*. The lesser petrosal nerve passes forward to the foramen ovale.

The abducent nerve bends sharply forward across the apex of the petrous bone, medial to the trigeminal ganglion. It is here that it leaves the posterior cranial fossa and enters the cavernous sinus.

The *arcuate eminence* is a rounded eminence found on the anterior surface of the petrous bone and is formed by the underlying *superior semicircular canal*.

The *tegmen tympani* is a thin plate of bone, a forward extension of the petrous part of the temporal bone that adjoins the squamous part of the bone. From behind forward, it forms the roof of the mastoid antrum, the tympanic cavity, and the auditory tube. It is important to realize that this thin plate of bone is the only major barrier separating infection in the tympanic cavity from the temporal lobe of the cerebral hemisphere.

The median part of the middle cranial fossa is formed by the body of the sphenoid bone (Fig. 2-5). In front is the *sulcus chiasmatis,* which is related to the optic chiasma and leads laterally to the *optic canal* on each side. Posterior to the sulcus is an elevation, the *tuberculum sellae.* Behind this elevation is a deep depression, the *sella turcica,* that lodges the *hypophysis cerebri.* The sella turcica is bounded posteriorly by a square plate of bone called the *dorsum sellae.* The superior angles of the dorsum sellae have two tubercles, called the *posterior clinoid processes,* which give attachment to the fixed margin of the tentorium cerebelli.

The cavernous sinus is directly related to the side of the body of the sphenoid (Figs. 2-5 and 2-6). It carries in its lateral wall the third and fourth cranial nerves

 Figure 2-6

Coronal section through the body of the sphenoid, showing the hypophysis cerebri and cavernous sinuses. Note the position of the internal carotid artery and cranial nerves.

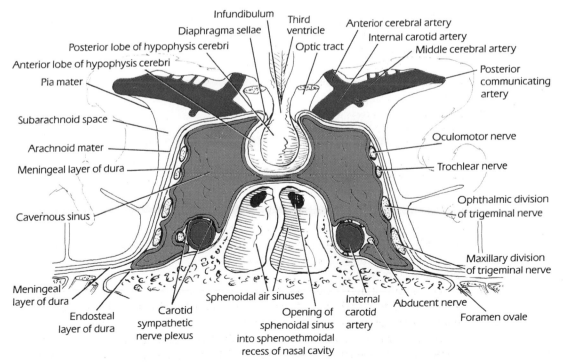

and the ophthalmic and maxillary divisions of the fifth cranial nerve (Fig. 2-6). The internal carotid artery and the sixth cranial nerve pass forward through the sinus.

Posterior Cranial Fossa

The posterior cranial fossa is very deep and lodges the parts of the hindbrain, namely, the *cerebellum, pons,* and *medulla oblongata.* Anteriorly, the fossa is bounded by the superior border of the petrous part of the temporal bone; posteriorly, by the internal surface of the squamous part of the occipital bone (Fig. 2-5). The floor of the posterior fossa is formed by the basilar, condylar, and squamous parts of the occipital bone and the mastoid part of the temporal bone.

The roof of the fossa is formed by a fold of dura, the *tentorium cerebelli,* which intervenes between the cerebellum below and the occipital lobes of the cerebral hemispheres above (Fig. 2-7).

The *foramen magnum* occupies the central area of the floor and transmits the medulla oblongata and its surrounding meninges, the ascending spinal parts of the accessory nerves, and the two vertebral arteries.

Figure 2-7

Interior of the skull, showing the dura mater and its contained venous sinuses. Note the connections of scalp veins and venous sinuses.

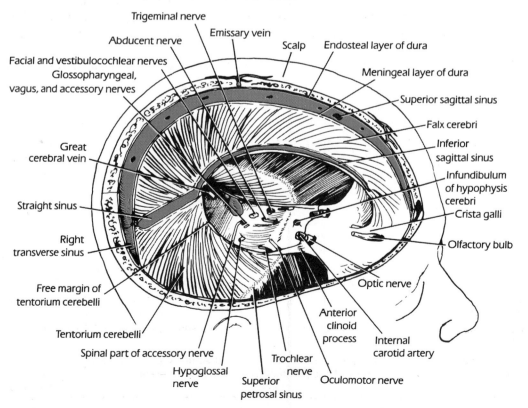

The *hypoglossal canal*, situated above the anterolateral boundary of the foramen magnum (Fig. 2-5), transmits the *hypoglossal nerve*.

The *jugular foramen* lies between the lower border of the petrous part of the temporal bone and the condylar part of the occipital bone. It transmits the following structures from front to back: the *inferior petrosal sinus*, the *ninth, tenth, and eleventh cranial nerves*, and the large *sigmoid sinus*. The inferior petrosal sinus descends in the groove on the lower border of the petrous part of the temporal bone to reach the foramen. The sigmoid sinus turns down through the foramen to become the *internal jugular vein*.

The *internal acoustic meatus* pierces the posterior surface of the petrous part of the temporal bone. It transmits the vestibulocochlear nerve and the motor and sensory roots of the facial nerve.

The *internal occipital crest* runs upward in the midline posteriorly from the foramen magnum to the *internal occipital protuberance*; to it is attached the small *falx cerebelli* over the occipital sinus.

On each side of the internal occipital protuberance there is a wide groove for the *transverse sinus* (Fig. 2-5). This groove sweeps around on either side, on the internal surface of the occipital bone, to reach the posterior inferior angle or corner of the parietal bone. The groove now passes onto the mastoid part of the temporal bone, where the transverse sinus becomes the *sigmoid sinus*. The *superior petrosal sinus* runs backward along the upper border of the petrous bone in a narrow groove and drains into the sigmoid sinus. As the sigmoid sinus descends to the jugular foramen, it deeply grooves the back of the petrous bone and the mastoid part of the temporal bone. Here, it lies directly posterior to the mastoid antrum.

Table 2-1 summarizes the main anatomic features on the floor of the cranial fossae.

Table 2-1   Summary of Main Anatomic Features on the Floor of the Cranial Fossae

Features	Location	Relevance
Anterior cranial fossa		
Orbital plates of frontal bone	Above orbits	Separate frontal lobes of cerebral hemispheres from eyes
Frontal crest	Midline internal surface of frontal bone	Attachment of falx cerebri
Crista galli	Upward midline bony projection	Attachment of falx cerebri
Cribriform plate of ethmoid bone	Midline	Perforations transmit olfactory nerves
Slit alongside cribriform plate	Close to midline	Transmits anterior ethmoidal nerve
Anterior clinoid processes	Medial ends of lesser wings of sphenoid bone	Attachment of free borders of tentorium cerebelli

(continued)

Table 2-1   *(continued)*

Features	Location	Relevance
Middle cranial fossa		
Median part		
Sulcus chiasmatis	Body of sphenoid bone between two optic canals, anterior to tuberculum sellae	Related to optic chiasma
Sella turcica	Deep fossa on body of sphenoid bone between cavernous sinuses	Lodges pituitary gland
Dorsum sellae	Square plate of bony part of sphenoid	Posterior clinoid processes give attachment to fixed borders of tentorium cerebelli
Lateral part		
Optic canal	Lesser wing of sphenoid bone	Transmits optic nerve, ophthalmic artery, and meninges
Superior orbital fissure	Slit between lesser and greater wings of sphenoid bone	Transmits lacrimal, frontal, trochlear, oculomotor, nasociliary, and abducent nerves; superior ophthalmic vein
Foramen rotundum	Greater wing of sphenoid bone	Transmits maxillary nerve
Foramen ovale	Greater wing of sphenoid bone	Transmits mandibular nerve and lesser petrosal nerve
Foramen spinosum	Greater wing of sphenoid bone	Transmits middle meningeal artery and vein
Foramen lacerum	Apex of petrous part of temporal bone	Transmits internal carotid artery from carotid canal to enter cavernous sinus
Trigeminal impression	Upper border of petrous part of temporal bone near apex	Occupied by trigeminal ganglion
Arcuate eminence	Anterior surface of petrous part of temporal bone	Formed by underlying superior semicircular canal
Tegmen tympani	Forward extension of petrous part of temporal bone	Forms thin roof for mastoid antrum, tympanic cavity, and auditory tube
Posterior cranial fossa		
Foramen magnum	Central part of floor in occipital bone	Transmits medulla oblongata, meninges, spinal parts of accessory nerves, and two vertebral arteries
Hypoglossal canal	Above anterolateral boundary of foramen magnum	Transmits hypoglossal nerve
Jugular foramen	Between petrous part of temporal bone and occipital bone	Transmits inferior petrosal sinus, glossopharyngeal, vagus, and accessory nerves, and sigmoid sinus
Internal acoustic meatus	Posterior surface of the petrous part of the temporal bone	Transmits vestibulocochlear and facial nerves
Groove for transverse venous sinus	Internal surface of occipital bone	Lodges transverse venous sinus

The Meninges

The brain and spinal cord are surrounded by three membranes, or meninges: the *dura mater*, the *arachnoid mater*, and the *pia mater*.

Dura Mater of the Brain

The dura mater is conventionally described as two layers, the endosteal layer and the meningeal layer (Fig. 2-7). These are closely united except along certain lines, where they separate to form venous sinuses.

The *endosteal layer* is nothing more than the ordinary periosteum covering the inner surface of the skull bones. It *does not extend* through the foramen magnum to become continuous with the dura mater of the spinal cord. Around the margins of all the foramina in the skull it becomes continuous with the periosteum on the outside of the skull bones. At the sutures it is continuous with the sutural ligaments.

The *meningeal layer* is the dura mater proper. A dense, strong fibrous membrane covering the brain, it is continuous through the foramen magnum with the dura mater of the spinal cord. It provides tubular sheaths for the cranial nerves as the latter pass through the foramina in the skull. Outside the skull the sheaths fuse with the epineurium of the nerves.

The meningeal layer sends inward four septa, which divide the cranial cavity into freely communicating spaces lodging the subdivisions of the brain. The function of these septa is to restrict rotatory displacement of the brain.

The *falx cerebri* is a sickle-shaped fold of dura mater that lies in the midline between the two cerebral hemispheres (Fig. 2-7). Its narrow end in front is attached to the internal frontal crest and the crista galli. Its broad posterior part blends in the midline with the upper surface of the tentorium cerebelli. The superior sagittal sinus runs in its upper fixed margin; the inferior sagittal sinus runs in its lower concave free margin; and the straight sinus runs along its attachment to the tentorium cerebelli.

The *tentorium cerebelli* is a crescent-shaped fold of dura mater that roofs over the posterior cranial fossa (Figs. 2-7 and 2-8). It covers the upper surface of the cerebellum and supports the occipital lobes of the cerebral hemispheres. In front there is a gap, the *tentorial notch*, for the passage of the midbrain (Fig. 2-8), thus producing an inner free border and an outer attached or fixed border. The fixed border is attached to the posterior clinoid processes, the superior borders of the petrous bones, and the margins of the grooves for the transverse sinuses on the occipital bone. The free border runs forward at its two ends, crosses the attached border, and is affixed to the anterior clinoid process on each side. At the point where the two borders cross, the third and fourth cranial nerves pass forward to enter the lateral wall of the cavernous sinus (Fig. 2-9).

Close to the apex of the petrous part of the temporal bone, the lower layer of the tentorium is pouched forward beneath the superior petrosal sinus to form a recess for the trigeminal nerve and the trigeminal ganglion.

The falx cerebri and the falx cerebelli are attached to the upper and lower surfaces of the tentorium, respectively. The straight sinus runs along its attachment

Figure 2-8

Diaphragma sellae and tentorium cerebelli. Note the position of the venous sinuses.

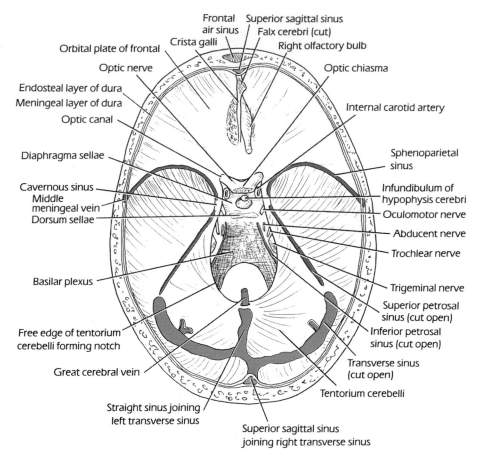

to the falx cerebri, the superior petrosal sinus along its attachment to the petrous bone, and the transverse sinus along its attachment to the occipital bone (Fig. 2-8).

The *falx cerebelli* is a small, sickle-shaped fold of dura mater that is attached to the internal occipital crest and projects forward between the two cerebellar hemispheres. Its posterior fixed margin contains the occipital sinus.

The *diaphragma sellae* is a small, circular fold of dura mater that forms the roof for the sella turcica (Fig. 2-6). A small opening in its center allows passage of the stalk of the hypophysis cerebri.

● **Figure 2-9**

Lateral view of the interior of the skull, showing the falx cerebri, tentorium cerebelli, brain stem, and trigeminal ganglion.

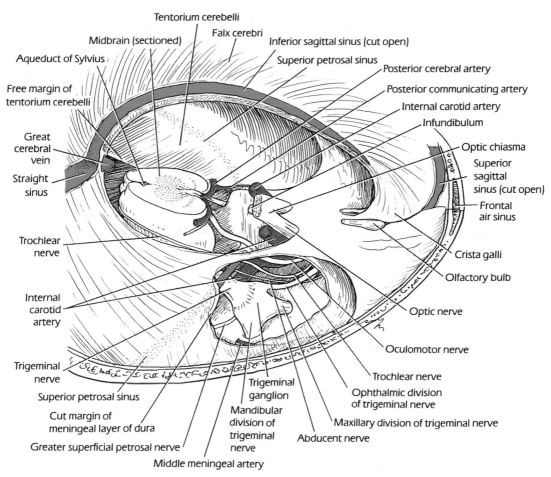

Dural Nerve Supply

Branches of the trigeminal, the vagus, and the first three cervical nerves and branches from the sympathetic system pass to the dura.

The dura possesses numerous sensory endings. The dura is sensitive to stretching, which produces the sensation of headache. Stimulation of the sensory endings of the trigeminal nerve above the level of the tentorium cerebelli produces referred pain to an area of skin on the same side of the head. Stimulation of the dural endings below the level of the tentorium produces referred pain to the back of the neck and the back of the scalp along the distribution of the greater occipital nerve.

Dural Arterial Supply

Numerous arteries supply the dura mater from the internal carotid, maxillary, ascending pharyngeal, occipital, and vertebral arteries. From the clinical standpoint, the most important of these arteries is the middle meningeal artery, which is commonly damaged in head injuries.

The *middle meningeal artery* arises from the maxillary artery in the infratemporal fossa. It enters the cranial cavity and runs forward and laterally in a groove on the upper surface of the squamous part of the temporal bone. To enter the cranial cavity, it passes through the foramen spinosum to *lie between the meningeal and endosteal layers* of dura (Fig. 2-10). The anterior (frontal) branch deeply grooves or tunnels the anteroinferior angle of the parietal bone, and its course corresponds roughly to the line of the underlying precentral gyrus of the brain. The posterior (parietal) branch curves backward and supplies the posterior part of the dura mater.

The *meningeal veins* lie in the endosteal layer of dura. The middle meningeal vein follows the branches of the middle meningeal artery and drains into the pterygoid venous plexus or the sphenoparietal sinus.

Arachnoid Mater of the Brain

The arachnoid mater is a delicate, impermeable membrane covering the brain and lying between the pia mater internally and the dura mater externally (Fig. 2-11). It is separated from the dura by a potential space, the *subdural space*, and from the pia by the *subarachnoid space*, which is filled with *cerebrospinal fluid*.

The arachnoid bridges over the sulci on the surface of the brain, and in certain situations the arachnoid and pia are widely separated to form the subarachnoid cisternae. The *cisterna cerebellomedullaris* lies between the inferior surface of the cerebellum and the roof of the fourth ventricle. The *cisterna pontis* lies on the anterior surface of the pons and the medulla oblongata. The *cisterna interpeduncularis* lies between the two cerebral peduncles. All the cisternae are in free communication with each other and with the remainder of the subarachnoid space.

In certain areas the arachnoid projects into the venous sinuses to form *arachnoid villi*. The arachnoid villi are most numerous along the superior sagittal sinus. Aggregations of arachnoid villi are referred to as *arachnoid granulations* (Fig. 2-12). Arachnoid villi serve as sites where the cerebrospinal fluid diffuses into the bloodstream.

The arachnoid is connected to the pia mater across the fluid-filled subarachnoid space by delicate strands of fibrous tissue.

It is important to remember that structures passing to and from the brain to the skull or its foramina must pass through the subarachnoid space. All the cerebral arteries and veins lie in this space, as do the cranial nerves. The arachnoid fuses with the epineurium of the nerves at their point of exit from the skull. For the optic nerve, the arachnoid forms a sheath that extends into the orbital cavity through the optic canal and fuses with the sclera of the eyeball (Fig. 6-38). Thus, the subarachnoid space extends around the optic nerve as far as the eyeball (see p. 382).

Figure 2-10

Right side of the head, with the meningeal layer of the dura exposed. The skull bones and periosteal layer of dura have been removed to reveal the middle meningeal artery and vein.

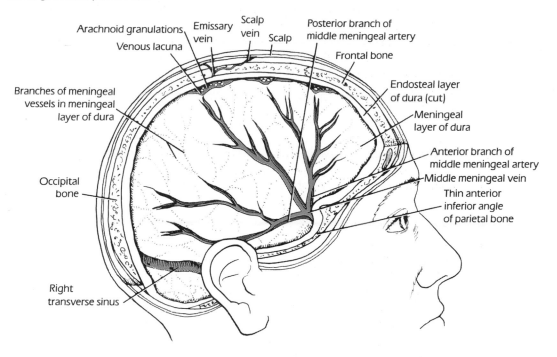

The *choroid plexuses* within the lateral, third, and fourth ventricles of the brain produce the *cerebrospinal fluid*. It escapes from the ventricular system of the brain through the three foramina in the roof of the fourth ventricle and so enters the subarachnoid space. It now circulates both upward over the surfaces of the cerebral hemispheres and downward around the spinal cord. The spinal subarachnoid space extends down as far as the *second sacral vertebra*. Eventually, the fluid enters the bloodstream by passing into the arachnoid villi and diffusing through their walls.

In addition to removing waste products associated with neuronal activity, the cerebrospinal fluid provides a fluid medium in which the brain floats. This mechanism effectively protects the brain from trauma.

Pia Mater of the Brain

The pia mater is a vascular membrane that closely invests the brain, covering the gyri and descending into the deepest sulci (Fig. 2-12). It extends over the cranial nerves and fuses with their epineurium. The cerebral arteries entering the substance of the brain carry a sheath of pia with them.

Figure 2-11

Right side of the head, with the arachnoid mater covering the cerebrum and cerebellum exposed. The periosteal and meningeal layers of dura have been removed.

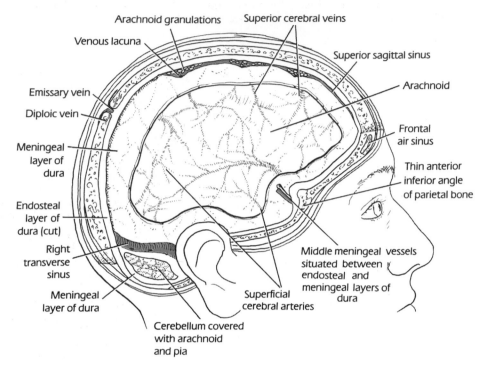

The pia mater forms the *tela choroidea* of the roof of the brain's third and fourth ventricles, and it fuses with the ependyma to form the choroid plexuses in the brain's lateral, third, and fourth ventricles.

The Venous Blood Sinuses

The venous sinuses of the cranial cavity are situated between the layers of the dura mater (Figs. 2-6, 2-7, and 2-8). They are lined with endothelium, and their walls are devoid of muscular tissue. They contain no valves. They receive tributaries from the various parts of the brain, from the diploë, from the orbit, and from the internal ear.

The *superior sagittal sinus* occupies the upper fixed border of the falx cerebri (Fig. 2-7). It begins in front at the foramen cecum, where it occasionally receives a vein from the nasal cavity. It runs backward, grooving the vault of the skull, and at the internal occipital protuberance it deviates to one or the other side (usually

Figure 2-12

Superior view of the head with the roof of the skull (calvarium) removed. On the left, a large portion of the meningeal layer of the dura has been removed to expose the underlying arachnoid mater. On the right, large portions of the meningeal layer of dura and arachnoid mater have been removed, revealing the cerebral blood vessels in the subarachnoid space and the cerebral cortex covered with pia mater.

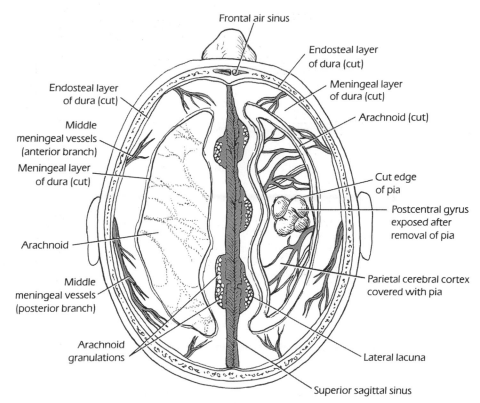

the right) and becomes continuous with the corresponding transverse sinus. The sinus communicates through small openings with two or three irregularly shaped *venous lacunae* on each side. Numerous arachnoid villi and granulations project into the lacunae, which also receive the diploic and meningeal veins (Fig. 2-12).

The superior sagittal sinus receives in its course the *superior cerebral veins*. At the internal occipital protuberance it is dilated to form the *confluence of the sinuses* (Fig. 2-8). Here, the superior sagittal sinus usually becomes continuous with the right transverse sinus; it is connected to the opposite transverse sinus and receives the *occipital sinus*.

The *inferior sagittal sinus* occupies the free lower margin of the falx cerebri. It runs backward and joins the *great cerebral vein* at the free margin of the tentorium cerebelli, to form the *straight sinus* (Fig. 2-8). The inferior sagittal sinus receives a few cerebral veins from the medial surface of the cerebral hemisphere.

The *straight sinus* occupies the line of junction of the falx cerebri with the tentorium cerebelli (Fig. 2-8). It is formed by the union of the inferior sagittal sinus with the great cerebral vein. It ends by turning to the left (sometimes to the right), to form the transverse sinus.

The *transverse sinuses* are paired structures that begin at the internal occipital protuberance (Figs. 2-8 and 2-10). The right sinus is usually continuous with the superior sagittal sinus; the left, continuous with the straight sinus. Each sinus occupies the attached margin of the tentorium cerebelli, grooving the occipital bone and the posteroinferior angle of the parietal bone. The transverse sinuses receive the superior petrosal sinuses, inferior cerebral and cerebellar veins, and diploic veins. They end by turning downward as the sigmoid sinuses.

The *sigmoid sinuses* are a direct continuation of the transverse sinuses. Each sinus turns downward and medially and grooves the mastoid part of the temporal bone, where it lies behind the mastoid antrum. The sinus then turns forward and downward through the posterior part of the jugular foramen, to become continuous with the superior bulb of the internal jugular vein.

The *occipital sinus* is a small sinus occupying the attached margin of the falx cerebelli. It commences near the foramen magnum, where it communicates with the vertebral veins and drains into the confluence of sinuses.

The *cavernous sinuses* are situated in the middle cranial fossa on each side of the body of the sphenoid bone (Fig. 2-6). Numerous trabeculae cross their interior, giving them a spongy appearance (hence the name). Each sinus extends from the superior orbital fissure in front to the apex of the petrous part of the temporal bone behind.

The internal carotid artery, surrounded by its sympathetic nerve plexus, runs forward through the cavernous sinus (Fig. 2-6). The abducent nerve also passes through the sinus. The internal carotid artery and the nerves are separated from the blood by an endothelial covering.

The third and fourth cranial nerves and the ophthalmic and maxillary divisions of the trigeminal nerve run forward in the lateral wall of the cavernous sinus (Fig. 2-6). They lie between the endothelial lining and the dura mater. The *tributaries* are the superior and inferior ophthalmic veins, the cerebral veins, the sphenoparietal sinus, and the central vein of the retina.

The sinus drains posteriorly into the superior and inferior petrosal sinuses, and inferiorly into the pterygoid venous plexus.

The two sinuses communicate with each other by means of the *anterior* and *posterior intercavernous sinuses*, which run in the diaphragma sellae in front and behind the stalk of the hypophysis cerebri (Fig. 2-6). Each sinus has an important communication with the facial vein through the superior ophthalmic vein.

The *superior* and *inferior petrosal sinuses* are small sinuses situated on the superior and inferior borders of the petrous part of the temporal bone on each side (Fig. 2-7). Each superior sinus drains the cavernous sinus into the transverse sinus, and each inferior sinus drains the cavernous sinus into the internal jugular vein.

Clinical Notes

Fractures of the Skull

Fractures of the skull are very common in the adult, but much less so in the young child. The infant skull has bones that are more resilient than those in the adult skull, and they are separated by fibrous sutural ligaments. In the adult, the inner table of the skull is particularly brittle. Moreover, the sutural ligaments begin to ossify during middle age.

The type of fracture that occurs in the skull will depend on the age of the patient, the severity of the blow, and the area of skull receiving trauma. The *adult skull* may be likened to an eggshell in that it possesses a certain limited resilience, beyond which it splinters. A severe, localized blow will produce a local indentation, often accompanied by splintering of the bone. Blows to the vault often result in a series of linear fractures that radiate out through the thin areas of bone. The petrous parts of the temporal bones and the occipital crests strongly reinforce the base of the skull and tend to deflect linear fractures.

In the *young child*, the skull may be likened to a table-tennis ball, in that a localized blow produces a depression without splintering. This common type of circumscribed lesion is referred to as a *"pond" fracture.*

Fractures of the anterior cranial fossa may damage the cribriform plate of the ethmoid bone. This usually results in tearing of the overlying meninges and underlying mucoperiosteum. The patient will have *epistaxis* and *cerebrospinal rhinorrhea.* Fractures involving the orbital plate of the frontal bone will result in hemorrhage beneath the conjunctiva and into the orbital cavity, causing *exophthalmos.* The frontal air sinus may also be involved, with hemorrhage into the nose.

Fractures of the middle cranial fossa are common, because this fossa is the weakest part of the base of the skull. Anatomically, this weakness is due to the presence of numerous foramina and canals in this region; the cavities of the middle ear and the sphenoidal air sinuses are particularly vulnerable. The leakage of cerebrospinal fluid and blood from the external auditory meatus is common. The seventh and eighth cranial nerves may be involved as they pass through the petrous part of the temporal bone. The third, fourth, and sixth cranial nerves may be damaged if the lateral wall of the cavernous sinus is torn. Blood and cerebrospinal fluid may leak into the sphenoidal air sinuses and then into the nose.

Fractures of the posterior cranial fossa may cause blood to escape into the nape of the neck deep to the postvertebral muscles. Some days later, it tracks between the muscles and appears in the posterior triangle, close to the mastoid process. The mucous membrane of the roof of the nasopharynx may be torn, and blood may escape there. In fractures involving the jugular foramen, the ninth, tenth, and eleventh cranial nerves may be damaged. The strong bony walls of the hypoglossal canal usually protect the hypoglossal nerve from injury.

Fractures of the Facial Bones

Signs of fractures of the facial bones include deformity, ocular displacement, and abnormal movement accompanied by crepitation and malocclusion of the teeth.

Anesthesia or paresthesia of the facial skin will follow fracture of bones through which branches of the trigeminal nerve pass to the skin.

Fractures of the nasal bones are very common. Although most of these are simple fractures and can be reduced under local anesthesia, some involve severe injuries to the nasal septum that require careful treatment under general anesthesia.

Fractures of the maxilla commonly result from a direct anteroposterior blow to the face. Malocclusion of the teeth, enophthalmos, and anesthesia of the cheek and upper lip (involvement of the infraorbital nerve) are frequent physical findings. (See "blowout" fractures of the maxilla, p. 87).

The *zygoma or zygomatic arch* may be fractured by a blow to the side of the face. Although it may occur as an isolated fracture, as from a blow from a clenched fist, it may be associated with multiple other fractures of the face, as often seen in automobile accidents.

Fractures of the Mandible

The mandible is horseshoe-shaped and forms part of a bony ring with the two temporomandibular joints and the base of the skull. Traumatic impact is transmitted around the ring, causing a single fracture or multiple fractures of the mandible, often far removed from the point of impact.

Injuries to the Brain

Injuries to the brain result from displacement and distortion of the neuronal tissues at the moment of impact. The brain may be likened to a log soaked with water floating submerged in water: It is floating in the cerebrospinal fluid in the subarachnoid space and is capable of a certain amount of anteroposterior movement, which is limited by the attachment of the superior cerebral veins to the superior sagittal sinus. The falx cerebri limits lateral displacement of the brain. The tentorium cerebelli and the falx cerebelli also restrict displacement of the brain.

It follows from these anatomic facts that blows to the front or back of the head lead to displacement of the brain, which may produce severe cerebral damage, stretching and distortion of the brain stem, and stretching and even tearing of the commissures of the brain.

Development of the Skull

The development of the skull is so complex that only those aspects that are important from a medical standpoint are considered here.

The skull consists of a protective case around the brain, the *neurocranium*, and the skeleton of the jaws. Initially, these parts are represented by a sheet of condensed mesenchyme that later may become converted into membrane, bone, or cartilage. In some areas the cartilage undergoes endochondral ossification, while in others it persists as cartilage throughout life. The neurocranium may be divided into the cartilaginous part and the membranous part.

The *cartilaginous neurocranium* is the basal region of the developing skull. In the earliest stages, it extends as a plate from the anterior part of the skull to the anterior border of the foramen magnum. Later, cartilaginous plates appear on either side, eventually forming the wings of the sphenoid bone. Each auditory vesicle becomes surrounded by cartilage, and a cartilaginous capsule develops around each olfactory pit. By the middle of the third month of prenatal life, the base of the skull is a unified mass of cartilage known as the *chondrocranium*. Ossification of the chondrocranium begins early in the third month, and most of the bones have two or more centers of ossification.

The *membranous neurocranium* ultimately forms the large, flat bones of the vault of the skull, namely, the *frontals, parietals, squamous portion of the occipital*, and the *squamous temporals*, and also smaller bones, the *lacrimals* and *nasals*. Thus, the bones that form the greater part of the sides and roof of the skull are intramembranous in origin. To allow for the rapid increase in size of the developing brain, these bones grow at their margins, and their curvature is modified by the process of bone resorption on the inner surface and new bone deposition on the outer surface.

Most of the bones of the skull are ossified by the time of birth, but they are mobile on each other. Their mobility is most marked in the vault, and the ability to overlap provides the molding of the cranium that is so important during the process of childbirth.

The Neonatal Skull

When compared with the adult skull, the neonatal skull shows a disproportionately large size of the cranium relative to the face (Fig. 2-13). In childhood, the growth of the mandible, the maxillary sinuses, and the alveolar processes of the maxillae results in greatly increased facial length.

The bones of the skull are smooth and unilaminar, there being no diploë present. The bones of the vault are not closely knit at the sutures, as in the adult, but are separated by unossified membranous intervals called *fontanelles*. Clinically, the anterior and posterior fontanelles are most important and are easily examined in the midline of the vault.

The *anterior fontanelle* lies between four bones: the two halves of the developing frontal bones anteriorly and the two parietal bones posteriorly (Fig. 2-13). It is usually impossible clinically to palpate the anterior fontanelle after the child is 18 months old, because the four bones have enlarged to close the gap. The *posterior fontanelle*, lying between the squamous part of the occipital bone and the posterior edges of the parietal bones, closes by the end of the first year.

At birth the tympanic part of the temporal bone is present as a C-shaped tympanic ring (Fig. 2-13). The *tympanic membrane* is near the surface. Although the tympanic membrane is nearly as large as that in the adult, it faces more inferiorly. During childhood the tympanic plate grows laterally, forming the bony part of the meatus, and the tympanic membrane comes to face more directly laterally.

In the newborn the *mastoid process* is not developed, and the *facial nerve*, as it emerges from the stylomastoid foramen, is very close to the surface and thus may be damaged by forceps in a difficult delivery. Later, the mastoid process develops in response to the pull of the sternocleidomastoid muscle when the child moves his head.

Figure 2-13

Neonatal skull: (A) the anterior
aspect and (B) the lateral aspect.

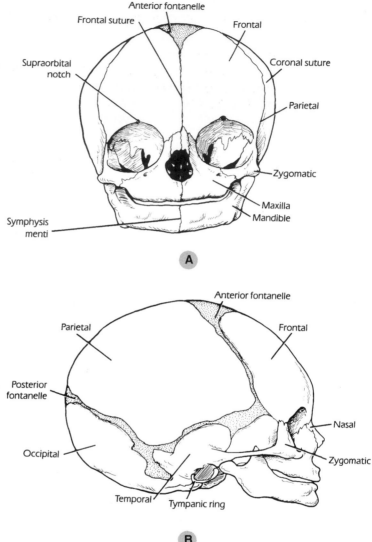

The mandible has right and left halves at birth, united in the midline with
fibrous tissue. The two halves fuse at the *symphysis menti* by the end of the
first year.

The *angle of the mandible* at birth is obtuse (Fig. 2-13), the head being placed
level with the upper margin of the body, and the coronoid process lying at a
superior level to the head. It is only after eruption of the permanent teeth that the
angle of the mandible assumes the adult shape and the head and neck grow so
that the head comes to lie higher than the coronoid process.

In old age, the size of the mandible is reduced when a person loses teeth. As
the alveolar part of the bone becomes smaller, the ramus becomes oblique in
position, so that the head is bent posteriorly.

Clinical Notes

A few of the more common congenital anomalies are briefly described below.

Cranioschisis

In cranioschisis the vault of the skull is open. This anomaly is usually associated with anencephaly. Occasionally it is combined with an open vertebral canal, *craniorachischisis.*

Parietal Foramina

Parietal foramina are localized defects of development in which symmetric foramina occur in the parietal bones. The condition is a mendelian dominant trait.

Ocular Hypertelorism

In ocular hypertelorism, the eyes are widely separated because of overgrowth of the lesser wing of the sphenoid.

Craniosynostosis

Craniosynostosis means premature fusion of some of the cranial sutures. If the sagittal suture is involved, the skull becomes elongated in anteroposterior diameter. If the coronal suture fuses early, the skull becomes turret-shaped because of the pushing upward of the parietal and frontal bones. This condition may lead to a rise in the cerebrospinal fluid pressure, which in turn may lead to mental retardation. Decompression of the skull by craniectomy, leaving the dura mater intact, may be required.

Plagiocephaly

The head is asymmetric in plagiocephaly, possibly because of irregular fusion of the cranial bones. This condition may be caused by excessive pressure on one part of the developing skull in utero; however, it is not caused by the molding that normally occurs during labor. The child develops perfectly normally, but the irregular shape of the skull persists.

Radiographic Appearance

The selected position of the skull relative to the film cassette will depend on the anatomic area that one wishes to demonstrate. This text will describe the appearance seen on a straight posteroanterior view and on a lateral view. Routine posteroanterior and lateral views of the skull for the study of the paranasal sinuses will also be described.

The *straight posteroanterior view* of the skull (Fig. 2-14) is taken with the subject's forehead and nose against the film cassette and the X-ray tube positioned behind the head, perpendicular to the film and in line with the external auditory meatus and the palpebral fissure. Unfortunately, in this position the petrous parts of the temporal bones are superimposed on the lower halves of the orbits.

The different parts of the vault of the skull are visible, as are the sagittal, coronal, and lambdoid sutures (Fig. 2-14). The frontal sinuses, the upper and lower

Figure 2-14

Posteroanterior radiograph of the skull.

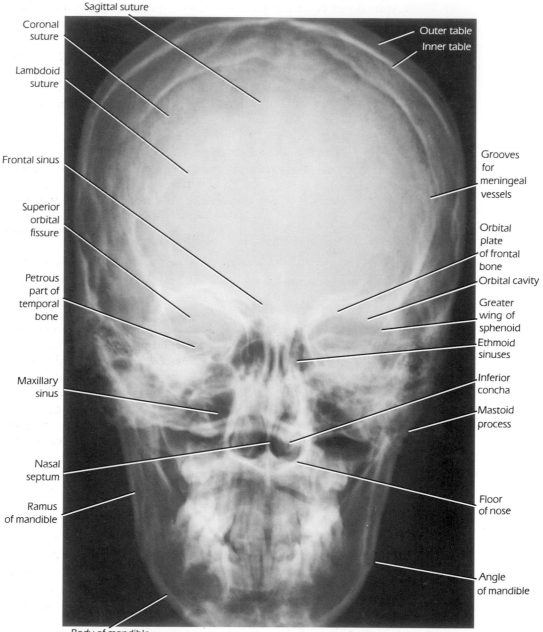

Sagittal suture

Coronal
suture

Lambdoid
suture

Outer table
Inner table

Frontal sinus

Grooves
for
meningeal
vessels

Superior
orbital
fissure

Orbital
plate
of frontal
bone

Orbital cavity

Petrous
part of
temporal
bone

Greater
wing of
sphenoid

Ethmoid
sinuses

Maxillary
sinus

Inferior
concha

Mastoid
process

Nasal
septum

Floor
of nose

Ramus
of mandible

Angle
of mandible

Body of mandible

margins of the orbit, the nasal septum and the conchae, the maxillary sinuses, and the maxillary teeth can be identified.

The rami and body of the mandible are easily recognized. The sphenoidal and ethmoidal air sinuses produce a composite shadow.

The *lateral view of the skull* (Fig. 2-15) is taken with the sagittal plane of the skull parallel with the film cassette. The X-ray tube is centered over the region of the sella turcica.

The different parts of the bones of the vault and base of the skull show clearly (Fig. 2-15). The zygomatic and maxillary bones, however, are superimposed on each other and are not clear. The coronal, squamosal (between the squamous part of the temporal bone and the parietal bone), and lambdoid sutures can be recognized. The inner and outer tables of the skull bones and the intervening diploë can be seen. Depressions on the inner table—commonly seen in children—are produced by the underlying cerebral convolutions.

The grooves produced by the anterior and posterior branches of the middle meningeal vessels may be seen running posteriorly across the parietal bones. A wide groove for the transverse sinus may also be identified as it crosses the occipital bone. Diploic vessels may be recognized as branching dark lines.

The pineal body, if calcified, can be seen as a small shadow above and behind the external auditory meatus.

Anteriorly, the frontal air sinuses appear clearly superimposed on each other. Behind them the two orbital plates of the frontal bones, which form the roofs of the orbits, can be seen. Behind these are the lesser wings of the sphenoid, the anterior clinoid processes, and the sella turcica. The curved lines of the greater wings of the sphenoid and the sphenoidal air sinuses should also be recognized.

Behind the sella turcica, the dorsum sellae and the posterior clinoid processes are clearly seen (Fig. 2-15). The two petrous parts of the temporal bones are superimposed and form a dense shadow between the middle and posterior cranial fossae. Translucent areas formed by the external auditory meatus and, behind them, the mastoid air cells can be identified. The auricle of the external ear frequently produces a curved shadow above the petrous parts of the temporal bones. The temporomandibular joint can be recognized in front of the external auditory meatus.

The nasal bones, the cribriform plate, the hard palate, the maxillary air sinus, and the teeth of the upper and lower jaws can all be seen. The ramus and body of the mandible, the hyoid bone, and the upper part of the cervical vertebral column should be identified.

The *posteroanterior view of the skull to visualize the paranasal sinuses* (Fig. 2-16) is taken with the forehead and nose against the film cassette and the X-ray tube positioned behind the head, but tilted slightly caudally. The frontal and ethmoid sinuses are well shown, but unfortunately the petrous parts of the temporal bones tend to obscure the maxillary sinuses (Fig. 2-16). The ethmoid bones are also superimposed on the sphenoidal sinuses.

The *lateral view of the skull to visualize the paranasal sinuses* (Fig. 2-17) is taken with the patient positioned in exactly the same manner as for a routine

Figure 2-15

Lateral radiograph of the skull.

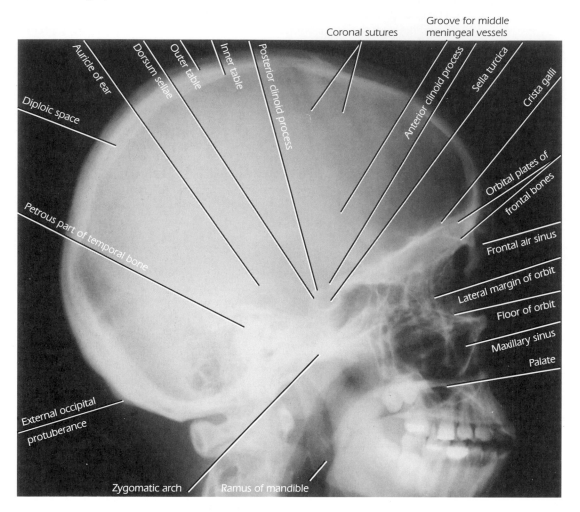

lateral radiograph. The sphenoidal and frontal air sinuses are well shown (Fig. 2-17). The ethmoidal and maxillary sinuses are also seen, but the bony trabeculae somewhat obscure the view.

Computed Tomography

Computed tomography (CT) is commonly used for the detection of intracranial lesions. The technique is safe for the patient and provides highly accurate information. CT relies on the same physics as conventional X-rays, in that structures are distinguished from one another by their ability to absorb energy from X-rays. The beams of X-rays, having passed through the region of the body under

Figure 2-16

Posteroanterior (Waters) radiograph of paranasal sinuses.

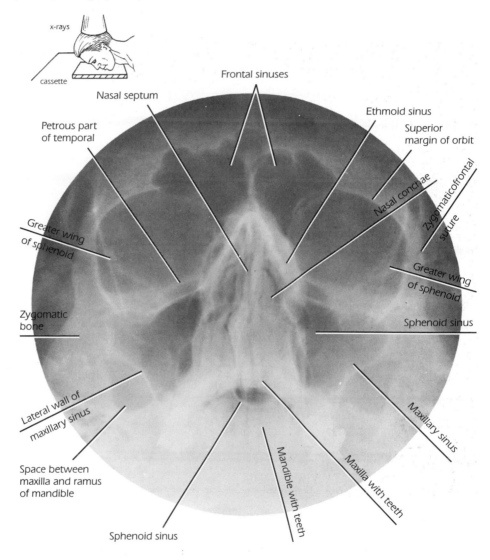

consideration, are collected by a special X-ray detector. The information is fed to a computer that processes the information, which is then displayed as a reconstructed picture on a television-like screen. Essentially, the observer sees an image of a thin slice through, for example, the head, which may then be photographed for later examination (Figs. 2-18 and 2-19). The procedure is quick, lasting only a few seconds for each slice, and most patients require no sedation.

Figure 2-17

Lateral radiograph of the paranasal sinuses.

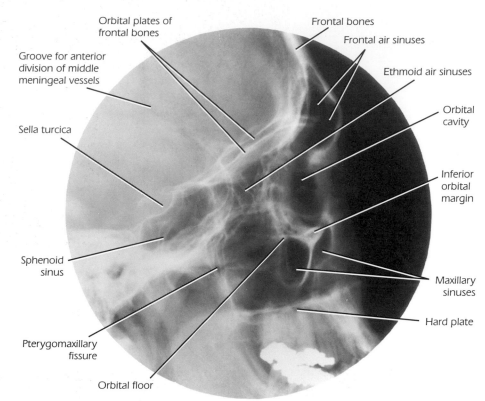

Orbital plates of
frontal bones

Groove for anterior
division of middle
meningeal vessels

Sella turcica

Sphenoid
sinus

Pterygomaxillary
fissure

Orbital floor

Frontal bones

Frontal air sinuses

Ethmoid air sinuses

Orbital
cavity

Inferior
orbital
margin

Maxillary
sinuses

Hard plate

Magnetic Resonance Imaging

The more recent technique of *magnetic resonance imaging* (MRI) uses the magnetic properties of the hydrogen nucleus excited by radiofrequency radiation transmitted by a coil surrounding the body part. The excited hydrogen nuclei emit a signal that is detected as induced electric currents in a receiver coil. MRI is absolutely safe to the patient, and because it provides better differentiation between different soft tissues, it can be more revealing than a CT scan. The reason for this is that some tissues contain more hydrogen in the form of water than do other tissues (Figs. 2-20 and 2-21).

Figure 2-18

CT scan of the skull using a horizontal cut (axial section) at the level of the orbital cavities and the tympanic cavities. The eyeball can be clearly seen.

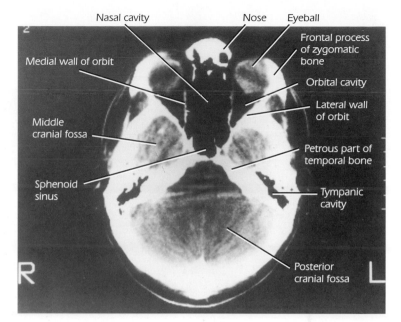

Figure 2-19

CT scan of the skull using a horizontal cut (horizontal section) showing the structure of the brain.

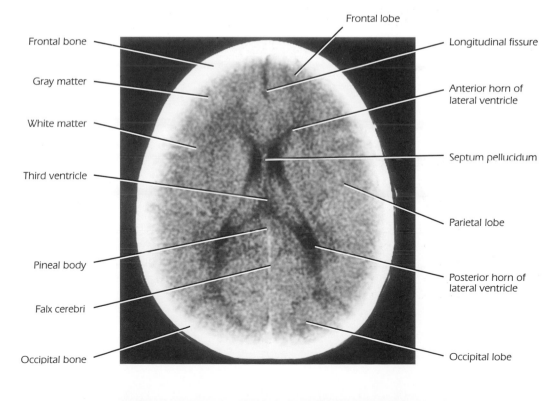

Figure 2-20

MRI of the skull using a sagittal cut (sagittal section) showing the structure of the brain.

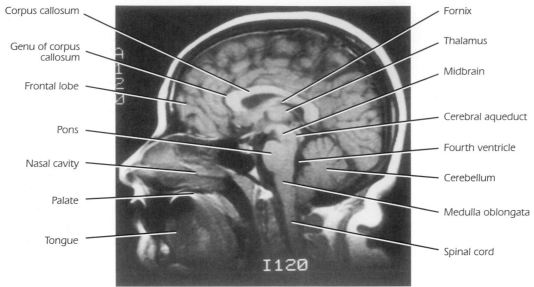

Corpus callosum

Genu of corpus callosum

Frontal lobe

Pons

Nasal cavity

Palate

Tongue

Fornix

Thalamus

Midbrain

Cerebral aqueduct

Fourth ventricle

Cerebellum

Medulla oblongata

Spinal cord

I120

 Figure 2-21

MRI of the skull using a coronal cut (coronal section) showing the structure of the brain. Note the differentiation between gray and white matter.

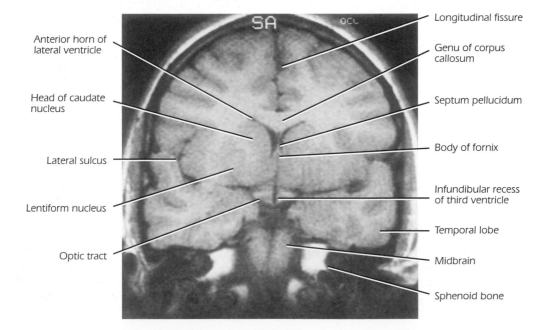

Anterior horn of lateral ventricle

Head of caudate nucleus

Lateral sulcus

Lentiform nucleus

Optic tract

Longitudinal fissure

Genu of corpus callosum

Septum pellucidum

Body of fornix

Infundibular recess of third ventricle

Temporal lobe

Midbrain

Sphenoid bone

CHAPTER 2
Clinical Problems

Answers on Page 57

1 A 32-year-old woman was struck in the face with a baseball while playing with her son. X-ray examination revealed multiple fractures of the bones around the orbit. Name the bones that form the orbital margin.

2 A 65-year-old man was found on ophthalmoscopic examination to have edema of both optic discs (bilateral papilledema) and congestion of the retinal veins. The cause of the condition was found to be a rapidly growing intracranial tumor. Using your knowledge of anatomy, explain the papilledema. Why does the patient exhibit bilateral papilledema?

3 A visiting neurosurgeon concluded his lecture on the "late effects of head injuries" by saying that the disabilities experienced by a patient are likely to be greater following damage to the dominant hemisphere than to the opposite hemisphere, and that the effect would be much greater in adults than in children. There is no question that this statement is true. What structures exist within the skull that are there clearly to limit damage to the cerebral hemispheres and other parts of the brain? Which blood vessels are damaged more commonly, the cerebral arteries or the cerebral veins? Are cranial nerves likely to be damaged in head injuries? If so, which ones are damaged most commonly, and what is the reason for their increased susceptibility?

4 A 12-year-old boy was admitted to a hospital for surgical correction of medial strabismus of the right eye. Twenty-four hours after the successful completion of the operation it was noted that his right eyeball was projecting forward excessively (proptosis) and the conjunctiva of the right eye was inflamed. A watery, purulent discharge could be expressed from beneath the eyelids. The ophthalmologist was greatly concerned, because he did not want the complication of cavernous sinus thrombosis to occur. What is the connection between infection of the eye and cavernous sinus thrombosis? Is cavernous sinus thrombosis a serious condition?

5 While performing an autopsy on a patient who had died of a meningioma, the pathologist explained to a group of residents that these tumors arise from the arachnoid mater. He observed that they occur in those areas where the arachnoid pierces the dura to form the arachnoid villi that project into the dural venous sinuses. He then asked the residents where they would expect to find meningiomas. Answer his question.

6 A 62-year-old woman was found, on examination, to have paralysis of the lateral rectus muscle of her left eye; the left pupil was dilated but reacted slowly to light, and there was some anesthesia of the skin over the left side of the forehead. A carotid arteriogram revealed the presence of an aneurysm of the right internal carotid artery situated in the cavernous sinus. Using your knowledge of anatomy, explain the clinical findings on physical examination.

7 At childbirth the fetal head becomes molded so that the parietal bones commonly override each other and the occipital bone. Explain how this change is possible.

8 A routine physical examination of a 10-year-old boy showed a complete absence of both clavicles. It was possible for the child to approximate the tips of his shoulders to each other below his chin. Neither trapezius muscle had clavicular fibers. Examination of the skull showed an abnormally large transverse diameter of the cranium, so that the whole skull appeared globular in shape. Examination of the mother showed that she had exactly the same condition. What is your diagnosis? Is any treatment necessary?

9 While playing baseball, a player was struck on the right side of the head with the ball. The player fell to the ground but did not lose consciousness. After resting for an hour and then getting up, he was seen to be confused and irritable. Later, he staggered and fell to the floor. On questioning, he was seen to be drowsy; twitching of the lower left half of his face and left arm was noted. A diagnosis of extradural hemorrhage was made. Which artery is likely to have been damaged? What is responsible for the drowsiness and muscle twitching?

10 A pediatrician was observing an 8-year-old girl playing with her toys. He noted that the child had perfectly normal use of her arms, but her legs were stiff and when she walked she tended to cross her legs and had a scissor-like gait. A diagnosis of cerebral diplegia secondary to birth injuries was made. Apparently, the child was born prematurely and she was a breech presentation. Using your knowledge of anatomy, explain what happens to the fetal skull bones during delivery. Why are the dural venous sinuses likely to be damaged at birth? Why is cerebral hemorrhage more likely to occur in a premature baby with a malpresentation?

11 A 48-year-old man complaining of a severe headache of 3 days' duration visited his physician. He said that the headache had started to become very severe about 1 hour after he hit his head on the mantelpiece after bending down to poke the fire. He was admitted to the hospital for observation. Three hours later, he was becoming mentally confused, and was developing a right-sided hemiplegia, opposite the side of the head injury. He had exaggeration of the deep reflexes and a positive Babinski response on the right side. Examination of the cerebrospinal fluid by lumbar puncture showed a raised pressure, with blood present in the fluid. X-ray examination showed no fracture of the skull. A diagnosis of subdural hematoma was made. What exactly is a subdural hematoma?

CHAPTER 2
Answers to Clinical Problems

1 The bones that form the orbital margin are the frontal, zygomatic, and maxillary bones.

2 The optic nerves are surrounded by sheaths derived from the pia mater, arachnoid mater, and dura mater. There is an extension of the intracranial subarachnoid space forward around the optic nerve to the back of the eyeball. A rise in cerebrospinal fluid pressure caused by an intracranial tumor will compress the thin walls of the retinal vein as it crosses the extension of the subarachnoid space (see p. 191). This will result in congestion of the retinal vein and bulging of the optic disc. Since both subarachnoid extensions are continuous with the intracranial subarachnoid space, both eyes will exhibit papilledema.

3 Loss of function of the dominant hemisphere results not only in loss of acquired skills of the dominant hand but also in loss of certain mental functions. The degree of disability depends on the degree of dominance of one hemisphere over the other. A child's brain possesses a degree of flexibility that is not present in the adult; so good recoveries can be expected in the young child.

The meninges and the cerebrospinal fluid afford a remarkable degree of protection to the delicate brain. The dural partitions limit the extent of brain movement within the skull.

The thin-walled cerebral veins are liable to be damaged during excessive movements of the brain relative to the skull, especially at the point where the veins join the dural venous sinuses. The thick-walled cerebral arteries are rarely damaged.

The long, small-diameter cranial nerves are particularly susceptible to damage during head injuries. The trochlear, abducent, and oculomotor nerves are commonly injured.

4 The anterior facial vein, the ophthalmic veins, and the cavernous sinus are in direct communication with one another. Infection of the skin of the face alongside the nose, ethmoidal sinusitis, and infection of the orbital contents may lead to thrombosis of the veins and, ultimately, cavernous sinus thrombosis. If untreated with antibiotics, this condition may be fatal, since the cavernous sinus drains many cerebral veins from the inferior surface of the brain.

5 Meningiomas arise from the arachnoid villi found along the dural venous sinuses. They are, therefore, most commonly found along the superior sagittal sinus and the sphenoparietal sinuses. They are rare below the tentorium cerebelli.

6 The internal carotid artery passes forward on the lateral surface of the body of the sphenoid within the cavernous sinus. An aneurysm of the artery may press on the abducent nerve and cause paralysis of the lateral rectus muscle. Further expansion of the aneurysm may cause compression of the oculomotor nerve and the ophthalmic division of the trigeminal nerve as they lie in the lateral wall of the cavernous sinus. This patient had left lateral rectus paralysis and paralysis of the left pupillary constrictor muscle resulting from involvement of, respectively, the abducent and oculomotor nerves. The slight anesthesia of the skin over the left side of the forehead resulted from pressure on the ophthalmic division of the left trigeminal nerve.

7 During the descent of the fetal head through the birth canal in labor, the fetal head becomes compressed and the bones of the calvarium overlap, a process known as molding. This process is possible because at this stage of bone growth each bone of the vault is separated by a wide area of membranous connective tissue.

8 This boy and his mother have cleidocranial dysostosis. This condition is caused by the inheritance of an autosomal dominant gene resulting in incomplete formation or absence of the clavicles. The membrane bones of the skull also are involved, causing the fontanelles to remain wide open. No treatment is necessary, because the excessive mobility of the shoulders is not a hindrance. However, in some cases the sternal or acromial ends of the clavicle may develop and exert pressure on the brachial plexus. In these cases, the offending bony fragments should be removed.

9 A minor blow to the side of the head may easily fracture the thin anterior part of the parietal bone or the squamous part of the temporal bone. The anterior branch of the middle meningeal artery commonly enters a bony canal in this region and is sectioned at the time of the fracture. The resulting hemorrhage causes the gradual accumulation of blood under pressure outside the meningeal layer of the dura mater. As the blood clot enlarges, pressure is exerted on the underlying brain, and symptoms of confusion and irritability become apparent. These are

followed later by drowsiness. Pressure on the lower end of the right precentral gyrus or motor area causes twitching of the facial muscles on the left, and later twitching of the left arm muscles. As the blood clot progressively enlarges, the intracranial pressure rises and the patient's condition deteriorates. The accurate placing of a burr hole in the skull and the tying off of the middle meningeal artery will save the patient's life.

10 During the descent of the fetal head through the birth canal in labor, the bones of the calvarium overlap, a process known as molding. If this process is excessive or takes place too rapidly, as in malpresentations or in premature deliveries (when a small fetus is born rapidly), the falx cerebri receives an abnormal strain. This stress involves the superior sagittal sinus, especially if the anteroposterior compression is excessive, and the sinus may tear where it joins the transverse sinus. The great cerebral vein also may tear. The result is either a subarachnoid or a subdural hemorrhage, with accompanying brain damage.

11 A subdural hematoma is an accumulation of blood clot in the interval between the meningeal layer of dura and the arachnoid mater. It results from tearing of the superior cerebral veins at their point of entrance into the superior sagittal sinus. The cause is usually a blow to the front or the back of the head, causing extreme anteroposterior displacement of the brain within the skull.

The Orbital Cavity

CHAPTER OUTLINE

Introduction

The orbital cavities are a pair of large bony sockets that contain the eyeballs, their associated muscles, nerves, vessels, and fat, and most of the lacrimal apparatus. Each cavity is pear-shaped and its apex is directed posteriorly, medially, and slightly upward; the stalk of the pear lying within the optic canal (Fig. 3-1). The medial wall runs anteroposteriorly parallel to the sagittal plane; the lateral wall diverges at an angle of about 45 degrees. Seven individual bones form the orbit— namely, the maxilla and palatine, the zygomatic and sphenoid, the frontal, the ethmoid, and the lacrimal bones (Fig. 3-1).

Orbital Margin

The strong orbital margin (or rim) is quadrilateral in shape with rounded corners. In the adult the orbital margin is wider than it is high (Fig. 3-1). The *supraorbital margin* is formed by the frontal bone, having a sharp lateral two-thirds and a rounded medial third. At the junction of the two areas is the *supraorbital notch or foramen** for passage of the supraorbital vessels and nerve (Fig. 3-1). The sharp *infraorbital margin* is formed laterally by the zygomatic bone and medially by the maxilla. The *lateral margin*, the strongest part of the orbital margin, is formed by the frontal process of the zygomatic bone below and the zygomatic process of the frontal bone above (Fig. 3-1). The suture between the two bones can be easily felt in the living subject. The *medial margin* is formed above by the maxillary process of the frontal bone and below by the lacrimal crest of the frontal process of the maxilla (Fig. 3-1). The upper part of the medial margin is indistinct and its lower half is sharp and easily felt.

Walls of the Orbital Cavity

The walls of the orbital cavity are lined with periosteum and consist of a roof, a floor, and a medial and a lateral wall.

The *apex* of the orbital cavity is at the medial end of the superior orbital fissure.

Roof

The concave roof or superior wall is formed by the orbital plate of the frontal bone and to a small extent by the lesser wing of the sphenoid posteriorly (Fig. 3-2). Anteromedially the roof is invaded by the frontal air sinus. Anterolaterally there is a slight depression, the *lacrimal fossa*, for the orbital part of the lacrimal gland. Medial to the supraorbital notch and 4 mm behind the orbital margin is a small depression or spine for the pulley of the superior oblique muscle (Fig. 3-2).

The roof of the orbit is thin and fragile and in old age portions of the roof may be absorbed. The roof separates the orbital cavity from the anterior cranial fossa and the frontal lobe of the cerebral hemisphere (Fig. 3-4).

* Sometimes the ligament binding the nerve and vessels to the notch is ossified.

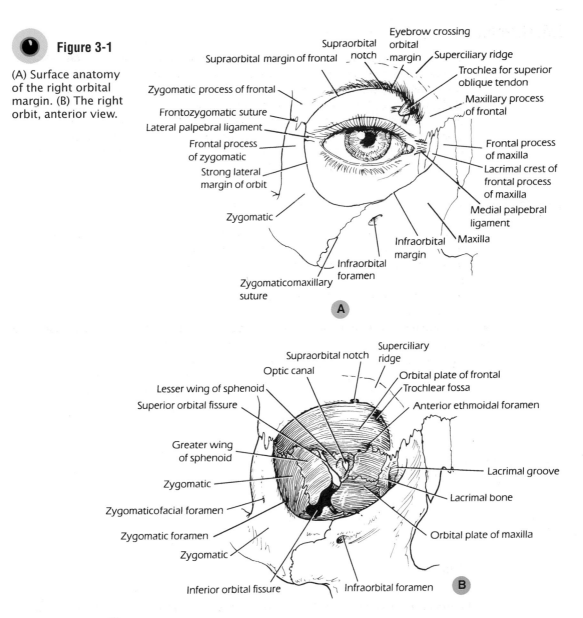

Figure 3-1

(A) Surface anatomy of the right orbital margin. (B) The right orbit, anterior view.

Floor

The thin floor or inferior wall is formed largely by the orbital plate of the maxilla, and also by the orbital surface of the zygomatic and the small orbital process of the palatine bone (Fig. 3-2). The orbital plate of the maxilla separates the orbital cavity from the maxillary sinus (Fig. 3-4). The floor is continuous with the lateral wall anteriorly but is separated from it posteriorly by the *inferior orbital fissure* (Fig. 3-1). Running forward from the fissure is the *infraorbital groove* (Fig. 3-2). At about the midpoint of the floor the infraorbital groove becomes the *infraorbital canal,* which opens onto the face as the *infraorbital foramen* (Fig. 3-3).

Figure 3-2

(A) Roof of the right and left orbits. (B) Floor of the right orbit.

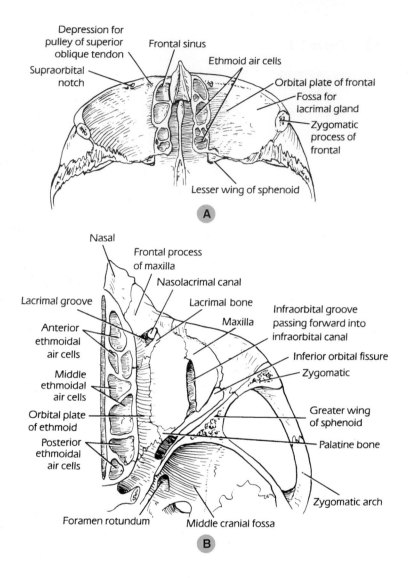

Lateral Wall

The lateral wall is the thickest wall (Fig. 3-4). The anterior third is formed by the zygomatic bone, which separates the orbit from the temporal fossa. The posterior two-thirds is formed by the greater wing of the sphenoid bone and it separates the orbit from the temporal lobe of the brain in the middle cranial fossa (Fig. 3-2). The lateral wall and roof are continuous anteriorly but they are separated posteriorly by the *superior orbital fissure* (Fig. 3-1). The superior orbital fissure communicates with the middle cranial fossa. Just posterior to the orbital margin, on the frontal process of the zygoma, is a small prominence, the *marginal tubercle*, to which is attached from before backward the aponeurosis of the levator palpebrae superioris, the lateral palpebral ligament, and the lateral check ligament.

Figure 3-3

Medial wall of the right orbit. The maxillary sinus is also shown.

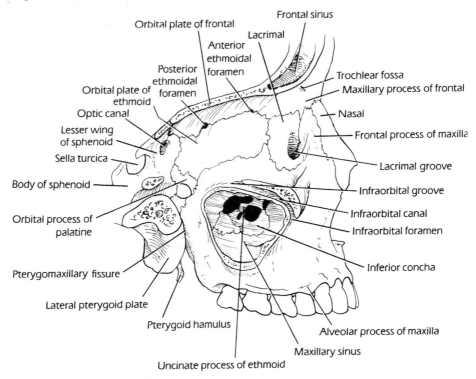

Medial Wall

The very thin medial wall is formed by four bones (Fig. 3-3). From anterior to posterior, these are the frontal process of the maxilla, the lacrimal bone, the orbital plate of the ethmoid, and a small part of the body of the sphenoid (Fig. 3-3). The orbital plate of the ethmoid forms the largest part of the medial wall. It is almost rectangular in shape, and the very thin bone separates the orbital cavity from the ethmoidal sinuses. On the anterior part of the medial wall is the *lacrimal groove* for the lacrimal sac (Fig. 3-3). The lacrimal groove is formed by the lacrimal bone posteriorly and the frontal process of the maxilla anteriorly. The groove is bounded in front and behind by the *anterior and posterior lacrimal crests*. Below, the lacrimal groove is continuous with the *nasolacrimal canal*, which leads inferiorly into the nasal cavity (Fig. 3-1).

Table 3-1 summarizes the walls of the orbit.

Openings into the Orbital Cavity and the Structures That Pass Through Them · · ·

The main *orbital opening* lies anteriorly and is bounded by the orbital margin.

The *optic canal*, which lies in the lesser wing of the sphenoid, is related medially to the body of the sphenoid (Fig. 3-1). It is situated close to the apex of the

Figure 3-4

(A) Coronal section of skull showing orbital cavities. Note the position of the ethmoidal sinuses and maxillary sinuses. (B) Apex of the right orbital cavity showing the superior orbital fissure, optic canal, the fibrous ring for the origins of the recti muscles, and the positions of the nerves entering the orbital cavity.

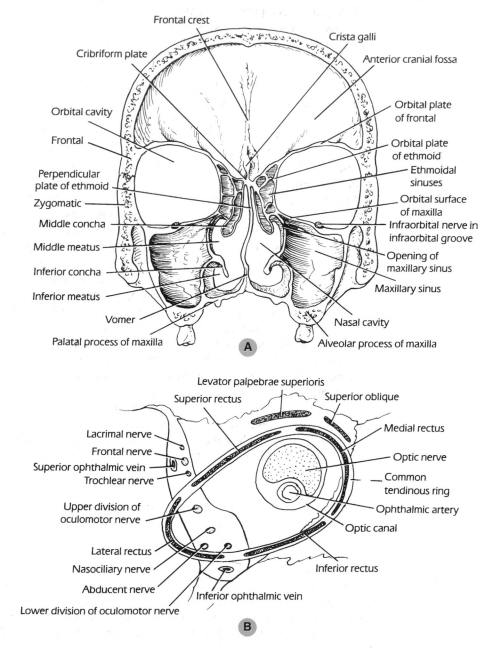

Table 3-1 Summary of the Walls of the Orbit

Walls	Bony Structures Forming the Walls
Roof	Orbital plate of frontal bone, and lesser wing of sphenoid
Floor	Orbital plate of maxilla, orbital surface of zygomatic, orbital process of palatine
Lateral wall	Zygomatic, and greater wing of sphenoid
Medial wall	Frontal process of maxilla, lacrimal bone, orbital plate of ethmoid, and body of sphenoid

orbit. Measuring 4 to 10 mm long, it connects the middle cranial fossa with the orbital cavity. The optic canal transmits the optic nerve with its sleeve of meninges, and extension of the subarachnoid space, and the ophthalmic artery with its surrounding sympathetic plexus (Fig. 3-4). The ophthalmic artery is the first branch of the internal carotid after it leaves the cavernous sinus.

The *superior orbital fissure*, lying between the lesser and greater wings of the sphenoid, connects the middle cranial fossa with the orbital cavity (Fig. 3-1). It lies between the roof and lateral walls of the orbit. The widest part of the fissure is at its medial end. About midway on the lower edge of the fissure is a small, sharp spine for the lateral rectus muscle. Bridging the medial end of the superior orbital fissure and attached to this spine is the *common tendinous ring* of origin for the four rectus muscles (Fig. 3-4). Passing through the superior orbital fissure, from lateral to medial, are the lacrimal nerve, the frontal nerve, and the trochlear nerve; and within the tendinous ring, the upper and lower divisions of the oculomotor nerve, the nasociliary nerve, and the abducent nerve (Fig. 3-4). The superior ophthalmic vein passes back through the lateral part of the superior orbital fissure to enter the cavernous sinus.

The *inferior orbital fissure* lies between the greater wing of the sphenoid and the maxilla (Fig. 3-1). It connects the pterygopalatine and infratemporal fossae with the orbital cavity. It is closed in the living subject by the periorbita and the muscle of Müller (see p. 67). The fissure transmits the maxillary nerve, which immediately changes its name to infraorbital nerve. It also permits passage of the zygomatic nerve, branches of the pterygopalatine ganglion, and the inferior ophthalmic vein, which drains into the pterygoid venous plexus.

The *ethmoidal foramina* lie in the frontoethmoidal suture or in the frontal bone (Fig. 3-3). They are situated where the roof joins the medial wall. The *anterior ethmoidal foramen* opens into the anterior cranial fossa at the lateral edge of the cribriform plate of the ethmoid bone. It transmits the anterior ethmoidal nerve and artery. The *posterior ethmoidal foramen* traverses the ethmoid bone. It transmits the posterior ethmoidal nerve and artery, which supply the ethmoidal sinuses.

The *zygomaticofacial and zygomaticotemporal foramina* are small foramina that lie on the lateral wall of the orbit (Fig. 3-1). The zygomaticofacial foramen lies close to the junction of the lateral wall and floor and transmits the zygomaticofacial nerve. The zygomaticotemporal foramen lies above the latter foramen close to the sphenozygomatic suture. It transmits the zygomaticotemporal nerve.

Relations of the Bony Orbit

Superior Relations

The roof, formed by the orbital plate of the frontal bone, contains between its two laminae anteromedially, the frontal air sinus (Fig. 3-3). Occasionally the ethmoid air cells also invade the roof. Superior to the roof are the meninges and the frontal lobe of the cerebral hemisphere.

Inferior Relations

Inferior to the floor lies the maxillary air sinus (Fig. 3-4). The infraorbital nerve and blood vessels lie within the infraorbital canal.

Lateral Relations

The lateral wall separates the orbital cavity anteriorly from the temporal fossa containing the temporalis muscle, and posteriorly from the middle cranial fossa, the meninges, and the temporal lobe of the cerebral hemisphere.

Medial Relations

The medial wall separates the orbital cavity, from anterior to posterior, from the nasal cavity, the ethmoidal sinuses, and the sphenoid sinus (Fig. 3-4).

The Periorbita or Orbital Periosteum (Orbital Fascia)

The periorbita is the periosteum of the bones that form the walls of the orbit. It is loosely attached to the bones and is continuous through the foramina and fissures with the periosteum covering the outer surfaces of the bones (Fig. 3-5). In the case of the superior orbital fissure, the optic canal, and the anterior ethmoidal canal, it becomes continuous with the endosteal layer of the dura mater. At places where it passes through foramina and also at sutures, it tends to be adherent to bone. At the optic canal the periorbita is also attached to the dural sheath of the optic nerve. At the orbital margin it becomes continuous with the periosteum on the external surface of the skull. Here it also gives rise to sheets that enter the eyelids to form the *orbital septum* (Fig. 3-5). A process is also given off to hold the trochlea for the superior oblique tendon in position. At the lacrimal groove it splits to enclose the lacrimal sac and continues inferiorly to form the periosteum of the nasolacrimal canal. Yet another extension of this fascia is said to enclose the lacrimal gland.

Posteriorly, around the optic canal and the medial end of the superior orbital fissure the periorbita is thicker to form a fibrous ring, the *common tendinous ring*, which gives origin to the tendons of the four rectus muscles (Fig. 3-4).

The periorbita receives its sensory innervation from the branches of the trigeminal nerve that lie within the orbital cavity.

Figure 3-5

Sagittal section of the orbital cavity showing the continuity of the tarsal plates, the orbital septa, the periosteum, the periorbita, and the periosteal layer of the dura. Note the fusion of the periosteal layer of dura with the meningeal layer of dura at the optic canal, the forward extension of the meninges, and the subarachnoid space to the back of the eyeball.

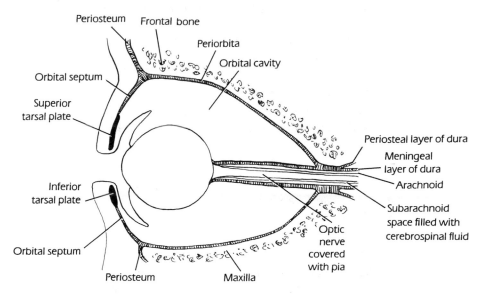

Orbital Muscle (Muscle of Müller)

The orbital muscle is a thin layer of smooth muscle that bridges the inferior orbital fissure. It is embedded in the fascia of the periorbita and is regarded as a vestigeal muscle, because its function is unknown. It receives its nerve supply from the sympathetic nerves.

Effect of Age on the Orbital Cavity

At birth the orbital cavities are relatively large and the orbital margins are ossified and strong and protect the eyeball during parturition. In the young child the orbital cavities look more laterally than do those in an adult. The superior and inferior orbital fissures are wider in a child and later become narrowed with the growth of the greater wing of the sphenoid. In the child the distances between the orbits are small and they move apart later with the development and expansion of the frontal and ethmoidal sinuses. In old age, bony absorption occurs and this may result in holes appearing in the roof, lateral wall, and medial wall.

Sex Differences in the Orbital Cavities $\cdots\cdots\cdots\cdots\cdots\cdots\cdots\cdots\cdots$

Until puberty the orbital cavities are almost identical in the two sexes. There-
after, the female orbits remain rounder, and the bones are smoother than in the
male.

Surface Anatomy of the Orbital Region $\cdots\cdots\cdots\cdots\cdots\cdots\cdots\cdots$

Superciliary Ridges

This is a prominent ridge above the upper margin of the orbit (Fig. 3-1). Deep to
the ridge on either side of the midline lie the frontal air sinuses.

Eyebrow

The medial end of the eyebrow lies below the medial end of the supraorbital
margin and the lateral end lies above the margin (Fig. 3-1).

Orbital Margins

The frontal, maxillary, and zygomatic bones forming the margins can easily be
felt (Fig. 3-1). The *frontozygomatic suture* can be clearly felt along the lateral
margin.

The *supraorbital notch* (if present) can be palpated at the junction of the
medial third and lateral two-thirds of the superior margin (Fig. 3-1). The supraorbital nerve can sometimes be rolled in the notch.

The *trochlea* of the superior oblique tendon can be felt with the fingertip
within the superomedial part of the orbital margin (Fig. 3-1).

The *lateral palpebral ligament* can be felt on firm but deep pressure between
the lateral bony margin of the orbit and the lateral end of the palpebral fissure
when the subject's eye is closed (Fig. 3-1). Its attachment to the orbital margin
lies just inferior to the frontozygomatic suture and is commonly marked by a
small bony marginal tubercle.

The *medial palpebral ligament* can be felt between the medial bony margin
of the orbit and the palpebral fissure (Fig. 3-1). The lower free border of the ligament can be more easily felt if the eyelids are gently pulled laterally.

The *anterior lacrimal crest*, the *lacrimal groove*, and the *posterior lacrimal
crest* can be easily felt along the medial part of the orbital margin.

The *infraorbital foramen* lies about 5 mm below the lower margin of the orbit
(Fig. 3-1). Its sharp upper margin can be recognized on deep pressure with the
fingertip.

**Clinical
Notes**

Close Relationship Between Orbit and Eyeball

The bony orbit, apart from the large anterior opening, is virtually a closed socket
for the eyeball. This fact, together with the relatively small amount of space
between the orbital walls and the eyeball, means that an expanding lesion within
the orbit will quickly cause proptosis. Moreover, the limited space between the

eyeball and the orbital margin severely restricts the removal of tumors. When diseased, the many important structures surrounding the orbit may extend into the orbital cavity to involve its contents. The intimate relationship between the growth of the eyeball and the growth of the orbital cavity is emphasized by the fact that enucleation of the eye in the child will result in impaired future growth of the orbit. The closeness of the two orbits in infants and their subsequent gradual separation due to growth of the sinuses may be forgotten by the physician, who may make an erroneous diagnosis of squint.

Congenital Abnormalities of the Orbit

Congenital abnormalities of the skull with resulting changes in the bones of the orbit and face may be associated with exophthalmos and with medial or lateral strabismus. Craniosynostosis, mandibulofacial dysostosis, development tumors, and defects of the orbital walls associated with meningocele and encephalocele are just a few such conditions.

Trauma to the Orbit

The orbital margin is very strong and not easily fractured. However, severe injury, as in automobile accidents, may involve the medial margin and the nose. Fractures of the superior margin may damage or displace the trochlea, producing symptoms of superior oblique paralysis. Fractures of the lateral margin involving the zygoma result in depression of the prominence of the cheek. Comminuted fractures of the lower margin also occur. So-called blow-out fracture of the floor and medial wall of the orbit is the most common result of blunt force to the face (see below). The bones that form the floor and medial wall are the thinnest bones in the orbit.

Penetrating Wounds

Sticks, pointed metal objects, umbrellas, and even surgical instruments may pierce the thin roof of the orbit and enter the cranial cavity and the frontal lobe of the brain. The thin medial wall has also been pierced by pointed objects.

Complications of Retrobulbar and Peribulbar Anesthesia

The small, crowded space between the bony orbital walls and the eyeball explains the possible complications following retrobulbar and peribulbar anesthesia (see pp. 322 and 323). Retrobulbar hemorrhage, with proptosis of the eye and increased intraocular pressure, is likely to occur if a too-sharp needle pierces the ophthalmic veins. Puncture of the meningeal sheath around the optic nerve, with subsequent diffusion of the anesthetic agent into the subarachnoid space, has been responsible for several reported cases of respiratory distress. The surgeon can minimize these complications if the tip of the advancing anesthetic needle, which is introduced into the orbit through the facial skin or through the conjunctiva, is kept away from the eyeball and is guided backward along the upper surface of the orbital floor. The use of a semisharp needle tip is also recommended. Peribulbar anesthesia using a $^5/_8$-inch needle rather than a $1^1/_2$-inch retrobulbar needle reduces the likelihood of hitting a blood vessel or penetrating the globe.

Air Sinuses

Infection of the air sinuses is the commonest cause of orbital cellulitis. The extremely thin medial orbital wall formed by the ethmoid bone is a common route by which infection enters the orbital cavity as the result of ethmoidal sinusitis.

The thin roof of the orbit with its overlying frontal sinus permits an expanding mucocele of that sinus to invade the orbital cavity.

The medial part of the floor of the orbit is a favorite site for a blow-out fracture involving the maxillary sinus. A severe blow to the eye causes the floor of the orbital cavity to buckle inferiorly into the maxillary sinus. Not only can this cause displacement of the eyeball inferiorly, with resulting symptoms of diplopia, but also the fracture may injure the infraorbital nerve, producing hypoesthesia of the skin of the cheek.

Tumors of the maxillary sinus may extend superiorly into the orbital cavity, causing proptosis.

The optic canal has a variable relationship with the sphenoid and ethmoidal sinuses. In most individuals, the body of the sphenoid and its contained sinus lie medial to the optic canal. In some subjects the sphenoid sinus and even the posterior ethmoidal sinus invade the lesser wing of the sphenoid and come to lie on the superior and lateral aspect of the optic canal.

Apex of the Orbital Cavity

The crowding together of important nerves passing through the superior orbital fissure and the optic canal makes this a very vulnerable site in occurrences of pathologic lesions. The symptoms and signs may include total ophthalmoplegia, blindness, and anesthesia of the cornea and the skin of the forehead and nose.

Periorbita

The loose attachment of the periorbita (periosteum) to the bones forming the walls of the orbit permits accumulation of blood and pus. However, one should remember the firm attachment of the periorbita to the margins of the various foramina and fissures when performing exenteration of the orbit.

Orbitalis Muscle (Muscle of Müller) and Exophthalmos

The orbitalis, a sheet of smooth muscle that bridges the inferior orbital fissure, is vestigeal and has no known function in humans. It was once believed to play a role in the exophthalmos caused by thyrotoxicosis (the increased bulk of the orbital contents, especially the extraocular muscles and fat, is now accepted as the cause of exophthalmos in this condition).

Figure 3-6

Frontal view of the right eye showing possible skin incisions used in the surgical approach to the orbit.

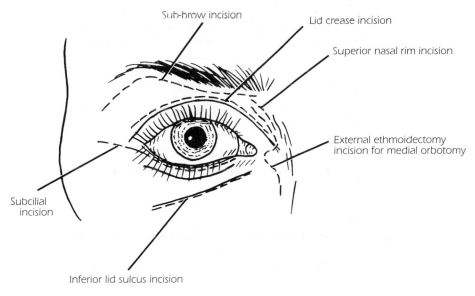

Sub-brow incision

Lid crease incision

Superior nasal rim incision

External ethmoidectomy incision for medial orbotomy

Subcilial incision

Inferior lid sulcus incision

Surgical Approaches to the Orbit

Figure 3-6 shows some of the common skin incisions made in surgical approaches to the orbit. In the superior approaches, the supraorbital notch is an important landmark because it marks the exit of the supraorbital nerve and artery. The attachment of the trochlea for the superior oblique muscle must be preserved if possible. The inferior approaches involve less important anatomic structures and fewer blood vessels are encountered.

Radiology ·

Computed Tomography (CT)

This technique permits visualization of considerable detail of the orbital cavity and its contents (Fig. 3-7). The walls of the orbital cavity, fascial planes, the eyeball, the extraocular muscles, and the large blood vessels can all be recognized. Contrast enhancement by intravenous injection of an iodine-containing compound enables one to visualize neoplasms and inflammatory tissue. This is the most common imaging modality used when evaluating the bones of the orbit, especially following trauma.

Figure 3-7

CT scan of the skull at the level of the orbital cavities and the tympanic cavities. The walls of the orbit and the eyeball can be seen.

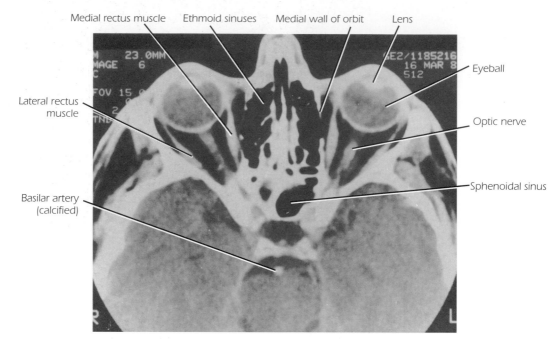

Magnetic Resonance Imaging (MRI)

This method provides better differentiation between soft tissues (Fig. 3-8). It is useful to delineate fine structures such as the optic nerve or muscles.

Ultrasonography

The use of high-frequency sound directed through the orbit provides a technique permitting visualization of soft tissue. In A-scan ultrasonography the sound waves are reflected at tissue interfaces and converted into an electric potential that is displayed on a cathode ray oscillograph. The optic nerve, the eyeball, the extraocular muscles, orbital fat, and pathologic lesions can all be visualized. In B-scan ultrasonography one can view a sectional representation of the eye (Fig. 3-9).

Figure 3-8

MRI showing the contents of the orbital and cranial cavities. Note that the eyeballs, the optic nerves, the optic chiasma, and the extraocular muscles can be identified.

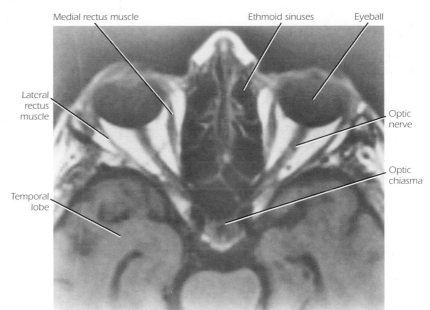

Medial rectus muscle   Ethmoid sinuses   Eyeball

Lateral rectus muscle

Optic nerve

Optic chiasma

Temporal lobe

 Figure 3-9

Ultrasonogram of the orbital cavity showing the posterior wall of the eyeball, the optic nerve, and the extraocular muscles. The retrobulbar fat can also be identified. The sound from the transducer penetrated the upper eyelid above the limbus and passed through the sclera, the ciliary body, the vitreous body, and the posterior wall of the eyeball. (Courtesy of Dr. J. S. Zacharia.)

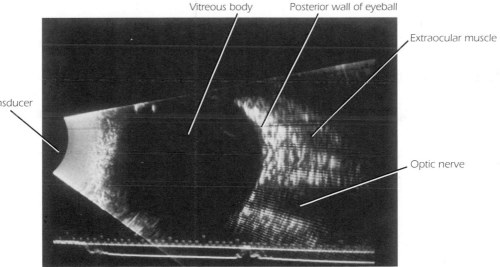

Vitreous body   Posterior wall of eyeball

Extraocular muscle

Sound transducer

Optic nerve

CHAPTER 3
Clinical Problems

Answers on Page 76

1 A group of children were playing with a bow and arrow. Suddenly, one child screamed and ran to his mother with an arrow projecting from his right eye. On examination the ophthalmologist found a wooden arrow had penetrated the upper eyelid and was directed upward, backward, and medially. Using your knowledge of anatomy, describe the structures that the arrow might have penetrated, having entered the orbital cavity.

2 A 34-year-old man with a swelling above the lateral margin of the right orbit consulted his physician. He said that he had had the swelling for many years and that it was gradually enlarging. On examination, a fluctuant, mobile swelling about 1 inch in diameter and confined to the soft tissue was seen about half an inch above the outer third of the right orbital margin. The physician made a diagnosis of a dermoid cyst, which was removed under a local anesthetic. Using your knowledge of anatomy, state the sensory innervation of the skin in this area. Indicate where you would infiltrate the nerve trunk with a local anesthetic agent.

3 A man aged 62 years presented with a swelling of the left upper eyelid and a complaint of double vision. He had a long history of chronic sinusitis. According to the patient, the double vision had started about 6 months previously. On examination, a tense, fixed cystic swelling could be felt deep to the medial third of the right upper eyelid. On asking the patient to look directly forward, the physician observed that the right eyeball was obviously displaced downward and laterally. Using your knowledge of anatomy, make a diagnosis and explain the signs and symptoms.

4 A 25-year-old woman driving her automobile was hit head on by another car that had crossed the center divide. She was not wearing her seat belt and her head was thrown forward, shattering the windshield. Three days later, on recovering consciousness in the intensive care unit, she complained of double vision. Careful examination revealed that her right cornea appeared to be displaced a little inferiorly compared to the left. She complained of loss of skin sensation and showed extensive bruising of her right cheek. Using your knowledge of anatomy, explain the signs and symptoms.

5 A 10-year-old girl was brought to her physician because of pain, redness, and swelling of her left eye. The pain worsened when she moved her eye. On examination, her right eye appeared normal, while the upper and lower lids of her left eye showed redness and edema of the skin, and the conjunctiva was markedly injected. Both eyelids were tender to touch and there was evidence of slight proptosis. She had a mild pyrexia (99°F); apart from stating that she was recovering from a prolonged severe cold, she and her parents said her general health had been good. Using your knowledge of anatomy, explain the proptosis. Explain the connection, if any, between her cold and her eye problem.

6 A 45-year-old man who was thrown from his motorcycle sustained multiple fractures of his face. Three weeks later it was noted that he had a slight proptosis of his right eye. A sonogram clearly showed a retrobulbar hematoma. Two months later, the space-occupying lesion had partially resolved. Six months later, the proptosis had disappeared and the sonogram showed no evidence of the hematoma. In fractures involving the bones of the walls of the orbital cavity, where does blood commonly accumulate?

7 Following a powerful forehand drive from his opponent during a game of tennis, a 30-year-old man received a severe direct blow to the left eye from the tennis ball. When he was examined in the emergency room, the left side of his face was found to be contused and swollen. The physician decided to wait a few days, to allow the swelling to subside, before assessing the full extent of the injury. In the interval he had a routine posteroanterior and lateral skull radiograph. Ten days later, the man was complaining of diplopia and was unable to rotate his left eye upward. He also had hypoesthesia of the skin below his left orbit. Using your knowledge of anatomy, make a diagnosis and explain the signs and symptoms.

8 An infant is born 10 weeks prematurely and is noted to have a cystic mass in the medial third of the superior right orbit. The mass pulsates and displaces the baby's eye downward and laterally. Using your knowledge of anatomy, explain the findings.

9 Tumors of the orbit can occur anywhere in the orbital cavity. Prior to the advent of CT and MRI, the location of such masses was deduced from the pattern of proptosis and displacement of the eye. Where in the orbit would a mass be in order to cause the following types of proptosis: axial (straight ahead), downward and medial displacement of the eye, downward and lateral displacement of the eye, lateral displacement of the eye, and upward displacement of the eye?

CHAPTER 3
Answers to Clinical Problems

1 A posteroanterior and a lateral radiograph of the child's head showed that the point of the arrow had traversed the thin roof of the orbit formed by the orbital plate of the frontal bone. In its passage it had pierced the periorbita, the frontal air sinus, and the meninges (including the subarachnoid space) and was situated in the frontal lobe of the right cerebral hemisphere.

2 The sensory innervation of the skin of the forehead in this area is the supraorbital branch of the frontal nerve, a branch of the ophthalmic division of the trigeminal nerve. The supraorbital nerve emerges from the orbital cavity by curving around the supraorbital notch or passing through the supraorbital foramen. The notch and foramen can be felt at the junction of the medial third and outer two-thirds of the superior orbital margin. It is here that you would infiltrate the nerve with the anesthetic.

3 The diagnosis was mucocele of the frontal sinus, which results from a blockage of the opening of the frontal sinus into the middle meatus of the nose by hypertrophied mucous membrane secondary to chronic frontal sinusitis. Normally, the frontal air sinus during development invades the orbital plate of the frontal bone, which forms the roof of the orbital cavity. The blocked air sinus fills with mucus and erodes the bony roof of the orbit. The expanding cyst then pushes down the periorbita and the eyeball, causing double vision.

4 This woman, who was fortunate to survive the accident, received a severe blow to her right eye and right maxilla. She sustained a blow-out fracture of the maxilla, which was confirmed on radiographic examination. The roof of the maxillary sinus was displaced downward away from the orbital cavity, allowing herniation of the right eyeball downward into the sinus, hence the diplopia. The infraorbital nerve passing forward in the infraorbital groove and canal received damage that caused loss of skin sensation over the cheek.

5 This patient had orbital cellulitis secondary to an acute infection of her ethmoidal air sinuses. The prolonged cold was complicated by the spread of the infection into the ethmoid sinuses. The infection had then invaded the soft tissues of the orbital cavity. The inflammatory reaction of the orbital contents had caused edema and swelling of the extraocular muscles; thus, movements of the eyeball worsened the orbital pain. The edema of the retrobulbar tissues in the confined bony space had resulted in proptosis. The inflammatory reaction had extended forward through the orbital septum to produce the redness and swelling of the eyelids.

6 The periorbita or periosteum lining the bones that form the walls of the orbital cavity is loosely attached to the bones except at the foramina or fissures, where it becomes continuous with the periosteum covering the outer surface of the bones. Blood or pus can easily accumulate between the periorbita and the bone, bulging into the orbital cavity and causing proptosis.

7 This patient had a blow-out fracture of his left maxillary sinus caused by the blunt trauma of the tennis ball on the eyeball, resulting in the inferior displacement of the floor of the orbit. The orbital contents had herniated downward into the sinus, causing the diplopia. The fracture of the floor of the orbit also damaged the infraorbital nerve—which explained the hypoesthesia of the facial skin. The patient's inability to rotate the eyeball superiorly was confirmed by a "forced duction" test, performed under local anesthesia, in which it was found impossible to rotate the eye upward with forceps. This meant that the inferior rectus muscle was entrapped between the bony fragments in the orbital floor. The X-rays confirmed the fracture and showed multiple spicules of bone projecting upward into the left orbital cavity and downward into the maxillary sinus.

8 This infant has an encephalocele or meningomyelocele due to incomplete closure of the fissure between the maxillary process of the frontal bone and the frontal process of the maxilla. Part of the frontal lobe of the brain has herniated through this bony defect into the orbit and has displaced the eye, causing pulsating exophthalmos.

9 In general, because there is only one large opening of the orbit (i.e., anteriorly), orbital masses cause proptosis and displacement of the eye in the direction opposite to their location. Therefore, optic nerve tumors cause axial proptosis, lacrimal gland tumors cause downward and medial displacement, dermoid tumors occurring supernasally will cause downward and lateral displacement, tumors arising from the medial rectus muscle or the ethmoid sinus will cause lateral displacement, and tumors arising from the inferior rectus muscle or the maxillary sinus will cause upward displacement.

The Paranasal Sinuses

CHAPTER OUTLINE

Introduction

A knowledge of the anatomy of the paranasal sinuses is important in understanding symptomatology in the ophthalmic setting. Many patients complaining of ocular pain consult the ophthalmologist. While a complete ophthalmologic examination is, of course, necessary to rule out true ocular or orbital causes of this symptom, the sensation of pain frequently arises from disease in the adjacent sinuses. For example, frontal sinusitis causes ocular pain, particularly on movement. It is important to differentiate this condition from the type of ocular pain with movement associated with retrobulbar neuritis. The close relationship that exists between the paranasal sinuses and the orbit, together with the fact that in many individuals these sinuses are separated from the orbital contents only by paper-thin bone, explains how inflammatory or neoplastic conditions can rapidly spread from one area into the other.

The paranasal sinuses are cavities in the interior of the maxilla, frontal, sphenoid, and ethmoid bones (Fig. 4-1). They vary considerably in size and shape in different individuals and at different ages. Lined with mucoperiosteum and filled with air, they communicate with the nasal cavity through relatively small apertures.

The mucus produced by the glands in the mucous membrane moves into the nasal cavity by the action of the cilia of the lining pseudostratified columnar ciliated epithelium. Drainage of the mucus is also assisted by the siphon action created during the blowing of the nose. The function of the sinuses is to act as resonators to the voice, and also to reduce the weight of the skull. When the apertures of the sinuses are blocked or the sinuses become filled with fluid, the quality of the voice changes markedly.

Maxillary Sinuses

The paired maxillary sinuses, usually the largest of the paranasal sinuses, are situated in the bodies of the maxillae (Figs. 4-1 and 4-2). The cavity of each sinus is pyramid-shaped; its base forms part of the lateral wall of the nose. Its apex extends laterally into the zygomatic process of the maxilla. The roof of the sinus is formed by the orbital plate of the maxilla and contains the infraorbital nerve and blood vessels (Fig. 4-2). The floor is formed by the alveolar process and lies about 1.25 cm below the level of the floor of the nose (Fig. 4-2). The apexes of the roots of the two premolar and the three molar teeth may produce conical projections on the sinus floor (Fig. 4-2). Sometimes the bone separating the sinus from the teeth is very thin; occasionally, it is absent. The anterior wall is related to the face and contains the canals for the anterior and middle superior alveolar nerves (branches of the infraorbital nerve) and blood vessels. The posterior wall is related to the infratemporal fossa and contains the posterior superior alveolar nerves (branches of the maxillary nerve) and blood vessels.

It is interesting to note that the medial wall or base not only is formed by the maxilla, but also receives contributions from the uncinate process of the ethmoid, the inferior concha (this is a separate bone), and the vertical plate of the palatine bone (Fig. 4-3).

Figure 4-1

(A) Bones of the face, showing regions where pain is experienced in sinusitis. (B) Positions of paranasal sinuses relative to the face.

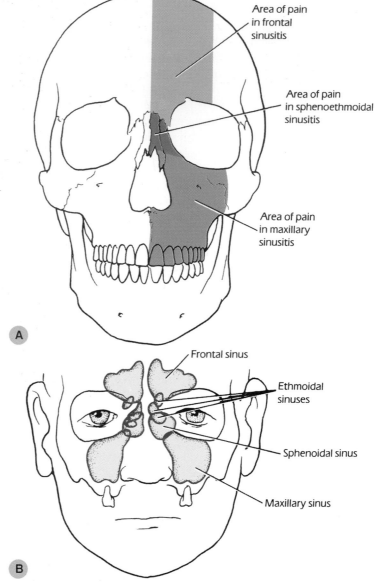

The cavity of the maxillary sinus is commonly indented by bony ridges and septa, so that the sinus may be completely or incompletely divided into two parts.

The maxillary sinus communicates with the nose through an opening in the superior part of its base (Figs. 4-3 and 4-4). A single small opening or small openings pierce the hiatus semilunaris and discharge into the middle meatus of the nose (Fig. 4-4).

Figure 4-2

(A) Position of the paranasal sinuses relative to the anterior cranial fossa. (B) Coronal section through the nasal cavity, showing the ethmoidal and maxillary sinuses.

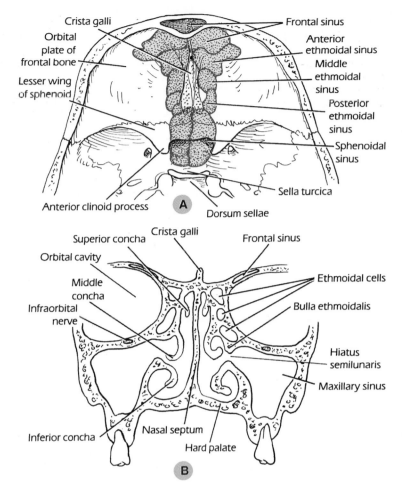

Nerve Supply

The mucous membrane is supplied by the infraorbital nerve and the anterior, middle, and posterior superior alveolar nerves.

Blood Supply

The arterial supply is from the anterior and posterior superior alveolar branches of the infraorbital and maxillary arteries, respectively. The veins drain through the ostium and join the venous plexuses in the nose.

Lymphatic Drainage

The vessels pass through the ostium and drain into the submandibular nodes.

Figure 4-3

(A) Parasagittal section through the anterior part of the skull, showing the right orbit and the medial wall of the right maxillary sinus. Note the thin plate of bone that separates the maxillary sinus from the cavity of the orbit. (B) Coronal section through the body of the sphenoid bone, showing the sphenoidal air sinuses, the hypophysis cerebri, and the cavernous sinuses. Note the position of the internal carotid artery and the cranial nerves.

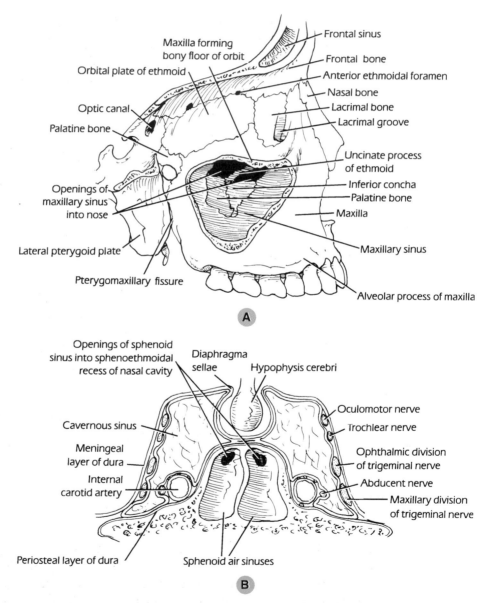

Figure 4-4

(A) Lateral wall of the right nasal cavity. (B) Lateral wall of the right nasal cavity; the superior, middle, and inferior conchae have been partially removed to show openings of the paranasal sinuses and the nasolacrimal duct into the meati.

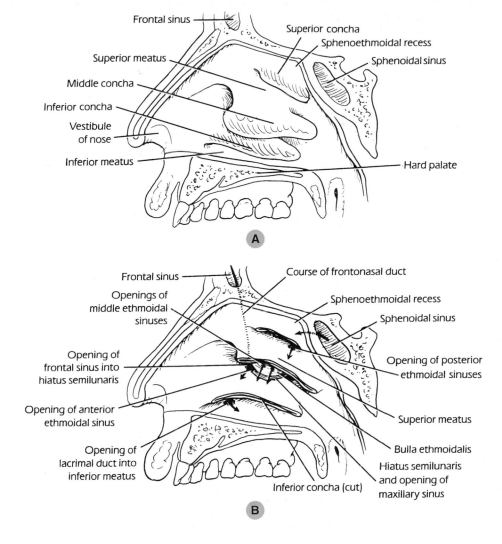

Frontal Sinuses

The two frontal sinuses lie within the frontal bone (Figs. 4-1 and 4-2). They are separated from each other by a bony septum, which frequently deviates from the median plane. Each sinus is roughly triangular in shape, extending upward above the medial end of the eyebrow and backward into the medial part of the roof of the orbit (Fig. 4-2). The frontal sinus often contains bony partitions that incompletely divide the cavity into a number of recesses.

The extent of development of the frontal sinus varies considerably. In some individuals one sinus may develop excessively and cross the midline to lie one in front of the other. In other individuals the vertical or the horizontal parts of the sinus may be absent or poorly developed. Rarely, the sinus is so large that it invades adjacent bones.

The anterior wall of the frontal sinus is related to the skin of the forehead and the supraorbital and supratrochlear nerves (Fig. 4-1). The thin posterior wall is related to the meninges and the frontal lobe of the cerebral hemisphere. The floor of the sinus is related to the orbit and the nose.

The frontal sinus communicates with the nose through the frontonasal duct or the ethmoidal infundibulum (Fig. 4-4). These structures open into the hiatus semilunaris in the middle meatus, close to the openings of the anterior ethmoidal sinuses and the maxillary sinus.

Nerve Supply

The mucous membrane is supplied by a branch from the supraorbital nerve as it passes through the supraorbital notch or foramen.

Blood Supply

The arterial supply is from the supraorbital and anterior ethmoidal arteries. The veins drain into the venous plexuses of the nose and into the supraorbital vein.

Lymphatic Drainage

The lymphatic vessels drain into the submandibular nodes.

Sphenoidal Sinuses

The two sphenoidal sinuses lie within the body of the sphenoid bone (Figs. 4-2 and 4-3). Of all the air sinuses, the sphenoidal vary most in their extent and development. Although the sphenoidal sinus may be limited to the sphenoid bone, in some individuals it may extend into the pterygoid processes or greater wing of sphenoid and may encroach on the basilar part of the occipital bone. It may even partially surround the optic canal in the lesser wing of the sphenoid. The two sphenoidal sinuses are usually separated by a vertical median septum, which is often deviated to one or the other side of the midline (Fig. 4-3). Quite commonly, one sinus is much larger than the other and extends across the midline to lie in front of or behind the other sinus.

The anterior wall of the sphenoidal sinus is related to the nasal cavity and to the ethmoidal sinuses (Fig. 4-4). The posterior wall is related to the posterior cranial fossa and the pons. Laterally lies the cavernous sinus, containing the internal carotid artery and the abducent nerve (Fig. 4-3). In front of the cavernous sinus the sphenoidal sinus is related laterally to the orbital cavity. Superiorly, the sinus is related to the hypophysis cerebri, the optic nerves, and the optic chiasma (Fig. 4-3). Inferiorly, the sinus is related to the nasopharynx and the pterygoid canal (Fig. 4-4).

The sphenoidal sinus opens into the nasal cavity into the sphenoethmoidal recess above the superior concha (Fig. 4-4).

Nerve Supply

The mucous membrane is supplied by the posterior ethmoidal nerves and the orbital branches of the pterygopalatine ganglion.

Blood Supply

The arterial supply is from the posterior ethmoidal arteries. The veins drain into the posterior ethmoidal veins.

Lymphatic Drainage

The lymphatic vessels drain into the retropharyngeal nodes.

Ethmoidal Sinuses

The ethmoidal sinuses consist of a honeycomb of air cells that lie within the ethmoid bone between the nose and the orbit (Figs. 4-1 and 4-2). They are not necessarily confined to the ethmoid bone but may invade the frontal, maxillary, lacrimal, sphenoid, and palatine bones. The number of air cells is very variable; there may be as few as three large cells or as many as 18 small cells. The ethmoid cells are commonly grouped together as anterior, middle, and posterior.

The ethmoidal sinuses are related superiorly to the anterior cranial fossa, the meninges, and the frontal lobe of the cerebral hemisphere (Fig. 4-2). Inferiorly lies the nose. Laterally, the sinuses are related to the orbital cavity. Medially lies the nose. The sinuses are separated from all these structures by paper-thin bone, and it is for this reason that infection of the ethmoidal sinuses can easily spread into the orbit causing orbital cellulitis.

The anterior group of air cells communicates with the nose through one or more openings into the ethmoidal infundibulum or the frontonasal duct (Fig. 4-4). They thus discharge into the middle meatus of the nose. The middle group of air cells open by one or more openings on or above the ethmoidal bulla into the middle meatus of the nose (Fig. 4-4). The posterior group of air cells, which lie close to the optic canal, open by one orifice into the superior meatus of the nose (Fig. 4-4).

Nerve Supply

The ethmoidal air cells are supplied by the anterior and posterior ethmoidal nerves and the orbital branches of the pterygopalatine ganglion.

Blood Supply

The arterial supply is from the anterior and posterior ethmoidal arteries and the sphenopalatine artery. The veins correspond to the arteries.

Lymphatic Drainage

The lymphatic vessels of the anterior and middle groups of air cells drain into the submandibular nodes; those of the posterior group drain into the retropharyngeal nodes.

The paranasal sinuses and their site of drainage into the nose are summarized in Table 4-1.

Development of the Paranasal Sinuses

The paranasal sinuses develop as diverticula from the nasal mucosa. At birth they are rudimentary or absent. At the time of the eruption of the permanent teeth and again at puberty, the sinuses increase rapidly in size.

Clinical Notes

Sinusitis

Infection of the paranasal sinuses is a common complication of nasal infections. Rarely, the cause of maxillary sinusitis is extension from an apical dental abscess.

The maxillary sinus is particularly susceptible to infection, because its drainage orifice through the hiatus semilunaris is vulnerably positioned near the roof of the sinus. In other words, the sinus has to fill with fluid before it can effectively drain when the person maintains an upright position.

The frontal sinus drains into the hiatus semilunaris close to the orifices of the ethmoidal and maxillary sinuses on the lateral wall of the nose. Thus, it is not surprising that a patient with frontal sinusitis nearly always has a maxillary sinusitis, or even an ethmoidal sinusitis.

The extreme thinness of the medial wall of the orbit relative to the ethmoidal air cells has been emphasized. Ethmoidal sinusitis is the commonest cause of orbital cellulitis. The infection can easily spread through the paper-thin bone.

Table 4-1   The Paranasal Sinuses and Their Site of Drainage into the Nose

Name of Sinus	Site of Drainage
Maxillary sinus	Middle meatus through hiatus semilunaris
Frontal sinus	Middle meatus via frontonasal duct or ethmoidal infundibulum
Sphenoidal sinuses	Sphenoethmoidal recess
Ethmoidal sinuses	
Anterior group	Middle meatus via ethmoidal infundibulum or frontonasal duct
Middle group	Middle meatus on or above bulla ethmoidalis
Posterior group	Superior meatus

Note that maxillary and sphenoidal sinuses are usually present in rudimentary form at birth, enlarge appreciably after the eighth year, and are fully formed in adolescence.

Physical Examination of the Paranasal Sinuses

The maxillary, frontal, and ethmoidal sinuses can be palpated clinically for areas of tenderness. The maxillary sinus can be examined by pressing one's finger against the anterior wall of the maxilla below the inferior orbital margin; pressure over the infraorbital nerve may reveal increased sensitivity. Because the bony walls are relatively thin, directing a beam of a flashlight either through the roof of the mouth or through the cheek in a darkened room will enable the examiner to determine whether or not the maxillary sinus is full of inflammatory exudate rather than air.

The frontal sinus can be examined by pressing one's finger upward beneath the medial end of the superior orbital margin. It is here that the relatively thin floor of the frontal sinus is closest to the surface. In a similar manner, the ethmoidal sinuses can be palpated by pressing one's finger medially against the medial wall of the orbit.

Referred Pain from the Paranasal Sinuses

The maxillary sinus is innervated by the infraorbital nerve and the anterior, middle, and posterior superior alveolar nerves. Pain from the sinus is referred to the upper jaw, including the teeth, as well as to the skin of the cheek.

The frontal sinus is innervated by the supraorbital nerve, which also supplies the skin of the forehead and scalp as far back as the vertex. Therefore, it is not surprising that patients with frontal sinusitis have pain referred over this area.

Variation in Size of the Paranasal Sinuses, Relative to the Orbital Boundaries and the Optic Canal

The extreme variations in the size of the frontal, ethmoidal, and sphenoidal sinuses have been emphasized. Invasion of the bony boundaries of the optic canal by the sphenoidal and ethmoidal sinuses could result in spread of infection from these sinuses to the optic nerve, causing retrobulbar neuritis.

Surgical intrusion in the treatment of chronic sinusitis or mucoceles could result in damage to the orbital contents or to the optic nerve.

Blow-out Fractures of the Maxilla

A severe blow to the eye may cause the floor of the orbit to buckle downward into the maxillary sinus. Apart from diplopia, the additional damage to the infraorbital nerve crossing in the roof of the sinus may result in loss of sensation to the cheek and upper lip.

Ethmoidal Fractures

Trauma to the eye, often negligible, can cause a fracture and inward buckling of the ethmoid bone into the ethmoidal sinuses. The volume of the orbit is expanded and the eye may sink back into the orbit, producing enophthalmos.

CHAPTER 4
Clinical Problems

Answers on Page 89

1 Following a severe cold, a patient complained of a frontal headache and a dull, aching pain on the right side of his face. What anatomic structures are likely to become secondarily infected from the nose? Explain the distribution of the pain.

2 A 58-year-old man who had suffered from chronic sinusitis for many years was seen by an otolaryngologist. After an extensive workup it was decided to operate on his sphenoidal air sinuses to improve the drainage. After the operation, the patient complained that he could not see with his right eye. Using your knowledge of anatomy, explain how this serious complication could occur.

3 Following a bicycle accident, an 18-year-old girl was diagnosed as having a blow-out fracture of her right maxilla, resulting in diplopia and right-sided enophthalmos. During the surgical procedure to restore the bony fragments of the floor of the right orbit, the facial and ophthalmic surgeons discussed the boundaries of the maxillary sinus. Using your knowledge of anatomy, describe the bones that form the walls of the maxillary sinus.

4 A 27-year-old man was punched in the right eye and sustained a bruise in the medial portion of the right lower lid and the nose, as well as a bloody nose. Two days later, after blowing his nose, he noticed that the right lower and upper eyelids swelled up and his eye bulged forward. Frightened by the experience, he sought the assistance of his ophthalmologist. Using your knowledge of the anatomy of the region, explain the mechanism of his injury and findings.

CHAPTER 4
Answers to Clinical Problems

1 The patient was suffering from a frontal and maxillary sinusitis on the right side. The supraorbital nerve supplies not only the frontal sinus but also the skin of the scalp as far back as the vertex. The pain is commonly referred to this area. The maxillary sinus is innervated by the infraorbital nerve, which also supplies the facial skin. The pain is referred to the skin of the face, and also commonly to the upper teeth.

2 The sphenoidal sinuses are the most variable in extent of all the paranasal sinuses. While in some individuals they may be small and limited to the body of the sphenoid bone, in others they may invade other parts of the sphenoid, or even the basilar part of the occipital bone. In some individuals, the sinus has invaded the lesser wing of the sphenoid and surrounded the optic canal, with only a paper-thin layer of bone separating the mucous membrane of the sinus from the optic nerve. In these circumstances, chronic sinusitis has been known to cause a retrobulbar neuritis. More important, the optic nerve is at great risk in these patients during surgery on the sinus.

3 The pyramid-shaped maxillary sinus has a base, an apex, and four walls. The base is formed by the maxilla, the ethmoid, the inferior concha, and the vertical plate of the palatine bone. The apex lies within the zygomatic process of the maxilla. The roof is formed by the orbital plate of the maxilla; the floor, by the alveolar process of the maxilla. The anterior wall faces the face and is formed by the maxilla; the posterior wall is formed by the back of the maxilla and is related to the infratemporal fossa.

4 This patient had sustained a fracture of the medial orbital wall (i.e., ethmoid bone) of the right eye. Such a fracture requires little force because the bone is paper thin. The bone buckled inward into the ethmoidal sinus and a communication between the sinus and the orbit was established. Ethmoidal mucosal injury leads to bleeding in the sinus and bloody discharge from the nose. When such patients sneeze or blow their nose, air can track from the nose into the orbit via the ethmoidal sinus and cause massive swelling of the lids and proptosis of the eyeball. This benign condition usually resolves as the air is absorbed into the bloodstream over several days. Patients who suffer such fractures should be cautioned against blowing their nose, sneezing, or traveling in airplanes.

The Ocular Appendages

The Eyebrows

The eyebrows lie at the junction of the forehead and the upper lid. The medial end of each arch usually lies just inferior to the orbital margin, while the lateral end lies above the orbital margin (Fig. 5-1). The hairs are thick and directed horizontally laterally. Several muscles of facial expression are inserted into the skin, permitting movement of the eyebrows. Raising of the eyebrows is accomplished by contracting the frontalis muscle; lowering of the eyebrows, by contracting the orbital part of the orbicularis oculi; drawing the eyebrows medially, by contracting the corrugator supercilii muscle. All these muscles are supplied by the seventh cranial nerve.

The eyebrows receive an *arterial supply* from the supraorbital and supratrochlear branches of the ophthalmic artery. The corresponding *veins* drain into the angular vein and so enter the facial vein. The *lymphatic drainage* of the lateral end is into the superficial parotid nodes; from the medial end, into the submandibular nodes.

Clinical Notes

Alopecia Areata and Hypothyroidism

Like all other hair-bearing areas of skin, the eyebrows are subject to a number of dermatologic diseases. For example, *alopecia areata* is a trophic disorder in which patches of hair are lost. In *hypothyroidism* the loss of hair in the outer third of the eyebrow is easily recognized.

Lacerations

The eyebrow is usually burst open as the result of a blunt object striking the skin against the underlying frontal bone. The skin wound may gape open, owing to

Figure 5-1

Surface anatomy of the right orbital margin, showing positions of the eyebrow, eyelids, and trochlea of the superior oblique tendon.

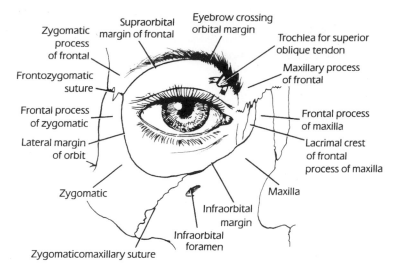

the pull of muscles. The eyebrow should be closed in layers starting with the muscle (frontalis, corrugator supercilii, or orbicularis oculi), followed by the subcutaneous tissue and finally the skin. The position of the hairs guides the approximation of the cut edges.

The Eyelids

Function and General Arrangement

The eyelids protect the eye from injury and excessive light by their closure. By blinking, they also assist in the distribution of tears over the anterior surface of the eyeball and their exit into the drainage system at the medial angle of the eye.

Each eyelid is divided by a horizontal furrow, the *superior palpebral sulcus*, into an *orbital* and a *tarsal* part (Fig. 5-2). The sulcus of the upper eyelid is formed by the insertion of the aponeurotic fibers of the levator palpebrae superioris into the skin. The sulcus of the lower eyelid, which is less obvious, is produced by a few connections between the skin and the orbicularis oculi muscle.

In addition, in old people, two sulci are often seen just below the inferior orbital margin. They are known as the *lateral or malar sulcus* and the *medial or naso-jugal sulcus*. They are produced by the skin being tethered to the underlying periosteum.

The upper eyelid (Fig. 5-2) is larger and more mobile than the lower. The eyelids meet at the *medial* and *lateral angles* (or *canthi*). The *palpebral fissure*, the elliptical opening between the eyelids, is the entrance into the conjunctival sac. When wide open, the fissure forms laterally an angle of about 60 degrees, but medially it is rounded. In whites and blacks, the lateral angle is about 2 mm higher than the medial angle; in Orientals, the lateral angle is about 5 mm higher than the medial. In whites and blacks, the palpebral fissure is widest at the junction of the medial third with the lateral two-thirds; in Orientals, the fissure is

Figure 5-2

(A) Right eye, showing parts of the eyelids and sulci. Note that with the eye open, the upper lid just covers the upper margin of the cornea. (B) Right eye with lids everted to show the conjunctival sac, and lacus lacrimalis, and the caruncula lacrimalis. Note the position of the tarsal glands beneath the conjunctiva and the puncta lacrimalia.

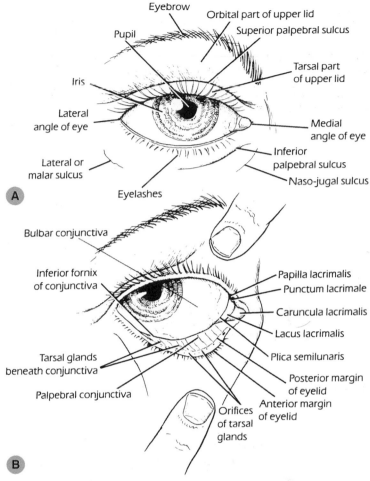

widest halfway along its length. In Orientals the medial angle is overlapped by a vertical skin fold, the *epicanthus*.

When the eye is closed, the upper eyelid completely covers the cornea of the eye. When the eye is open and looking straight ahead, the upper lid just covers the upper margin of the cornea (Fig. 5-2). The lower lid lies just below the cornea when the eye is open and rises only slightly when the eye is closed.

The lateral angle of the eye is directly in contact with the eyeball, whereas the medial rounded angle lies about 6 mm medially from the eyeball (Fig. 5-2). Here the two eyelids are separated by a small triangular space, the *lacus lacrimalis*, in the center of which is a small, pinkish elevation, the *caruncula lacrimalis*. A semilunar fold, called the *plica semilunaris*, lies on the lateral side of the caruncle.

The margin of each eyelid is about 2 mm thick and 30 mm long. The lateral five-sixths of the eyelid margin, the ciliary portion, has squared edges. The medial one-sixth of the margin, the lacrimal portion, has rounded edges. About 5 mm from the medial angle there is a small elevation, the *papilla lacrimalis* (Fig. 5-2). On the summit of the papilla is a small hole, the *punctum lacrimale*, which varies in size from approximately 0.4 to 0.8 mm in diameter; the punctum leads into the *canaliculus lacrimalis*. The papilla lacrimalis projects into the lacus, and the punctum and canaliculus serve to carry tears down into the nose.

The *eyelashes*, which are short, curved hairs, are present on the margins of the eyelids from the lateral angle of the eye to the lacrimal papilla (Fig. 5-2). They are longer and more numerous on the upper lid and curve upward, while those of the lower lid curve downward; they are arranged in double or triple rows. Just in front of the posterior edge of the margin of the lids are the orifices of the *tarsal glands* (*meibomian glands*). The tarsal glands number about 20 to 25 in each lid, and can be seen as yellowish lines on the inner surface of the everted eyelid (Fig. 5-3). The orifices of the tarsal glands mark the site of junction between the skin

Figure 5-3

(A) Complete eversion of the upper eyelid of the right eye, made possible by stiffness of the superior tarsal plate; the lower eyelid is pulled downward. Note the orifices of the tarsal glands and the puncta lacrimalia; note also the branches of the posterior conjunctival arteries. (B) Posterior view of the eyelids with the palpebral fissure nearly closed. Note the tarsal glands with their short ducts and orifices. In this diagram the palpebral conjunctiva has been removed to show the tarsal glands in situ.

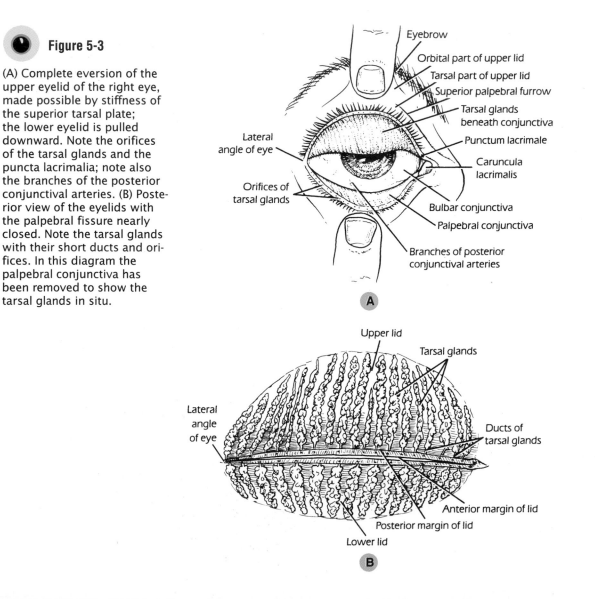

and the conjunctiva. A grayish line or slight sulcus can sometimes be seen running along the eyelid margin between the eyelashes and the openings of the tarsal glands. This represents the line of demarcation between the anterior portion of the eyelid formed by the skin and orbicularis oculi muscle and the posterior portion formed by the tarsus and the conjunctiva. This line can be important surgically, because it serves as a plane along which the eyelid may be split with minimal scarring.

Structure

From superficial to deep, each eyelid consists (Fig. 5-4) of 1) skin, 2) subcutaneous tissue, 3) striated muscle fibers of the orbicularis oculi, 4) orbital septum

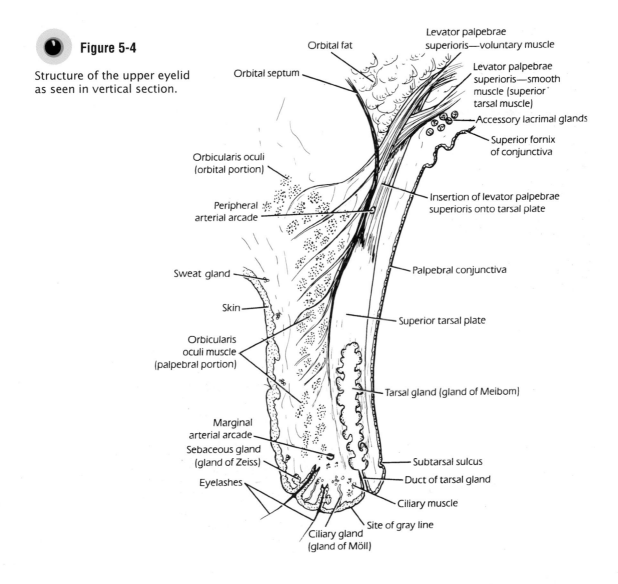

Figure 5-4

Structure of the upper eyelid as seen in vertical section.

and tarsal plates, 5) smooth muscle, and 6) conjunctiva. The upper lid also receives the insertion of the levator palpebrae superioris muscle.

Skin

The skin is very thin and easily folds. For a full examination of the skin of the eyelids, the eye should be closed to erase the folds.

Microscopic examination of the skin shows many small hairs with sebaceous glands and small sweat glands. The epidermis contains numerous melanocytes. At the margin of the lid the dermis becomes denser and the papillae are higher. The skin becomes continuous with the conjunctiva just in front of the posterior edge at the site of the orifices of the tarsal glands (meibomian glands) (Fig. 5-4).

The *eyelashes* are short, thick, curved (Fig. 5-4), and more numerous on the upper eyelid (150 in the upper lid and 75 in the lower). They are commonly darker than the scalp hairs, do not become gray with age, and are replaced every 100 to 150 days. The hair follicles are arranged in two or three rows along the anterior edge of the eyelids and do not possess erector pili muscles. The *sebaceous glands of Zeis* open into each follicle.

Behind and between the follicles, modified sweat glands, the *ciliary glands of Moll*, open into the follicles or onto the eyelid margin.

Subcutaneous Tissue

The subcutaneous tissue is very loose and rich in elastic fibers. In whites, it is almost devoid of fat.

Orbicularis Oculi

The *orbicularis oculi muscle* (Figs. 5-4 and 5-5) is a flat, elliptical muscle that surrounds the orbital margin (Fig. 5-6) extending onto the temporal region and cheek (orbital part); it also extends into the eyelids (palpebral portion) and farther, behind the lacrimal sac (lacrimal portion). It is composed of striated muscle.

 Figure 5-5

Photomicrograph of a vertical section of the upper eyelid at its free margin. Portions of an eyelash follicle and its associated sebaceous gland are visible at the left. Portions of a tarsal gland can be seen on the right. Note the bundles of fibers of the orbicularis oculi muscle. (H&E; × 40.)

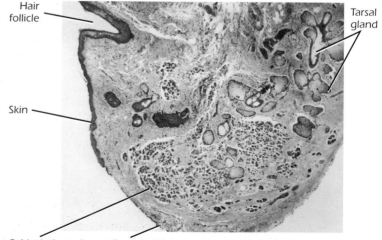

Figure 5-6

(A) The different parts of the orbicularis oculi muscle. Note the medial palpebral ligament and the lateral palpebral raphe. (B) Horizontal section through the lacrimal sac, showing the lacrimal portion of the orbicularis oculi muscle.

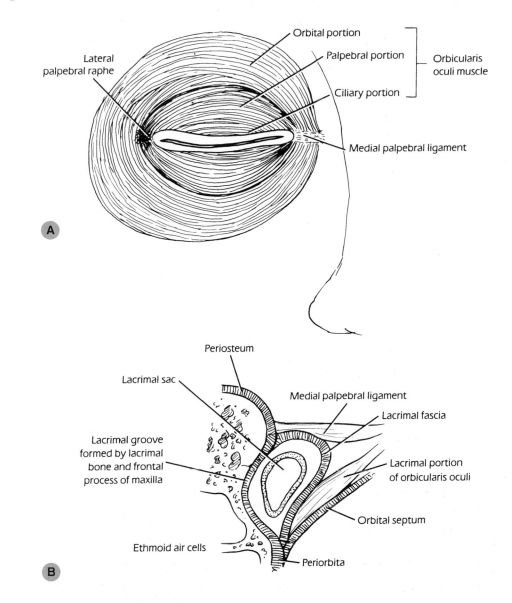

The *palpebral portion of the orbicularis oculi muscle* consists of thin bundles of fibers that arise from the medial palpebral ligament (Fig. 5-6); they are attached to the superficial and deep surface of the ligament, but not to its lower margin. The fibers also arise from the neighboring bone. The fibers sweep laterally and concentrically across the eyelids and in front of the orbital septum. At the lateral angle of the eye, the fibers interlace at the *lateral palpebral raphe*. At the lid margin there is a small group of fine muscle fibers, known as the *ciliary muscle*.

Beneath the orbicularis oculi muscle lies a thin layer of connective tissue containing the blood vessels and nerves of the eyelid.

Nerve Supply   Temporal and zygomatic branches of the facial nerve enter the deep surface of the muscle from the lateral side.

Action   The orbital portion of the orbicularis oculi muscle pulls on the skin of the forehead, temple, and cheek like a pursestring and draws it toward the medial angle of the orbit. The skin is thrown into prominent folds, which overlap the eyelids and add protection to the underlying eye. This part of the muscle is largely under voluntary control, although it may be made to contract reflexly.

The palpebral portion closes the eyelids so that the upper lid is lowered and the lower lid is raised. Its action is both voluntary and involuntary. The blinking reflex ensures that a film of tears wipes over the cornea. The reflex is initiated by drying of the cornea. When strongly contracted, both lids are pulled medially.

The lacrimal portion pulls the eyelids medially and also pulls on the lacrimal fascia to dilate the lacrimal sac. The action on the sac provides the pumping mechanism for the tears. It also helps to position the puncta lacrimalia so that they are applied to the eyeball or the lacus lacrimalis.

The entire muscle has an important role in facial expression. The antagonist muscle to the orbital portion is the frontal belly of the occipitofrontalis muscle; that of the palpebral portion is the levator palpebrae superioris.

Orbital Septum and Tarsal Plates

The fibrous framework of the eyelids is formed by a membranous sheet, the *orbital septum* (Figs. 5-4 and 5-7). This is attached to the orbital margin, where it is continuous with the periosteum (periorbita). The orbital septum separates the eyelids from the contents of the orbital cavity. The orbital septum lies posterior to the medial palpebral ligament. On the lateral side of the orbit, it lies posterior to the lateral raphe of the orbicularis oculi, but anterior to the lateral palpebral ligament.

The tarsal plates consist of dense fibrous tissue and give the eyelids firmness and shape. The *tarsal plate of the upper lid* is much larger than the lower and is crescent-shaped (Fig. 5-7). It measures about 10 mm in height at the center and gradually narrows toward its ends. Attached to its upper edge are the orbital septum and the smooth muscle fibers of the levator palpebrae superioris.

The *tarsal plate of the lower lid* is smaller, measuring about 5 mm in height at the center and gradually narrowing toward its ends. Attached to its lower edge is the orbital septum.

The *medial palpebral ligament* attaches the medial ends of the tarsi to the lacrimal crest and the frontal process of the maxilla (Fig. 5-7). The ligament has an indefinite upper border but a thick and prominent lower border. The medial palpebral ligament lies anterior to the lacrimal sac.

The *lateral palpebral ligament* attaches the lateral ends of the tarsi to the marginal tubercle on the orbital margin formed by the zygomatic bone. It is a poorly

Figure 5-7

The right orbital margin, with the orbital septum and the superior and inferior tarsal plates in position. Note the relationship between the medial palpebral ligament and the lacrimal sac; note also the tendinous fibers of the levator palpebrae superioris piercing the orbital septum in the upper eyelid.

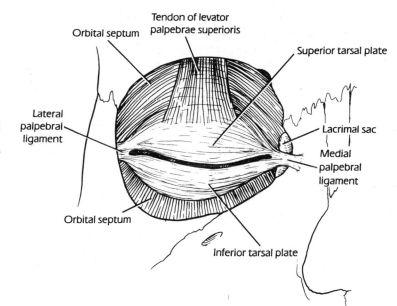

developed ligament. This ligament must not be confused with the lateral palpebral raphe (Fig. 5-6), which lies superficial to the lateral palpebral ligament and consists of the interlacing fibers of the palpebral part of the orbicularis oculi muscle.

The *orbital septum*, described above, is perforated by the nerves and blood vessels that exit from the orbital cavity to reach the face and scalp, and by the aponeurotic fibers of the levator palpebrae superioris.

The *tarsal glands* (meibomian glands) are embedded within the substance of the tarsal plates (Figs. 5-3, 5-4, and 5-5). There are about 20 to 25 in each lid, arranged in a single row, and the ducts discharge their secretion onto the eyelid margin. When the eyelid is everted, they can be seen as long yellow structures beneath the conjunctiva. The tarsal glands are modified sebaceous glands consisting of a long central canal surrounded by 10 to 15 acini (Fig. 5-4). The mouths of the ducts are lined with stratified squamous epithelium and the cells of the acini are polyhedral cells. The tarsal gland secretion is oily in consistency and prevents the overflow of tears. It also helps to make the closed eyelids airtight. The oily material forms the external layer of the precorneal tear film and hinders rapid evaporation of tears.

Smooth Muscle

The smooth muscle forms the superior and inferior tarsal muscles. The *superior tarsal muscle* is continuous above with the levator palpebrae superioris and below it is attached to the upper edge of the tarsal plate of the upper lid (Fig. 5-4). The function of the superior tarsal muscle is to raise the upper lid and assist the striated muscle of the levator palpebrae superioris. The *inferior tarsal muscle* is attached to the lower margin of the inferior tarsal plate of the lower eyelid and connects it to the fascial sheath of the inferior rectus muscle. The function of the inferior tarsal muscle is to lower the lower lid. The two tarsal muscles are inner-vated by sympathetic nerves from the superior cervical sympathetic ganglion.

Conjunctiva

The conjunctiva is a thin mucous membrane that lines the eyelids and is reflected at the *superior and inferior fornices* onto the anterior surface of the eyeball (Fig. 5-8). It thus covers part of the sclera, and its epithelium is continuous with that of the cornea. At the margin of the eyelid, the conjunctiva continues into the skin along the posterior margin of the openings of the tarsal glands. Here the thinner, nonkeratinized squamous epithelium of the conjunctiva changes into the keratin-ized stratified squamous epithelium of the epidermis. A shallow groove on the back of the lid, the *subtarsal sulcus*, lies about 2 mm from the posterior edge of the lid margin. The sulcus tends to trap small foreign particles introduced into the conjunctival sac and thus is clinically important.

The richly vascular conjunctiva lining the eyelids gives the back of the lids a reddish or pinkish color. The extreme thinness of the conjunctiva enables the examiner to see the underlying tarsal glands as yellowish streaks (Fig. 5-3).

The area of the conjunctiva that covers the upper tarsal plate is strongly bound down to it in its entire extent. The conjunctiva covering the lower tarsal plate is adherent only to its upper half.

The detailed structure of the conjunctiva is discussed on page 109.

 Figure 5-8

Sagittal section of the eyelids and anterior portion of the eyeball showing the conjuncti-val sac and the different parts of the conjunctiva.

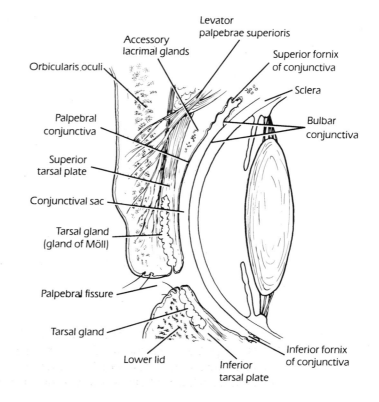

Levator Palpebrae Superioris

The upper lid, as distinct from the lower lid, contains the insertion of a powerful striated muscle, the levator palpebrae superioris (Fig. 5-8). The tendon of insertion is an aponeurosis that descends into the upper lid posterior to the orbital septum. Tendinous fibers then pierce the orbital septum and become attached to the anterior surface of the superior tarsal plate. Some of the fibers pass forward between the muscular bundles of the orbicularis oculi to attach to the skin. It is these latter fibers that produce the horizontal furrow of the upper lid.

The aponeurosis of the levator palpebrae superioris muscle is much wider than the muscle belly. The medial and lateral expansions are called *horns*. The lateral horn indents the lacrimal gland so that the gland appears to wrap around the lateral border of the aponeurosis (Fig. 5-15). This arrangement partially divides the lacrimal gland into a thin palpebral portion and a thick orbital portion. The lateral horn is attached to the marginal tubercle of the zygomatic bone along with the lateral palpebral ligament (Fig. 5-7). The medial horn fuses with the orbital septum and the medial palpebral ligament. The attachments of the medial and lateral horns serve to check the action of the muscle on the upper eyelid.

Arising from the inferior surface of the aponeurosis is a thin sheet of smooth muscle, the superior tarsal muscle (Fig. 5-4). This muscle is inserted into the upper edge of the superior tarsal plate. Arising from its superior surface is a layer of fascia that ascends behind the orbital septum to attach to the periosteum of the orbital rim.

The levator palpebrae superioris originates from the inferior surface of the lesser wing of the sphenoid above and anterior to the optic canal (see Fig. 8-16, page 247).

Nerve Supply   The main striated part of the levator palpebrae superioris is supplied by the superior branch of the oculomotor nerve. The smooth muscle (superior tarsal muscle) is supplied by sympathetic nerves from the superior cervical sympathetic ganglion.

Action   The levator palpebrae superioris raises the upper lid. Fear or excitement causes contraction of the smooth muscle (superior tarsal muscle), resulting in further elevation of the lid. Division of the cervical sympathetic paralyzes the smooth muscle, causing drooping of the upper lid (ptosis).

Fascial Spaces

A number of potential fascial spaces exist in the eyelids. These are named according to their position—the *subcutaneous, submuscular, pretarsal,* and *preseptal spaces* (Fig. 5-9).

Arterial Supply

The eyelids are supplied by the lateral and medial palpebral arteries (Fig. 5-10). The *lateral palpebral arteries* are derived from the lacrimal artery, which is a branch of the ophthalmic artery. The *medial palpebral arteries*, superior and inferior, arise from the ophthalmic artery below the trochlea of the superior oblique

Figure 5-9

Sagittal section of the upper eyelid, showing the different fascial spaces.

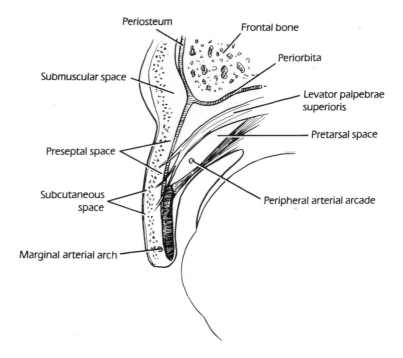

muscle. Having passed behind the lacrimal sac, they enter the eyelids. Each artery divides into two branches that pass laterally, forming two arches in each eyelid. The arches anastomose with the lateral palpebral arteries and with branches of the superficial temporal, transverse facial, and infraorbital arteries.

Venous Drainage

The veins of the eyelids, which are larger and more numerous than the arteries, drain medially into the ophthalmic and angular veins and laterally into the superficial temporal vein.

Lymphatic Drainage

The lymphatic vessels from the lateral two-thirds of the upper and lower lids drain into the superficial parotid nodes. Those from the medial angle drain into the submandibular nodes (Fig. 5-11).

Nerve Supply

The sensory nerve supply to the upper lids is from the infratrochlear, supratrochlear, supraorbital, and lacrimal nerves from the ophthalmic division of the trigeminal nerve (Fig. 5-11). The skin of the lower lid is supplied by the infratrochlear branch of the ophthalmic division of the trigeminal at the medial angle; the remainder of the lower lid is supplied by branches of the infraorbital nerve, the terminal portion of the maxillary division of the trigeminal nerve.

Figure 5-10

(A) The arterial supply of the upper and lower eyelids of the right eye. (B) Sagittal section of the upper eyelid and eyeball, showing the anterior and posterior conjunctival arteries and their connection to the anterior ciliary artery.

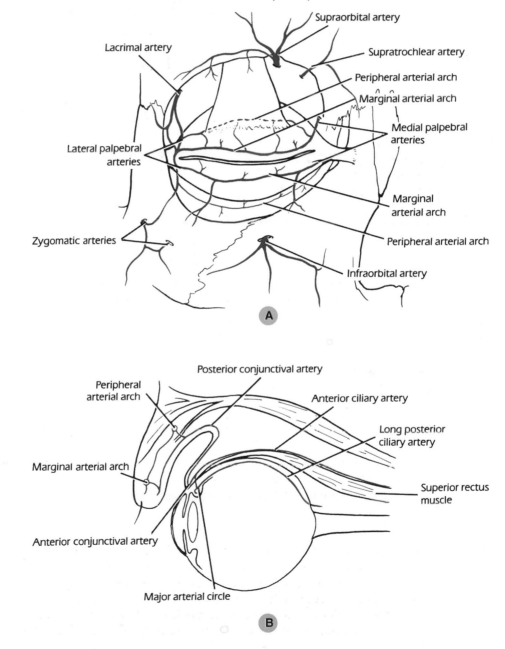

Figure 5-11

(A) The lymphatic drainage of the eyelids. (B) The sensory nerve supply to the eyelids.

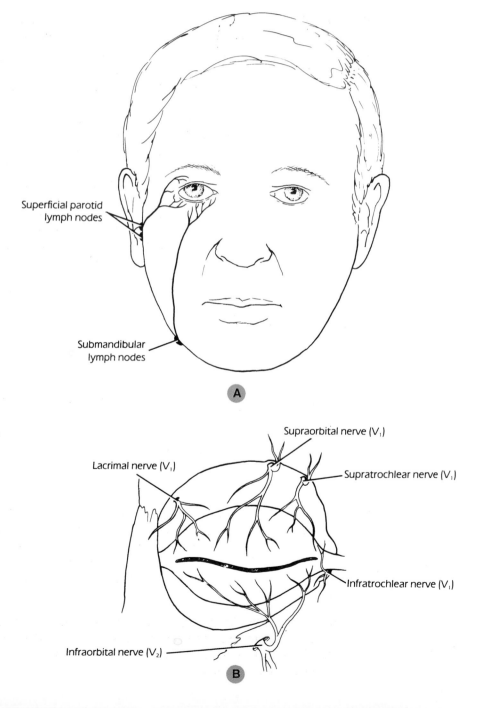

The orbicularis oculi muscle is innervated by the temporal and zygomatic branches of the facial nerve. The smooth muscle of the eyelids (superior and inferior tarsal muscles) are supplied by sympathetic nerve fibers from the superior cervical sympathetic ganglion.

Movements

The position of the eyelids at rest depends on the tone of the orbicularis oculi and levator palpebrae superioris muscles and the position of the eyeball. Normally, when a person is looking forward with the eyes open, the upper lid covers about half the width of the superior portion of the iris, while the lower lid crosses the lower edge of the cornea.

At times of fear or excitement, the palpebral fissure is further widened by the increased tone of the smooth muscle fibers of the superior tarsal muscle (part of the levator palpebrae superioris) and the inferior tarsal muscle.

One closes the eyelids by contracting the orbicularis oculi and relaxing the levator palpebrae superioris muscles. One opens the eye by contracting the levator palpebrae superioris, raising the upper lid. On looking upward, the levator palpebrae superioris contracts, and the upper lid moves with the eyeball. The lower lid rises slightly but lags behind the eyeball. The raising of the lower lid is believed to occur as the result of the pull of the conjunctiva, which is attached to the sclera and the lower lid.

On looking downward, both lids move, the upper lid continues to cover the upper part of the cornea, and the levator palpebrae superioris relaxes. The lower lid is pulled downward slightly by the conjunctiva, which is attached to the sclera and the lower lid. It is the contraction of the inferior rectus muscle that pulls the conjunctiva downward.

Clinical Notes

Lid Skin

The extreme thinness of the skin of the eyelids makes this skin very difficult to match grafting skin from other areas of the body. The presence of delicate, loose subcutaneous tissue permits the accumulation of blood resulting from trauma or of edema fluid secondary to nephrosis.

Lid Glands

Meibomian Gland Dysfunction   A relatively common condition occurring in middle-aged and elderly individuals, particularly fair-skinned persons, is occlusion of the tarsal gland openings. This results in a reduced outpouring of secretion or a qualitative change in the secretion, and adversely affects the tear film. In this condition, excessive evaporation of tears occurs and may lead to a dry eye state.

Chalazion   This is a localized, progressive, painless swelling of the lid resulting from chronic inflammation of a tarsal gland. Since the gland lies on the conjunctival surface of the tarsal plate, the swelling should be incised through the conjunctival surface of the lid.

Hordeolum (stye)   An external hordeolum is an acute infection of a lash follicle or a sebaceous gland (of Zeis) or a ciliary sweat gland (of Moll); all drain externally to the skin surface of the lid. An internal hordeolum is an acute infection of a tarsal gland (of Meibom). The tarsal glands usually drain through the conjunctival surface of the lid.

Lid Muscle

Paralysis of Orbicularis Oculi Muscle   Paralysis of the orbicularis oculi muscle from a lesion of the seventh cranial nerve prevents closure of the eye and permits the lower lid to sag away from the eyeball (ectropion). The puncta of the lacrimal canaliculi are no longer kept in the lacus lacrimalis, so that tears escape over the lower lid (epiphora). Senile weakness of the orbicularis may also cause the above conditions.

Paralysis of Levator Palpebrae Superioris Muscle   Paralysis of the levator palpebrae superioris from a lesion of the third cranial nerve, myasthenia gravis, or senile dehiscence of the aponeurosis produces severe drooping of the upper eyelid (ptosis) and loss of the superior palpebral fold and the horizontal furrow.

Paralysis of the superior tarsal muscle—a thin sheet of smooth muscle attached to the levator palpebrae superioris—can occur following a lesion of the cervical part of the sympathetic nervous system. A less severe form of ptosis occurs. When associated with constriction of the pupil and enophthalmos, this condition is known as Horner's syndrome.

Orbital Septum

The orbital septum separates the lid connective tissue spaces from the orbital contents. Not only does it serve to hold the orbital fat in position, but it forms a barrier to prevent infection from passing from the eyelids into the orbital cavity (or vice versa). Herniation of the orbital fat into the eyelid is most commonly seen in the elderly. The septum is weakest on the medial side of the lower lid.

Tarsal Plates

The tarsal plates, which consist of dense connective tissue, give the lids shape and support. To limit distortion of these plates and the eyelids as the result of scar tissue formation following surgery, the surgeon usually incises the plates in a vertical plane.

Fascial Spaces

The subcutaneous pretarsal and preseptal spaces of the lids are potential areas for accumulation of blood or inflammatory exudate. The preseptal space is not continuous with the potential space of the scalp beneath the epicranial aponeurosis, because the epicranial aponeurosis is fused to the periosteum at the orbital margin. Small communications may exist along the course of blood vessels and nerves.

Relationship Between the Cornea and the Palpebral Fissure

In an emergency, when the eyes reflexly close as a protective mechanism against trauma, chemicals, or fire, the last part of the cornea to be covered by the lids is just below the center. The damaged area may be even lower than expected, since the cornea tends to move upward with approaching danger. In the elderly, corneal damage may be more extensive because of poor tone of the orbicularis oculi.

Anesthetizing the Eyelids

The sensory nerves to the eyelids run in the areolar tissue beneath the orbicularis oculi muscle. To block these nerves, the local anesthetic must be injected deep to this muscle.

Splitting the Eyelid

Between the rows of eyelashes and the orifices of the tarsal glands on the lid margin lies the so-called *gray line*, or sulcus. The gray color is due to relative avascularity. The insertion of a scalpel blade into the gray line permits the scalpel to enter the submuscular connective tissue, enabling the surgeon to split the lid easily into anterior and posterior portions. The anterior portion consists of the skin, subcutaneous tissue, and the orbicularis oculi muscle; the posterior portion consists of the tarsal plates, orbital septum, and the conjunctiva. A minimal formation of scar tissue follows this procedure.

Lacerations

With lacerations of the eyelids, usually little or no tissue loss occurs and necrosis of lid tissue is rare because of the excellent blood supply to the lids. Debridement should be avoided to prevent ectropion.

Correct alignment of the posterior lid margin is essential to avoid deformity. The posterior lid margin suture should be placed first and its ends left long so that traction can be applied to preserve the alignment. Through-and-through lacerations are closed in layers, with the deepest layer consisting of the conjunctiva and the tarsal plate being sutured first. The muscle and skin are then sutured as a single layer.

Lacerations involving the lacrimal canaliculus require placement of a stent within the lumen. Lacerated medial or lateral palpebral ligaments must be repaired carefully.

Lacerations parallel with the lid margins can be closed with simple interrupted sutures. Since the pull of the orbicularis muscle is in line with the laceration, an unsightly scar is unlikely.

Reconstruction Following Excision of Tumors

In those cases where excision of a small tumor requires the removal of 25 percent or less of the eyelid margin, the skin incision can be closed directly provided there is not undue tension. When there is excessive laxity of the lids, as may be found in older patients, larger areas of the eyelids may be removed and the margins of the defect directly united. Great care is taken to ensure that the lid margin is accurately aligned to avoid deformity. Here again, the first suture is inserted into the posterior lid margin and the ends are left long for traction.

Larger tumors requiring the removal of much larger areas of the eyelids may require plastic surgery with rotational cheek skin flaps.

Conjunctiva

The conjunctiva is a thin mucous membrane that lines the eyelids and is reflected at the superior and inferior fornices onto the anterior surface of the eyeball (Fig. 5-8). The conjunctival epithelium is continuous with the epidermis of the skin at the lid margin and with the corneal epithelium at the limbus. The conjunctiva thus forms a potential space, the *conjunctival sac*, which is open at the palpebral fissure (Fig. 5-8).

General Arrangement

For purposes of description, the conjunctiva can be divided into three regions: 1) the palpebral conjunctiva, 2) the conjunctival fornices, and 3) the bulbar conjunctiva.

Palpebral Conjunctiva

This lining of the eyelids has already been described (see page 100). It is firmly attached to the posterior surfaces of the tarsal plates.

Conjunctival Fornices

The conjunctiva of the superior and inferior fornices forms transitional regions between the palpebral and bulbar conjunctivae. It is loosely attached to the underlying fascial expansions of the sheaths of the levator and recti muscles. Contraction of these muscles can pull the conjunctiva so that it moves with the eyelids and the eyeball. The looseness of the underlying connective tissue permits accumulation of edema fluids. The ducts of the lacrimal gland open into the lateral part of the superior fornix.

The superior fornix is situated about 10 mm from the limbus; the inferior fornix, about 8 mm from the limbus. Medially the fornices are absent and are replaced by the caruncle and the plica semilunaris. On the lateral side the fornices are extensive and lie about 14 mm from the limbus, thus extending posterior to the equator of the eyeball.

Bulbar (Ocular) Conjunctiva

This portion lies in contact with the eyeball (Fig. 5-8). It is thin and translucent, and the underlying white sclera is clearly visible. It is loosely attached by connective tissue to the sclera and the fascia bulbi covering the tendons of the recti muscles. About 3 mm from the cornea, the conjunctiva becomes more closely attached to the sclera and the fascia bulbi. The line along which fusion of the conjunctiva to the cornea occurs is called the *conjunctival limbus* (Fig. 5-12). It is situated about 1 mm anterior to the edge or limbus of the cornea, that is, the

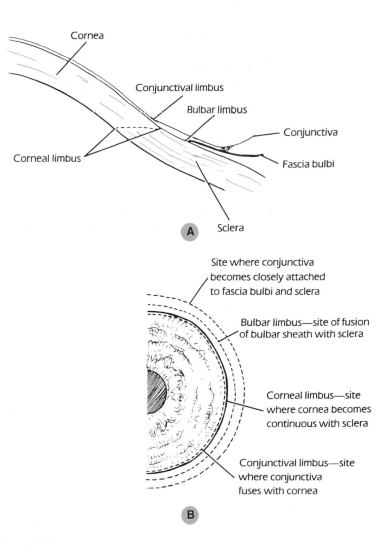

Figure 5-12

Diagrams showing the relationship between the attachment of the conjunctiva and the fascia bulbi to the cornea and sclera. (A) The corneal scleral junction in section. (B) The corneal scleral junction, anterior view. Note the positions of the conjunctival limbus, the corneal limbus, and the bulbar limbus.

junction between the cornea and the sclera. The bulbar sheath fuses with the sclera about 1.5 mm posterior to the corneal limbus (Fig. 5-12).

Structure

Histologically, the conjunctiva has an epithelial covering of stratified columnar cells consisting of two to five layers resting on a lamina propria of loose connective tissue (Fig. 5-13). At the limbus there is a change to stratified squamous nonkeratinized epithelium, which is continuous with the epithelium covering the cornea. Also at the limbus, the lamina propria forms papillae, which are not seen elsewhere in the conjunctiva. On the posterior edge of the lid margin, along the posterior margin of the openings of the tarsal glands, the conjunctiva joins the skin (Fig. 5-4). Here the nonkeratinized squamous epithelium of the conjunctiva becomes continuous with the keratinized stratified squamous epithelium of the epidermis.

Figure 5-13

Photomicrographs of sections of the conjunctiva. (A) The epithelial covering and the loose connective tissue of the lamina propria. (H&E; × 200.) (B) Conjunctiva at the limbus (arrow); note the presence of papillae in the lamina propria. Note also the continuation of the conjunctival epithelium with the corneal epithelium. (H&E; × 200.) (C) The presence of scattered goblet cells in the conjunctival epithelium. (H&E; × 200.)

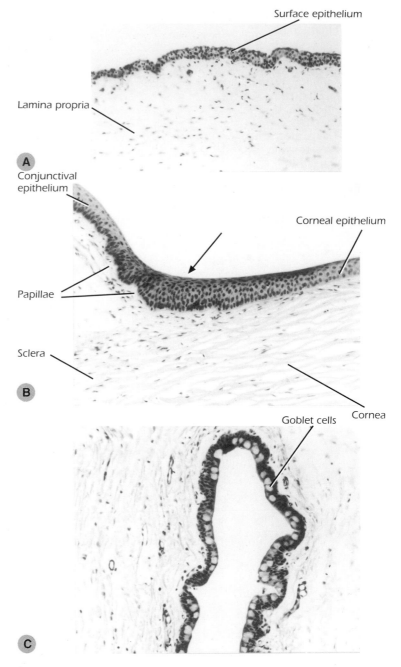

Goblet cells are found scattered along the surface of the conjunctiva, being most numerous inferonasally and present in greater number in children and young adults. Although they may occur singly, they are commonly found lining crypts. Their secretion is important contributing stability to the tear film.

Accessory Lacrimal Glands

Situated in the connective tissue of the conjunctiva, the accessory lacrimal glands (Fig. 5-4) are found scattered throughout the conjunctival sac. They may number as many as 50. They are similar to the lacrimal glands, and their ducts open to the free surface of the conjunctiva.

Conjunctival Submucosa

This consists of fine, delicate connective tissue (Fig. 5-13), which ends at the edges of the cornea. In its superficial part are large collections of lymphocytes, which are present in highest concentration in the fornices and are absent in the marginal conjunctiva. The deeper part of the submucosa contains denser fibrous tissue and the blood vessels, nerves, smooth muscle, and accessory lacrimal glands. The submucosa projects toward the surface epithelium at the limbus and at the lid margins to form conjunctival papillae.

Conjunctival Arteries

The arterial supply of the conjunctiva arises from the two palpebral arches in each eyelid and from the anterior ciliary arteries (Fig. 5-10). The palpebral arches are the large marginal and smaller peripheral, running respectively along the marginal and peripheral borders of the tarsal plates.

The large *marginal arch* runs 3 mm from the free border of the eyelid between the tarsal plate and the orbicularis oculi muscle (Fig. 5-10). Small branches pass from one arch to the other in front and behind the tarsal plates. It is the arteries on the posterior surface of the tarsal plates that supply the palpebral conjunctiva.

Branches from the *peripheral arch* supply the superior and inferior conjunctival fornices (Fig. 5-10). Many then run under the bulbar conjunctiva, forming the *posterior conjunctival arteries*, to supply the bulbar conjunctiva; these arteries then proceed toward the cornea. At the limbus they anastomose with the *anterior conjunctival arteries*, which are branches of the anterior ciliary arteries. The anterior ciliary arteries arise from the muscular branches of the ophthalmic artery to the rectus muscles (see page 280). Some persons have no peripheral arterial arch to the lower lid. In these subjects the marginal arch supplies the conjunctiva along with the anterior ciliary arteries.

Conjunctival Veins

The conjunctival veins are more numerous than the arteries. They accompany the arteries and drain into the palpebral veins or directly into the superior and inferior ophthalmic veins.

Conjunctival Lymph Drainage

The conjunctival lymph vessels are arranged as a superficial and a deep plexus in the submucosa. Those from the lateral side drain into the superficial parotid nodes; those from the medial side pass to the submandibular nodes.

Conjunctival Nerves

The sensory innervation of the bulbar conjunctiva is from the long ciliary nerves, which are branches of the nasociliary nerve, a branch of the ophthalmic division of the trigeminal nerve. Innervation of the superior palpebral conjunctiva and the superior fornix conjunctiva is from the frontal and lacrimal branches of the ophthalmic division of the trigeminal nerve. Sensory innervation of the inferior palpebral conjunctiva and that of the inferior fornix is laterally from the lacrimal branch of the ophthalmic division of the trigeminal nerve and medially from the infraorbital nerve from the maxillary division of the trigeminal nerve.

Lacrimal Caruncle

The lacrimal caruncle is a small, pinkish ovoid body (Fig. 5-2) situated in the lacus lacrimalis at the medial angle of the eye; it lies on the medial side of the plica semilunaris. The caruncle is an area of modified skin possessing a few fine, colorless hairs and sebaceous and sweat glands. It differs from skin in that it contains accessory lacrimal glands and the stratified squamous epithelium is non-keratinized. The *arterial supply* is from the superior medial palpebral arteries. The *lymphatic drainage* is into the submandibular lymph nodes. The *nerve supply* is from the infratrochlear branch of the nasociliary nerve.

Plica Semilunaris

The plica semilunaris is a halfmoon-shaped fold of the conjunctiva lying lateral to and partly under the caruncle (Fig. 5-2). The lateral margin is free and concave. Beneath the fold is a small space about 2 mm deep when the eye is looking medially. When the eye is looking laterally, the space practically disappears.

The epithelial covering resembles that of the conjunctiva and contains many goblet cells. The submucosa contains adipose tissue and some smooth muscle fibers. The connective tissue is highly vascular.

The plica semilunaris may represent the nictitating membrane of lower vertebrates. More probably it is a slack fold of conjunctiva to allow the eyeball to move fully laterally. No such fold exists on the lateral side of the eyeball, where the conjunctival fornix is extensive and permits the eyeball to move fully medially.

 Clinical Notes

Palpebral Conjunctiva Examination

This conjunctiva is thin, translucent (almost transparent), firmly attached to the deep surface of the tarsal plates, and very vascular. The thinness and transparency allow the examiner, by everting the lids, to visualize the yellowish tarsal glands arranged in rows embedded in the posterior surfaces of the tarsal plates. The many blood vessels can also be seen and examination of the palpebral conjunctiva is commonly used clinically in the diagnosis of anemia.

The firm attachment of the conjunctiva to the tarsal plates makes surgical separation of these structures, especially in the upper lid, extremely difficult.

Arterial Supply of the Bulbar Conjunctiva and Disease

The peripheral bulbar conjunctiva is supplied by the posterior conjunctival branches of the peripheral arterial arch. They extend forward to within 4 mm of the corneoscleral limbus. In the normal conjunctiva, they can only just be seen. In acute conjunctivitis these vessels dilate, and, because they are superficial, they appear bright red. Since they are situated in the connective tissue of the conjunctiva, they move with the conjunctiva and can be constricted with topical epinephrine.

Dilatation of the arteries and arteriolization of the conjunctival vessels can be seen when the venous drainage of the conjunctiva is reduced (see p. 289).

The central bulbar conjunctiva, that is, the area adjacent to the corneoscleral limbus, is supplied by the anterior conjunctival branches of the anterior ciliary arteries. The anterior conjunctival arteries give off superficial branches to form a *superficial conjunctival plexus* and a *deep episcleral plexus.*

In inflammatory disease of the cornea, the superficial conjunctival pericorneal plexus becomes dilated and the vessels appear bright red. Moreover, because they are superficial, they move with the conjunctiva and can be constricted with topical epinephrine.

In inflammatory disease of the iris or ciliary body or in closed-angle glaucoma, the deep episcleral pericorneal plexus becomes dilated. The vessels appear dull red because of their deep location. Since they are in the sclera, they do not move with the conjunctiva, but the redness disappears on pressure; they cannot be constricted with topical epinephrine.

In very severe inflammatory disease, all the arteries supplying the bulbar conjunctiva become dilated as the result of their profuse anastomotic connections.

Surgical Grasping of the Conjunctiva

The difficulty in grasping the palpebral conjunctiva with surgical forceps—which has already been noted—results from the firm tethering of the membrane to the tarsal plates.

The conjunctiva at the superior fornix is loosely attached by fascia to the fascia of the levator palpebrae superioris and the superior rectus muscles. Similarly, there is some connection between the inferior fornix and the fascia of the inferior rectus muscle.

Where the conjunctiva of the fornices is reflected onto the eyeball, it lies loose and can be easily grasped with surgical forceps. In fact, it is here that the bulbar conjunctiva is incised, along with the bulba fascia, to perform tenotomy of the recti muscles.

About 3 mm from the corneoscleral limbus, the conjunctiva, the bulba fascia (Tenon's capsule), and the sclera become firmly united. Although it is difficult to raise a fold of conjunctiva at this site, at least a firm grip can be obtained with forceps. It is possible to separate the conjunctiva from the bulba fascia and the sclera right up to the corneoscleral limbus.

Surgical Site for Piercing the Eyeball in Glaucoma

The region between the bulbar limbus (attachment of the bulbar sheath to the sclera) about 1.5 mm posterior to the corneoscleral limbus and the conjunctival limbus (attachment of the conjunctiva to the cornea) about 1 mm anterior to the corneoscleral limbus is a common surgical site for piercing the eyeball in the treatment of glaucoma.

Lacrimal Apparatus

The lacrimal apparatus consists of the lacrimal gland, which secretes tears; the lacrimal lake; the lacrimal canaliculi; the lacrimal sac; and the nasolacrimal duct, which carries the tears into the nasal cavity (Fig. 5-14).

Lacrimal Gland

General Arrangement

The lacrimal gland consists of a large *orbital part* and a small *palpebral part*, which are continuous with each other around the lateral edge of the aponeurosis of the levator palpebrae superioris (Fig. 5-15).

The larger orbital part is almond-shaped and lies in the lacrimal fossa on the anterior and lateral part of the roof of the orbit, just within the margin of the orbit (Fig. 5-14). The superior surface is convex and related to bone. The inferior surface lies above the aponeurosis of the levator palpebrae superioris, and more laterally, above the upper margin of the lateral rectus muscle. The anterior border is related to the orbital septum, and the posterior border is in contact with the orbital fat.

The smaller palpebral part (about one-third the size of the orbital part) lies below the aponeurosis of the levator palpebrae superioris and extends into the upper eyelid. The superior surface is therefore related to the aponeurosis; the inferior surface lies in contact with the lateral part of the superior fornix of the conjunctiva, through which the gland can be seen when the eyelid is everted.

The lacrimal gland has no definite capsule, but the periorbita is believed to split and enclose it.

The approximately 12 ducts of the gland pass from the orbital part through the palpebral part to open into the superior conjunctival fornix (Fig. 5-15). Additional ducts from the palpebral part open independently into the superior fornix.

In addition to the main lacrimal gland, numerous small accessory lacrimal glands are scattered around the conjunctival sac, especially in association with the conjunctival fornices (see page 111). The presence of these smaller glands is sufficient to keep the cornea moist should the main gland become nonfunctional as the result of disease or be surgically removed.

Structure

As seen with the light microscope, the lacrimal gland is a lobulated tubulo-acinar structure, the lobules separated from one another by loose connective tissue (Fig. 5-17). On section, the acini are seen as round or tube-shaped masses of columnar cells with central lumens. The smallest intralobular ducts are lined with a

Figure 5-14

(A) The formation of tears from the lacrimal gland and their passage across the front of the eye to drain into the nose. (B) A cross-section of the lacrimal sac showing its relationship to the medial palpebral ligament, the lacrimal part of the orbicularis oculi, the lacrimal fascia, and the periorbita lining the lacrimal groove. (C) The different drainage ducts connecting the conjunctival sac with the inferior meatus of the nose.

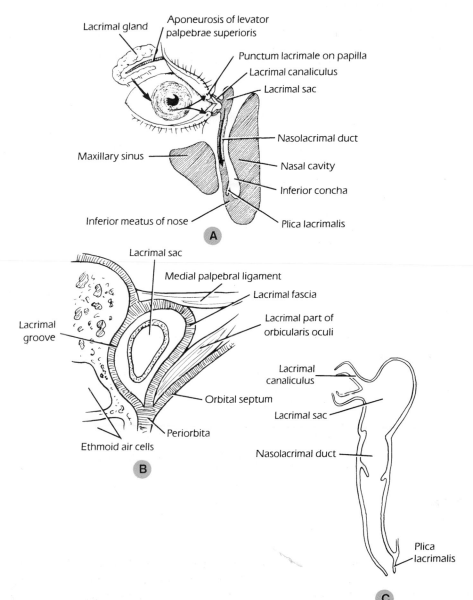

Figure 5-15

Sagittal section of the orbital and palpebral portions of the lacrimal gland, showing the relationship of the gland to the aponeurosis of the levator palpebrae superioris muscle and to the superior fornix of the conjunctiva.

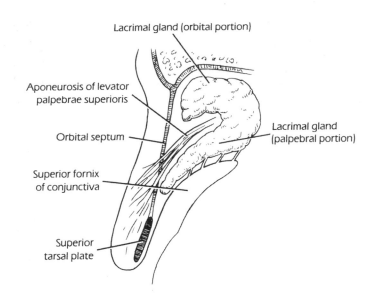

 Figure 5-16

The autonomic innervation of the lacrimal gland.

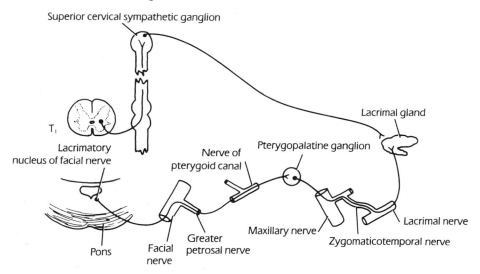

layer of low columnar or cuboidal cells and have myoepithelial cells at the periphery. The larger intralobular ducts have a two-layered epithelial lining.

    As seen with the electron microscope, the epithelial secretory cells of the acini are surrounded by a discontinuous layer of myoepithelial cells and rest on a basal lamina. The secretory cells are truncated-conical in shape (Fig. 5-18) and have microvilli on their apical or luminal surface. Laterally, the plasmalemma is

Figure 5-17

Photomicrograph of a section of the lacrimal gland, showing numerous secretory serous acini and an interlobular duct. (H&E; × 100.)

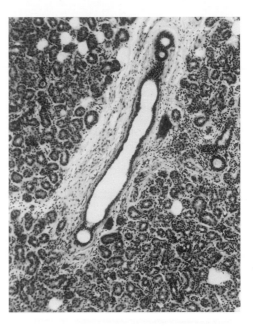

attached to that of adjacent cells by junctional complexes and scattered desmosomes. Narrow extensions of the acinar lumen that can sometimes be seen between adjacent secretory cells are referred to as canaliculi.

The secretory cell contains a basally located nucleus. The cytoplasm has a well-developed, rough-surfaced endoplasmic reticulum, a well-developed Golgi complex, moderate numbers of mitochondria, free ribosomes, lipid droplets, and vacuoles. Dominating the apical and middle regions of the cytoplasm are large numbers of secretory granules (Fig. 5-18).

The round or ovoid secretory granules are membrane-bound. The granules are either homogeneous or finely granular, and they vary considerably in their electron density. Different researchers have attempted to use the electron microscopic appearances of the granules to divide up the secretory cells into various categories. Some workers believe that the differences of the granules merely represent different stages in secretory activity in one or two distinct cell types. The predominance of dense granules suggests that most of the secretory cells are of the serous type. However, the staining of many of the secretory granules positively for acid mucopolysaccharides appears to indicate that mucus is also produced.

Arterial Supply

The lacrimal artery, a branch of the ophthalmic artery, enters its posterior border. The infraorbital artery, a branch of the maxillary artery, also sometimes supplies the gland. The *venous drainage* is into the ophthalmic vein. The *lymphatic drainage* joins that of the conjunctiva and passes to the superficial parotid lymph nodes.

Figure 5-18

Electron micrograph of an acinus of the human lacrimal gland, showing a lumen filled with secretion, surrounded by columnar epithelial secretory cells (SC). Numerous dark-staining secretory granules (SG and G) are present in the apical and middle regions of the cytoplasm. Several nuclei (N) are also seen. (× 4000.) (Courtesy of Fred Lightfoot.)

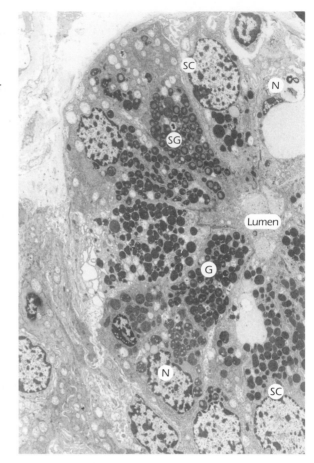

Nerve Supply

The lacrimal gland receives both autonomic and sensory nerve fibers.

The *parasympathetic* secretomotor nerve supply is derived from the *lacrimatory nucleus* of the facial nerve (Fig. 5-16). The preganglionic fibers reach the *pterygopalatine ganglion* (sphenopalatine ganglion) through the *nervus intermedius* and its *great petrosal branch* and through the *nerve of the pterygoid canal*. The postganglionic fibers leave the ganglion and join the maxillary nerve. They then pass into its *zygomatic branch* and the *zygomaticotemporal nerve*. They reach the lacrimal gland within the *lacrimal nerve*.

The *sympathetic* postganglionic fibers arise from the superior cervical sympathetic ganglion and travel in the plexus of nerves around the internal carotid artery. They join the *deep petrosal nerve*, the *nerve of the pterygoid canal*, the *maxillary nerve*, the *zygomatic nerve*, the *zygomaticotemporal nerve*, and, finally, the lacrimal nerve (Fig. 5-16).

The *sensory fibers* reach the lacrimal gland in the lacrimal nerve, a branch of the ophthalmic division of the trigeminal nerve.

Higher Nervous Control and Reflex Control of Lacrimal Secretion   The parasympathetic lacrimatory nucleus of the facial nerve is believed to receive afferent fibers from the hypothalamus through the *descending autonomic pathways* in the *reticular formation*. This may explain the nervous pathway involved in emotional responses when there is excessive production of tears, as in crying. A similar pathway, believed to connect the olfactory system with the lacrimatory nucleus, may account for the excessive tear production in response to certain olfactory stimuli. Reflex lacrimation secondary to irritation of the cornea or conjunctiva occurs following the passage of afferent nervous stimuli along the ophthalmic and maxillary divisions of the trigeminal nerve. The sensory nuclei of the trigeminal nerve are connected to the lacrimatory nucleus by internuncial neurons.

Lacrimal Secretion

The secretion produced by the acinar cells passes into the duct system, where it is thought that the lining cells modify its composition. The final watery secretion (tears) contains lysozyme (antibacterial enzyme), IgA (immunoglobulin), and beta-lysin (bactericidal protein), which serve as a defense against microorganisms. The lacrimal gland also secretes substances that affect the ocular surface by regulating epithelial cell turnover. Furthermore, hormones, particularly androgens, support lacrimal secretion and also suppress immunologic activity within the lacrimal glands. The main function of the tears is to keep the corneal epithelium moist, so that the surface epithelial cells have a medium in which to live, thus preserving the most important refractive mechanism of the eye. A secondary function is to lubricate the front of the eyeball so that it moves freely beneath the lids. (Lubrication may also be performed by the lipids excreted by the meibomian glands.)

Lacrimal Drainage

Punctum Lacrimale

The punctum lacrimale (Fig. 5-3) is a small round or oval orifice situated on the summit of a small projection, the *papilla lacrimalis*, at the medial end of the lid margin. The punctum is in line with the openings of the tarsal glands. Surrounding the punctum, the conjunctiva is somewhat avascular, so that the area appears pale red.

To visualize the puncta the lids have to be everted; the punctum of the upper lid is slightly medial to that of the lower lid. The upper punctum looks downward and backward; the lower punctum looks upward and backward. The tone of the orbicularis oculi muscle presses the puncta backward toward the lacus lacrimalis.

Lacrimal Canaliculi

Each canaliculus measures about 10 mm long and consists of a vertical and a horizontal portion (Fig. 5-14). The lacrimal canaliculi begin at the puncta and they pass almost vertically from the lid margin. After 2 mm they turn sharply medially. The upper canaliculus runs medially and downward; the lower one, medially and upward. At the junction of the vertical and horizontal portions the canaliculi are slightly dilated to form an *ampulla.*

The canaliculi now pierce the periorbita (lacrimal fascia) that encloses the lacrimal sac. The two channels now enter the lateral surface of the sac about 2.5 mm below its apex (Fig. 5-14). At the point of entrance the canaliculi are either separate or have united to form a common stem. A small diverticulum of the sac (the sinus of Maier) is situated at the site of entry.

The canaliculi lie behind the medial palpebral ligament and are surrounded by the fibers of the pars lacrimalis of the orbicularis oculi muscle.

The walls of the canaliculi are thin and elastic and are lined with stratified squamous epithelium.

During blinking of the eye the canaliculi are pulled medially, shortened, and compressed by the lacrimal part of the orbicularis oculi. This pumping action assists in dilatation of the lacrimal sac.

Lacrimal Sac

The lacrimal sac, measuring about 12 mm long, is situated in the lacrimal fossa formed by the lacrimal bone and the frontal process of the maxilla (Fig. 5-14). It is thus positioned in the anterior part of the medial wall of the orbit. The lacrimal sac, the blind upper end of the nasolacrimal duct, receives on its lateral side near its upper end the openings of the lacrimal canaliculi.

The lacrimal sac is enclosed by a fascial sheath, the *lacrimal fascia,* which is attached behind to the posterior lacrimal crest of the lacrimal bone and in front to the anterior lacrimal crest of the maxilla. The fascia is formed from the periorbita, which is the periosteum of the orbital bones.

Between the lacrimal sac and the lacrimal fascia is a venous plexus. The lacrimal fascia separates the sac from the medial palpebral ligament anteriorly and the lacrimal part of the orbicularis oculi posteriorly. The medial palpebral ligament covers only the upper part of the anterior aspect of the lacrimal sac (Figs. 5-6 and 5-7).

The upper half of the sac is related medially to the anterior ethmoidal sinuses (Fig. 5-6). The lower half is related medially to the anterior part of the middle meatus of the nose (Fig. 5-14).

The angular vein, formed by the union of the supratrochlear and supraorbital veins, and later becoming the facial vein, crosses the anterior surface of the medial palpebral ligament about 8 mm medial to the medial canthus and therefore lies in important anterior relationship to the lacrimal sac.

The wall of the lacrimal sac consists of fibroelastic tissue and is lined with two layers of columnar cells. Goblet cells are present.

Nasolacrimal Duct

The nasolacrimal duct, about 18 mm long, connects the lower end of the lacrimal sac with the inferior meatus of the nose (Fig. 5-14). It is narrower in the middle than at either end. The direction of the duct is downward, backward, and lateral. The duct is lodged in the bony nasolacrimal canal that lies between the maxillary sinus and the nasal cavity. The canal is formed by the maxilla, the lacrimal bone, and the inferior nasal concha.

The wall of the nasolacrimal duct is closely attached to the periosteum lining the canal. Within the walls is a venous plexus that is continuous above with that of the lacrimal sac and below with the veins of the nasal mucous membrane. The duct is lined with two layers of columnar epithelium; some of the cells are ciliated.

The nasolacrimal duct opens below into the anterior part of the inferior meatus of the nose (Fig. 5-14). The opening is guarded by a flap of mucous membrane called the *plica lacrimalis*, which, if well developed, serves as a valve preventing air from entering the lacrimal sac when one is blowing the nose.

Arterial Supply to the Lacrimal Sac and the Nasolacrimal Duct

The arteries are branches of the medial palpebral of the ophthalmic, the facial, the infraorbital from the maxillary, and the sphenopalatine arteries of the maxillary. The *nerve supply* is from the infratrochlear branch of the ophthalmic division of the trigeminal nerve and the anterior superior alveolar nerve, a branch of the maxillary division of the trigeminal nerve.

Tear Production

The normal tear formation necessary to keep the eye moist is provided by a continuous secretion from the accessory lacrimal glands scattered throughout the conjunctival sac. Excessive production of tears, as in crying, is due mainly to reflex nervous stimulation of the main lacrimal gland. Under normal conditions, tear production just exceeds that lost by evaporation; the remainder passes down the nasolacrimal duct.

Tear Distribution in the Conjunctival Sac

Tear fluid accumulates in the conjunctival fornices and the lacus lacrimalis. It also collects as a striplike collection of fluid between the posterior margin of the eyelids and the eyeball. The superior marginal strip overlaps the cornea for about 1 mm as a straight line. Should the upper lid be gently raised away from the eyeball, the tear fluid rises into the superior fornix.

The inferior marginal strip rises up over the cornea for about 1 mm as the result of surface tension. Similarly, when the lower lid is pulled down from the eyeball, the level of the tear fluid sinks into the inferior fornix.

The capacity of the conjunctival sac is about 25 to 30 mL. When the volume of tears secreted exceeds this amount, clinical tearing results.

Tear Circulation and Drainage

Tears produced by the lacrimal gland and the scattered accessory lacrimal glands enter the conjunctival sac. The tear fluid is carried across the sac to the lacus lacrimalis. This process is brought about under the physical influence of capillarity and by the blinking movements of the eyelids. Most of the tears travel in the fornices of the sac and in the grooves between the lid margins and the eyeball.

Under normal conditions, the tear fluid does not pour down over the surface of the cornea, because this would interfere with the refraction of the eye. Periodically the upper lid blinks and wipes a thin film of tears across the cornea, thus preventing desiccation of its superficial cells. The oily secretion of the tarsal glands (and the sebaceous glands of the eyelashes) at the lid margin prevents the overflow of tears. Exaggerated tear production, as in crying, causes the tears to flow across the cornea and escape across the lower lid margin and flow down the skin of the cheek. Under these circumstances, the cornea ceases to function as an efficient lens.

During sleep, the lid margins are in apposition and the conjunctival sac is closed. The tears are drained from the lacus lacrimalis by the canaliculi. The puncta of the canaliculi are kept in contact with the lacus lacrimalis or with the eyeball (when the eyeball is medially rotated) by the tone of the orbicularis oculi in the eyelids. Tear fluid enters the canaliculi by capillarity. The orbicularis oculi is attached to the medial palpebral ligament, which is tethered to the lacrimal sac by fascia. The sudden contraction of the lacrimal part of the orbicularis oculi shortens and compresses the canaliculi and causes dilatation of the lacrimal sac, resulting in the tears being sucked into the sac. This combined mechanism is referred to as the pumping action of the orbicularis oculi.

The passage of tears down the wide-bored nasolacrimal duct occurs as the result of gravity and the evaporation of the fluid at the orifice into the nose, aided by the movement of air during inspiration and expiration.

Tear Film

The precorneal tear film is composed of three layers: 1) The thin, superficial oily layer, measuring about 0.9 to 0.2 μm, is produced predominantly by the tarsal (meibomian) glands and to a slight extent by the sebaceous glands (Zeis) and sweat glands (Moll); 2) the thick, watery layer, measuring about 6.5 to 7.5 μm, is secreted by the lacrimal glands; and 3) the *thin mucin*,* measuring about 0.5 μm, is secreted by the conjunctival goblet cells and from the lacrimal gland cells.

The thin, oily layer inhibits evaporation of the underlying watery layer. The watery layer contains the lysozyme, immunoglobulin, and beta-lysin and is the defense against invading organisms. The thin, deep mucin layer wets the microvilli of the corneal epithelium.

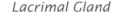

Clinical Notes

Lacrimal Gland

The *ducts*, which number about 12, originate mostly in the orbital part of the gland and then traverse the palpebral part of the gland to open into the superior

---

*Freeze substitution studies suggest that the mucin layer is much thicker than originally believed.

fornix of the conjunctival sac. It follows that surgical removal of the palpebral part of the gland will in most individuals destroy the drainage of the whole gland.

Obstruction to Secretions   The openings of the ducts into the conjunctival sac may be obstructed by scarring of the conjunctiva caused by erythema multiforme, ocular cicatricial pemphigoid, trachoma, and chemical burns.

Surgical Damage   Since the smaller palpebral part of the lacrimal gland lies within the upper lid, damage to it may occur during surgery to the upper lid.

Tumors   *Tumors* of the lacrimal gland are commonly benign, for example, mixed cell tumors and benign lymphoid hyperplasia. Less common tumors are malignant, for example, malignant lymphoma and adenocarcinoma. Benign tumors tend to grow slowly, causing fullness in the upper outer portion of the upper eyelid, with subsequent displacement of the eyeball. Malignant tumors tend to produce early erosion of the lacrimal fossa in the roof of the orbit, causing severe pain.

Dry Eyes   Drying of the conjunctiva and cornea results from a deficiency of the watery component of tears, as in disease of the main lacrimal gland or accessory lacrimal glands. It can also occur when there is a deficiency of the mucin component of tears, as in disease of the goblet cells of the conjunctiva in cases of hypovitaminosis A, Stevens-Johnson disease, chemical burns, and ocular cicatricial pemphigoid. As mentioned previously, dysfunction of the meibomian glands can lead to excessive evaporation of tears and to the dry eye state.

The outflow of tears in dry eyes can be restricted by reducing the size of the punctum lacrimale by plugs, by cautery, or by laser.

Lacrimation   Excessive production of tears may be caused reflexly, as in photophobia and inflammations of the conjunctiva, cornea, and ciliary body. Congenital glaucoma with corneal edema can also produce excessive tears.

Lacrimal Canaliculi

Passing a Probe   Probing of the drainage system requires a sound knowledge of the direction and length of the various ducts. For example, it should be remembered that each canaliculus passes vertically for about 2 mm before bending sharply medially at a right angle; 8 mm farther, the canaliculi enter the lacrimal sac. Gently pulling the eyelids laterally results in straightening of the canaliculus.

Lacrimal Sac

Inflammatory Disease   The lacrimal sac is located in the lacrimal fossa in the anterior part of the medial wall of the orbit. The upper part of the sac is covered anteriorly by the medial palpebral ligament. It follows that distention of the sac with inflammatory exudate or pus will cause a visible swelling below the lower border of the ligament. Moreover, an abscess or a fistula will point or open in this region.

Surgical Incisions   In making an incision through the skin close to the medial canthus of the eye in an anterior approach to the lacrimal sac, it is essential to avoid the angular vein. The angular vein, which is the upper part of the facial vein, is formed by the union of the supratrochlear and supraorbital veins. It descends across the anterior surface of the medial palpebral ligament lateral to the facial artery and about 8 mm medial to the medial canthus. The medial palpebral ligament may have to be divided to expose the sac fully. Bleeding from the venous plexus around the lacrimal sac may be troublesome.

The sac may also be approached from the nasal cavity via endoscopy.

Nasolacrimal Duct

Passing a Probe   In passing a probe downward, it should be remembered that the direction of the duct is downward backward and laterally; the duct is about 18 mm long. It opens below into the anterior part of the inferior meatus of the nose. The probe is inserted into the punctum of the upper lid, directed vertically and then medially into the lacrimal sac, then turned downward at right angles in the nasolacrimal duct to the inferior meatus. The end of the probe should then be visible within the nose.

CHAPTER 5
Clinical Problems

Answers on Page 128

1 A 20-year-old medical student went to his physician and complained of an acute tender area on the middle of his left lower eyelid. Examination revealed a localized red, indurated area on the eyelid margin. Closer examination showed a yellowish spot in the center of the swelling, indicating that the abscess was about to rupture. Gentle eversion of the lid showed no evidence of swelling on its posterior surface. What is the diagnosis? Which anatomic structure(s) is (are) involved in the inflammatory process? On which part of the margin of the lid does the abscess tend to point?

2 A 14-year-old boy was involved in a fight during school recess. Another much larger student hit him in the right eye with his fist. During the next hour both eyelids of the victim's right eye swelled up until he could barely see. Examination by the ophthalmologist revealed a bluish-red discoloration of both eyelids of his right eye with narrowing of the palpebral fissure. The discoloration extended to the forehead and the right cheek. Careful separation of the eyelids showed a localized hemorrhage of the inferolateral part of the bulbar conjunctiva. When the conjunctiva was gently moved with the tip of the examiner's little finger, the hemorrhage moved also. On asking the patient to look medially, the ophthalmologist could clearly see the posterior limit of the conjunctival hemorrhage. Does this patient have a simple "black eye," or is this a fracture of his anterior cranial fossa? What role does the orbital septum play in enabling one to distinguish between these lesions? Is the appearance of the conjunctival hemorrhage important in making a diagnosis?

3 A 75-year-old man complaining of a small nodule on the outer part of his right lower eyelid visited his physician. He said that he had noticed it about a year ago and was concerned about it now because it was gradually enlarging and had ulcerated. On examination, the nodule was about 4 mm in diameter and was ulcerated with pearly margins. It was noted that the base of the ulcer was tethered to deeper structures. Otherwise the right eye was normal in all respects. The superficial parotid lymph nodes were not palpable. What is your diagnosis? To what deep structures was the ulcer likely to be fixed? Would you expect the superficial parotid nodes to be enlarged in this patient?

4 A 3-month-old boy was taken to a pediatrician because his mother had noticed that his left eye watered excessively when he cried. Recently she noted that when she gently wiped his eye with a tissue, a yellowish, sticky fluid exuded into the medial corner. The infant was referred to an ophthalmologist, who confirmed the epiphora of the left eye and the emergence of pus into the lacus lacrimalis from the puncta when firm pressure was applied to the lacrimal sac. What is the diagnosis? What is the most likely cause in a child of this age? What are the anterior anatomic relations of the lacrimal sac? Describe the anatomy of the drainage passages and give the direction and length of each of the tubes.

5 In nephrosis one of the classic clinical findings is swelling of the eyelids that tends to be most pronounced in the morning. In heart failure, edema tends to be located in the skin of the lower part of the body and to be worse at night. Why is there this difference?

6 A 35-year-old man was getting off the back of a truck when it started to move. Having placed his feet on the ground, he grabbed a rail on the truck with his right hand and held on. The truck continued along the road for one block before it stopped. In the meantime, the man had been dragged along the road as he held on to the truck. He was seen in the emergency room in a state of shock, with cuts and abrasions to his legs. On careful examination of his right arm, a number of muscles were found to be weak or paralyzed. In addition, it was noted that the pupil of the right eye was constricted and that there was drooping of the right upper eyelid. The right eyeball seemed to be less prominent than the left. The skin of the right cheek felt warmer and drier, and was redder in color, than the left cheek. Using your knowledge of anatomy, explain the clinical findings. What is the precise cause of this patient's ptosis of the right upper eyelid?

7 A 10-year-old girl who was walking to school passed a group of workmen digging a hole in the road. A sudden gust of wind carried some dirt particles into the air, and she suddenly experienced pain in her right eye. Although she wiped her eye and repeatedly blew her nose, the discomfort persisted. On being examined by an ophthalmologist, she was found to have a small foreign body in her right conjunctival sac. Using your knowledge of anatomy, describe the different regions of the sac. What is the sensory nerve supply to the conjunctiva? Where do foreign bodies frequently lodge beneath the upper eyelid? In order to remove the foreign body from beneath the upper lid, the eyelid must be carefully everted. What structure within the upper lid preserves its shape and form and assists the ophthalmologist in keeping the lid everted?

8 A 36-year-old man was diagnosed as having an aneurysm of the right internal carotid artery at the point where it passes through the cavernous sinus. It was noted that the patient had severe ptosis of the right eye and lateral strabismus. Using your knowledge of anatomy, explain the clinical findings. Why is the degree of ptosis in this condition more severe than that found in Horner's syndrome? Is the levator palpebrae superioris muscle attached to other anatomic structures in addition to the superior tarsal plate?

9 A 40-year-old woman complaining of a painless swelling of the upper lid of her left eye attended her physician. She said she had had the swelling for about 2 years and it was gradually increasing in size. On examination, a beadlike swelling measuring about 3 mm in diameter could be felt in the substance of the lid. On eversion of the lid, the area of conjunctiva related to the swelling was dark red. On closer questioning, the patient admitted that sometimes she experienced blurred vision in the left eye. What is the diagnosis? Which anatomic structure is involved? If the swelling were to become infected, as it sometimes does, toward which surface of the eyelid would the abscess point? Which surface of the eyelid would you incise for drainage? How do you account for the blurring of vision?

10 A 35-year-old woman visited her physician because of repeated attacks of muscular weakness. On questioning, she admitted that she felt weak all the time but the sensation grew worse with activity. Her husband had recently noticed that her right eyelid tended to droop toward the end of the day. About 3 weeks ago, after extensive walking in a shopping mall, she experienced double vision. Her visit to the doctor was precipitated by a change in her voice, which was gradually becoming weak. On examination the patient was noted to have ptosis of the right eye. On being asked to look up to the ceiling for 2 or 3 minutes, the eyelid drooped even further. A period of rest restored the eyelid to its previous position. Following an intramuscular injection of neostigmine, the patient's eyelid returned to normal, and the strength of her voice improved. What is your diagnosis? Using your knowledge of anatomy, explain her ptosis of the right eye. What is the cause of the diplopia?

11 A 60-year-old woman visited her physician because she had noticed puffiness of her left lower eyelid. Her friends told her that it was getting worse, and that she should seek medical advice. She said that she had first seen the swelling 5 years earlier. On examination, the left lower eyelid looked normal, but at the junction with the cheek just above the orbital margin a soft tissue swelling could be detected on palpation. A diagnosis of orbital fat herniation was made. Using your knowledge of anatomy, explain how fat herniation can occur.

12 A frail 80-year-old man visited his ophthalmologist. He complained of soreness of his left eye and excessive tear formation that necessitated repeated wiping of the eye. On examination, both lower eyelid margins were turned out away from the eyeball; the condition was worse on the left eye. The palpebral and bulbar parts of the conjunctiva were red and injected, and the inferior punctum was away from the lacus lacrimalis and the marginal tear film. There was no previous history of eye disease. What is your diagnosis? Using your anatomic knowledge, explain the mechanism involved in normally keeping the eyelids in contact with the eyeball. Which muscle(s) is (are) responsible for pumping the tears out of the lacrimal sac into the nasal cavity?

13 A 54-year-old woman was seen by an ophthalmologist. She complained of repeated involuntary blinking in both eyes. The condition started 5 years ago and has become progressively worse, and she is now unable to read or drive. She heard that an injection of the botulinum toxin could help her. Explain the reason for administering this toxin and where you would inject it.

14 A 25-year-old man was in a motor vehicle accident and his face was thrown against the windshield. On recovery in the emergency department, it was noticed that his right eyelid was drooping and he was unable to raise it. Examination of the cranial nerves found nothing abnormal. What specific structure was damaged and how might the situation be rectified?

15 A 40-year-old black woman with sarcoidosis was seen by an ophthalmologist because of bulging of both eyes and eyelids. She was unable to produce tears and she said that her eyes felt dry and itchy. Physical examination revealed bilateral proptosis and downward and medial displacement of the eyes. The lateral third of each eyelid was found to be swollen. Using your knowledge of anatomy, name the structure most likely affected by the sarcoidosis.

16 Describe the path taken by a tear drop from secretion to excretion.

17 A 69-year-old woman complained of chronic tearing of her left eye, requiring constant wiping of tears from her cheek. Because of the disability, it is difficult for her to read and sew. Ophthalmic investigation revealed a blockage of the lacrimal drainage system at the junction of the lacrimal sac and the nasolacrimal duct. Surgery is planned to bypass the nasolacrimal duct. Where would you perform this bypass?

CHAPTER 5
Answers to Clinical Problems

1 The student had a hordeolum or stye of his left eye. The usual cause is a staphylococcal infection of the eyelash follicle, the sebaceous gland of Zeis, or the ciliary gland of Moll. The suppurative infection tends to point on the anterior part of the lid margin. Repeated multiple styes tend to occur as the result of spread of infection along the eyelid margin.

2 This schoolboy had a severe "black eye." In this boy's condition the contusion involved not only the eyelids but the skin of the cheek and forehead. In anterior cranial fossa fractures, the hemorrhage occurs into the orbital cavity and is limited anteriorly by the attachment of the orbital septum to the orbital margin. In such cases the discoloration tends to be circular. In fractures of the anterior cranial fossa, because the bleeding is deeply placed, it tends to be purplish from the start, whereas with a black eye the color is initially red.

Yes, the appearance of the hemorrhage has diagnostic importance. If the conjunctiva is traumatized in a so-called black eye, the hemorrhage tends to be localized and is into the conjunctiva, so that it moves with the conjunctiva. In fractures of the anterior cranial fossa the hemorrhage extends forward under the conjunctiva; there is no posterior edge, and the blood does not move with the conjunctiva.

3 Histologic examination of the neoplasm after surgical removal identified the lesion as a basal cell carcinoma. It was noted that the columnar cells had already extended through the subcutaneous tissue and were invading the orbicularis oculi muscle. Basal cell carcinomas spread slowly and usually by direct extension. Only very rarely are the regional lymph nodes involved. The lymph drainage of the lateral parts of both lids is into the superficial parotid nodes.

4 This boy was suffering from chronic dacrocystitis secondary to congenital obstruction of the nasolacrimal duct. The obstruction results from failure of the nasolacrimal duct to open up and drain into the inferior meatus of the nose (see Chap. 1, p. 15).

The lacrimal sac is related anteriorly to the medial palpebral ligament, fascia, the orbicularis oculi, and the skin; the angular vein crosses the palpebral ligament.

The drainage passages start at the puncta on the tip of the papilla lacrimalis. The canaliculi first pass vertically in the eyelids for about 2 mm and then turn sharply at right angles and run medially for about 8 mm to enter the lacrimal sac. The lower end of the lacrimal sac is connected to the inferior meatus of the nose by the nasolacrimal duct. This duct, which measures about 18 mm long, passes downward, backward, and slightly laterally. The detailed anatomy of the lacrimal passages is described on page 119.

5 The skin of the eyelids is very thin and stretches easily. The underlying subcutaneous tissue is delicate and very loose. Large quantities of edema fluid can accumulate in this loose connective tissue. In nephrosis, when there is a loss of large quantities of plasma proteins from the blood, fluid escapes from the blood capillaries and readily accumulates in the eyelids; the edema tends to be worse in the morning because of the subject's recumbent posture. In congestive heart failure, the high venous pressure on the right side of the heart raises the venous pressure at the venous end of the capillaries, especially in the dependent parts. Consequently, edema tends to occur in the legs and the scrotum. This is intensified by upright posture and therefore becomes worse toward the end of the day.

6 As a result of holding on to the moving truck with his right hand, this man had sustained a severe traction injury of the eighth cervical and first thoracic roots of the brachial plexus. The various paralyzed forearm and hand muscles were characteristic of Klumpke's paralysis. In this accident, the pull of the first thoracic nerve was so severe that the white ramus communicantes to the inferior cervical sympathetic ganglion was torn. This effectively cut off the preganglionic sympathetic fibers to the right side of the man's head and neck, causing a right-sided Horner's syndrome—demonstrated by 1) constriction of the pupil, 2) drooping of the upper lid, and 3) enophthalmos. The arteriolar vasodilatation, due to loss of sympathetic vasoconstrictor fibers, was responsible for the red, hot cheek on his right side. The dryness of the skin of his right cheek was due to the loss of the sympathetic secretomotor supply to the sweat glands. The precise cause of the right-sided ptosis of the upper eyelid was a paralysis of the smooth muscle of the levator palpebrae superioris (the superior tarsal muscle or Müller's muscle). This muscle is innervated by the sympathetic part of the autonomic nervous system.

7 The conjunctival sac is lined with conjunctiva, and this is arbitrarily divided into the following parts, which are continuous with one another: 1) the palpebral conjunctiva, lining the eyelids; 2) the conjunctival fornix, formed by the reflection of the conjunctiva onto the eyeball from the eyelids (it is absent on the medial side); and 3) the bulbar conjunctiva, which is attached to the eyeball.

The sensory nerve supply for the conjunctiva is derived superiorly from the supraorbital and supratrochlear nerves from the frontal branch of the ophthalmic division of the trigeminal nerve; inferiorly from the infraorbital branch of the maxillary division of the trigeminal nerve; medially from the infratrochlear branch of the nasociliary branch of the ophthalmic division of the trigeminal nerve; and laterally from the lacrimal branch of the ophthalmic division of the trigeminal nerve. The circumcorneal region of the bulba conjunctiva is supplied by the long ciliary nerves, which are branches of the nasociliary nerve, a branch of the ophthalmic division of the trigeminal nerve.

Foreign bodies frequently move around the conjunctival sac, and if they do not reach the lacus lacrimalis, they often lodge in the subtarsal sulcus, which runs close to and parallel with the posterior edge of the upper lid margin.

The superior tarsal plate, formed of dense fibrous tissue and semilunar in shape, serves as a skeleton to the upper lid to maintain its shape. It is easily recognized through the conjunctiva of the everted upper lid.

8 The aneurysm of the internal carotid artery was pressing on the right oculomotor nerve in the lateral wall of the cavernous sinus, causing complete paralysis of the striated muscle fibers of the levator palpebrae superioris and the medial rectus muscle. In Horner's syndrome, caused by a lesion of the sympathetic part of the autonomic system, the smooth muscle component of the levator palpebrae superioris—a small part of the levator muscle—is paralyzed. This results in the eyelid's drooping only 1 to 2 mm.

The aponeurosis of the levator muscle is attached not only to the anterior surface of the superior tarsal plate but also into the skin of the upper eyelid. Paralysis of the main part of this muscle results in loss of the superior palpebral fold and of the horizontal furrow.

In addition, the lateral and medial horns of the aponeurosis are attached to the bony margin of the orbital cavity. For further details, see page 101.

9 This woman had a chalazion of her left eye. The granulomatous lesion resulted in blockage of the neck of a tarsal gland (meibomian gland), and the gradual accumulation of secretion produced the small painless swelling. Acute infection of the gland would result in suppuration, and pointing would occur on the conjunctival surface of the eyelid. An abscess should be drained by a small incision over the gland through the conjunctiva. It must be remembered that the tarsal glands are embedded on the inner surface of the tarsal plates. Blurring of vision is caused by the swelling's distortion of the eyeball, causing astigmatism.

10 This woman was suffering from myasthenia gravis, which is an autoimmune disorder resulting in a reduced responsiveness of the postsynaptic membrane of the myoneural junction to acetylcholine. The condition frequently starts with weakness of the levator palpebrae superioris, causing ptosis. The diplopia is caused by the weakness of the extraocular muscles, so that conjugate movements of the eyeball are disrupted.

11 The orbital fat is kept in position within the orbit by the attachment of the orbital septum at its periphery to the periorbita of the orbital margin. However, several sites of potential weakness exist: 1) where the aponeurosis of the levator palpebrae superioris pierces the septum to pass to its insertion on the anterior surface of the superior tarsal plate and the skin; 2) where the blood vessels and nerves leave the orbital cavity to reach the eyelids; and 3) in the inferior eyelid, where the fascia of the inferior rectus muscle pierces the septum.

12 This rather feeble old patient was suffering from atonic ectropion. The eyelids are normally kept in contact with the eyeball by the tone of the orbicularis oculi muscle. In this patient, the muscle was weak in both eyes. In addition, the normal tone of this muscle keeps the superior and inferior puncta of the canaliculi dipping into the marginal tear film and the tear fluid in the lacus lacrimalis.

The so-called lacrimal pump is the mechanism by which the lacrimal canaliculi in the upper and lower eyelids are compressed and shortened and the lacrimal sac is opened up. This has a sucking action on the tear fluid in the lacus lacrimalis. The medial fibers of the palpebral part of the orbicularis oculi pull the eyelids medially, shortening and compressing the canaliculi. In addition, the lacrimal sac is pulled open by the attachment of the lacrimal part of the orbicularis to the fascia covering the sac.

13 Blepharospasm is an idiopathic disease with chronic, often intermittent contraction of the orbicularis oculi and frontalis muscles; it occurs most commonly in middle-aged women. These women may have severe visual and functional limitations due to the constant blinking. The most common treatment is to inject the botulinum A toxin, a neuromuscular blocking agent, into the affected muscles. It is important that the injection be confined to the muscles involved, as it may diffuse deeply and paralyze the levator palpebrae superioris or the extraocular muscles, producing drooping of the eyelid (ptosis) or strabismus.

14 In this patient the right levator palpebrae superioris muscle or its aponeurosis had been traumatized, resulting in ptosis or lid drooping. Usually the muscle or its aponeurosis is bruised and will recover within a few weeks. Permanent lid drooping from this cause is the result of laceration or disinsertion of the aponeurosis from the tarsal plate and requires surgical reattachment. Patients with traumatic ptosis are usually observed for at least 3 months after injury to enable maximal recovery of the levator before resorting to surgery.

15 Ophthalmic manifestations of sarcoid include eyelid and conjunctival deposits, iris nodules, retinal vascular changes, and lacrimal gland enlargement. The downward and medial displacement of the proptotic eye globes suggested enlargement or a tumor of the lacrimal glands. CT and MRI confirmed the presence of an enlarged lacrimal gland due to sarcoid infiltration. Bulging and drooping of the lateral third of both eyelids produced the diagnostic S-shaped lid sign. The dry eyes were due to the diminished tear production by the diseased lacrimal glands.

16 Tears are produced in the accessory lacrimal glands scattered throughout the conjunctival sac and in the main lacrimal gland. The tears stream across the cornea, providing it with lubrication, and accumulate in the lacus lacrimalis. The movement of the tears is assisted by the blinking movements of the eyelids. Although much of the tears are lost by evaporation, the remainder enter the upper and lower puncta lacrimalia, the lacrimal canaliculi, and the lacrimal sac. During blinking movements of the eyelids, the canaliculi are shortened and compressed by the lacrimal part of the orbicularis oculi. In the lacrimal sac, gravity pulls the tears into the nasolacrimal duct and they descend into the nose, where they evaporate or drain posteriorly into the nasopharynx and are swallowed. Exaggerated tear production causes the tears in the nose to descend, producing a "runny nose." In crying, the tears escape across the lid margin and flow down the skin of the cheek.

17 Dacryocystorhinostomy (DCR) is used to bypass the nasolacrimal duct. The lacrimal sac is opened, part of the nasal bone is removed, the nasal mucosa is incised, and the mucosa of the lacrimal sac and nasal cavity are sewn together. This technique allows the free flow of tears from the lacrimal sac into the nasal cavity just below the middle concha.

The Eyeball

Fascial Sheath of the Eyeball (Fascia Bulbi, Tenon's Capsule) · · · · · · · · · · · ·

The fascial sheath is a thin membrane that envelops the eyeball and separates it from the orbital fat (Fig. 6-1). It thus forms a socket for the eyeball. The inner surface of the sheath is smooth and shiny and is separated from the outer surface of the sclera by a potential space called the *episcleral space*. Crossing the space and attaching the fascial sheath to the sclera are numerous delicate bands of connective tissue. Attached to the outer surface of the fascial sheath are coarse trabeculae that run through the orbital fat.

Anteriorly, the fascial sheath is firmly attached to the sclera about 1.5 mm posterior to the corneoscleral junction. Posteriorly, the sheath fuses with the meninges around the optic nerve and with the sclera around the exit of the optic nerve. Close to the optic nerve the fascial sheath of the eyeball is pierced by the ciliary nerves and vessels (Fig. 6-2) and by the vortex (vorticose) veins.

The tendons of all six extrinsic muscles of the eye pierce the fascial sheath as they pass to their insertion on the eyeball (Figs. 6-1 and 6-2). At the site of perforation the fascial sheath is reflected along the tendons of these muscles to form on each a tubular sleeve. The superior oblique muscle sleeve extends as far as the trochlea; the inferior oblique muscle sleeve extends to the origin of the muscle on the floor of the orbit.

The tubular sleeves for the four recti muscles have important expansions. Those for the medial and lateral recti are strong and are attached to the lacrimal and zygomatic bones (Fig. 6-1). Because these expansions may limit the actions of these muscles on the eyeball, they are called the *medial and lateral check ligaments* (Fig. 6-2).

Thinner and less distinct expansions extend from the superior rectus tendon to that of the levator palpebrae superioris (Fig. 6-2), and from the inferior rectus to the inferior tarsal plate. Their exact functions are not known, although the superior expansion may ensure that the two muscles work in tandem when the individual looks upward. Similarly, the inferior expansion assists in pulling down the lower eyelid and maintaining an appropriate alignment of the lid with the globe when the person looks downward.

The inferior part of the fascial sheath of the eyeball is thickened and is continuous medially and laterally with the medial and lateral check ligaments (Fig. 6-2). This hammock-like arrangement of the fascial sheath constitutes what is known as the *suspensory ligament (of Lockwood)*. This thickened area receives contributions from the fascia of the inferior rectus and the inferior oblique muscles as they cross each other below the eyeball (see pages 249 and 252).

Function

The main function of the fascial sheath of the eyeball is to position and support the eyeball within the orbital cavity and permit the actions of the extrinsic muscles to produce movement of the eyeball. Very little movement takes place between the eyeball and the sheath. Thus, the eyeball and sheath move together on a bed of orbital fat.

Figure 6-1

(A) Sagittal section of the orbit, showing the arrangement of the fascia around the eyeball and the extraocular muscles. Note the position of the suspensory ligament.
(B) Horizontal section of the right orbit, showing the fascial arrangement. Note the check ligaments. Do not confuse the lateral palpebral raphe, which lies in front of the orbital septum and is part of the orbicularis oculi muscle (not shown), with the lateral palpebral ligament, which lies behind the orbital septum.

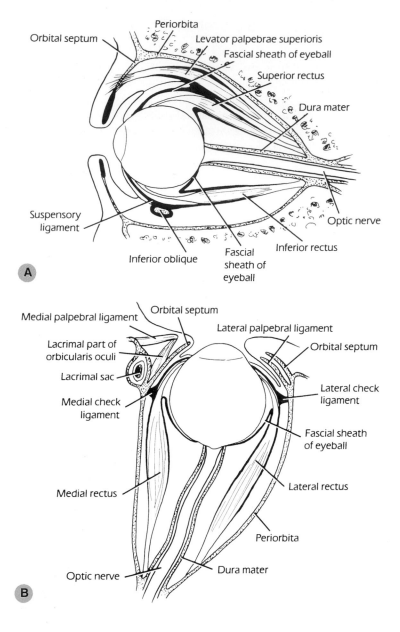

 Clinical Notes

Enucleation of the Eyeball

In situations where it is necessary to remove the eyeball, the fascial sheath of the eyeball should be preserved to serve as a socket for the prosthesis. Because the extraocular muscles have fascial sleeves that are continuous with the sheath of the eyeball, the socket will then move when the muscles contract. An external prosthesis (glass eye) resting on the conjunctiva, over the socket, will also move to some degree as the socket shifts.

Figure 6-2

(A) Fascial sheath of the eyeball after removal of the eyeball. Note how the tendons of the extrinsic muscles of the eyeball, nerves, and blood vessels pierce the sheath to reach the eyeball. (B) Coronal section of the right orbit, showing the relationship of the fascial sheath to the tendons of the extrinsic muscles —in particular, the superior rectus, the levator palpebrae superioris, the inferior rectus, and the inferior oblique. The black line representing the suspensory ligament has been excessively thickened to emphasize its presence.

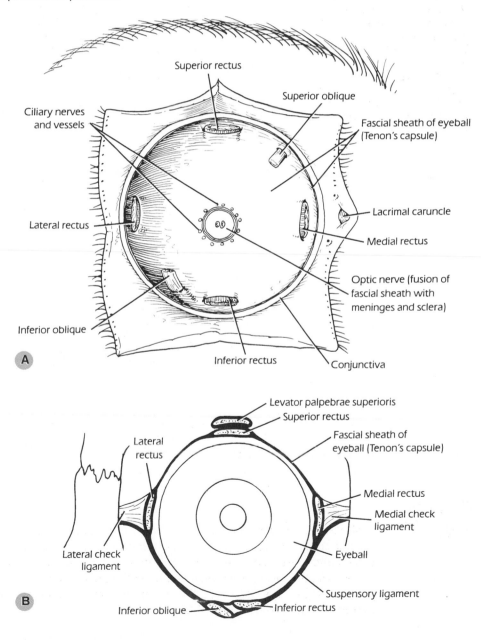

Recession and Advancement of the Inferior Oblique and Inferior Rectus Muscles

The close relationship existing between the suspensory ligament (thickening of the inferior part of the fascial sheath of the eyeball) and the tendons of the inferior oblique and inferior rectus muscles makes operations on these muscles very difficult and the results unpredictable.

Surgical Removal of the Maxilla

Extensive removal of the maxilla for the treatment of malignant disease is not accompanied by sagging of the eyeball. The reason for this is that the suspensory ligament is strong enough to provide the eyeball with adequate support from below.

Herniation of Orbital Fat

The various extensions of the fascial sheath of the eyeball through the orbital fat to the bony walls of the orbital cavity assist the orbital septum in preventing herniation of the fat into the eyelids.

The Eyeball

The eyeball is situated in the orbital cavity, a location that serves to protect it and provide a rigid bony origin for the six extrinsic muscles that produce ocular movement.

General Shape and Dimensions

The eyeball is made up of the segments of two spheres of different sizes placed one in front of the other (Figs. 6-3 and 6-4). The anterior, smaller segment is transparent and forms about one-sixth of the eyeball; it has a radius of curvature of about 8 mm. The posterior, larger segment is opaque and forms about five-sixths of the eyeball; it has a radius of about 12 mm.

The *anterior pole* of the eye is the center of curvature of the transparent segment, or *cornea*. The *posterior pole* is the center of the posterior curvature of the eyeball, and it is located slightly temporal to the optic nerve. The *geometric* or *optic axis* is a line connecting the two poles. The *equator* lies midway between the two poles (Fig. 6-4).

The *visual axis* is a line connecting the fovea centralis of the retina with the nodal point of the eye and continuing anteriorly through the cornea. Remember that, because the fovea centralis is temporal and slightly inferior to the posterior pole, the visual axis and the optic axis do not coincide (Fig. 6-3).

The anteroposterior diameter of the eye measures about 24 mm. Since the eyeball is slightly flattened in a vertical plane, the vertical diameter is about 23 mm; the horizontal diameter, about 23.5 mm.

The longer the anteroposterior diameter of the eye, the more myopic the eye is (i.e., light rays tend to be focused in front of the retina); conversely, the shorter the anteroposterior diameter of the eye, the more likely it is that the eye will be hyperopic (i.e., the light rays will be focused behind the plane of the retina). The actual focus is a result of a complex interplay involving the refracting power of

● **Figure 6-3**

Horizontal section through the eyeball at the level of the optic nerve. The optic axis and the axis of the eyeball are included.

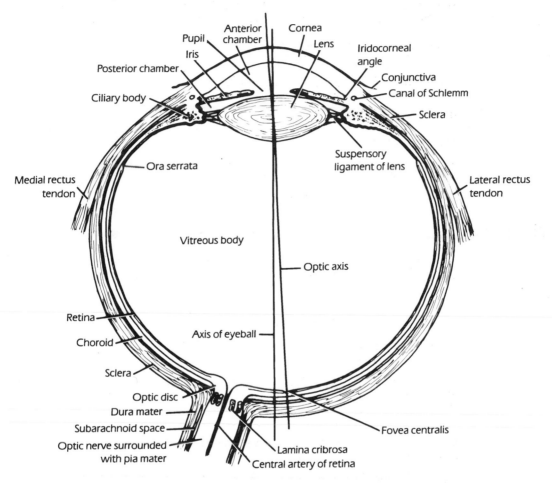

the cornea, which is dependent on its anterior curvature; the refracting power of the lens; and the length of the eyeball.

Position

The eyeball is situated in the anterior part of the orbital cavity, closer to the roof than the floor, and nearer the lateral than the medial wall. The orbital margins have a fairly constant relationship to the eyeball. Vertically, a straight edge applied to the superior and inferior orbital margins passes in contact with the cornea or slightly anterior to it. A horizontal straight edge applied to the lateral and medial margins reveals that about one-third of the eyeball lies anterior to it. Because the lateral orbital margin is the least prominent, it is consequently the lateral surface of the eyeball that is most exposed.

Figure 6-4

(A) Diagram of the eyeball, showing the poles and the equatorial and meridional planes. (B) Diagram of the front of the eyeball showing the distances between the insertions of the recti tendons and the corneoscleral junction or limbus. The seven anterior ciliary arteries are also shown. Note that there is only one anterior ciliary artery associated with the lateral rectus muscle.

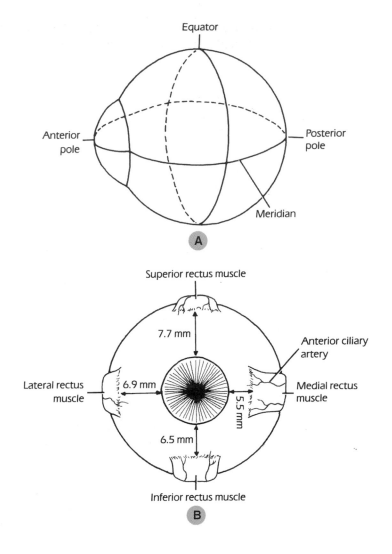

Exposure of the Eyeball to Trauma

Clinical Notes

Although the eyeball is reasonably well protected by the surrounding bony orbit, it is protected anteriorly only from large objects, such as tennis balls, which tend to strike the orbital margin but not the globe. The bony orbit provides no protection from small objects, such as golf balls, which may cause severe damage to the eye. Careful examination of the eyeball relative to the orbital margins shows that it is least protected from the lateral side. Rupture of the eyeball most commonly occurs from a blow directed from below and laterally.

Displacement of the Eyeball

A space-occupying mass within the cone formed by the extraocular muscles quickly causes forward displacement of the eyeball. An expanding mass outside the muscle cone has to be very large before displacement of the eyeball will occur. Moreover, the proptosis is usually asymmetric.

Layers of the Eyeball

The eyeball consists of three layers (Fig. 6-3), which from without inward are 1) the fibrous layer, 2) the vascular pigmented layer, and 3) the nervous layer.

Fibrous Layer

The fibrous layer is made up of a posterior, opaque part, the sclera, and an anterior, transparent part, the cornea (Fig. 6-3).

Sclera

The sclera forms the posterior five-sixths of the eyeball and is opaque (Fig. 6-3). In the adult the sclera is white (see also Fig. 8-23). In children, when the sclera is thin, the pigment cells of the choroid show through, giving the sclera a bluish tinge. In the elderly the sclera may have a yellowish tinge from the deposition of fat.

In the adult the sclera is about 1 mm thick posteriorly, thinning at the equator to 0.6 mm. It is thinnest, 0.3 mm, immediately posterior to the tendinous insertions of the recti muscles. At the corneoscleral junction the sclera is 0.8 mm thick. Anteriorly, the sclera forms the "white" of the eye and is covered with the fascial sheath of the eyeball and the conjunctiva. Posteriorly, the sclera is connected by delicate connective tissue to the fascial sheath of the eyeball. The outer surface of the sclera is smooth except where the tendons of the orbital muscles are attached to it (Fig. 6-4). The medial rectus inserts 5.5 mm posterior to the limbus; the inferior rectus, 6.5 mm; the lateral rectus, 6.9 mm; and the superior rectus, 7.7 mm. The insertions of the superior oblique and inferior oblique muscles are posterior to the scleral equator (see p. 251).

The sclera is perforated posteriorly about 3 mm medial and 1 mm above the posterior pole of the eyeball by the optic nerve. The site of this perforation is sometimes referred to as the *posterior scleral foramen*. Here the sclera is fused with the dural and arachnoid sheaths of the optic nerve. Where the optic nerve fibers pierce the sclera it is weakened and has a sieve-like appearance and is known as the *lamina cribrosa* (Fig. 6-3). One of the openings in the lamina is larger than the rest and transmits the central retinal artery and vein. Since the lamina cribrosa is a relatively weak area, it can be made to bulge outward by a rise in intraocular pressure, producing a cupped disc.

The sclera is also pierced by three groups of small apertures—anterior, middle, and posterior.

The anterior apertures are located at the insertion of the recti muscles and are for branches of the *anterior ciliary arteries* (Fig. 6-4). Each rectus muscle has two anterior ciliary arteries, with the exception of the lateral rectus muscle, which only has one.

The middle apertures are situated about 4 mm posterior to the equator of the eye and number about four or five. These are for the exit of the vortex veins (Fig. 6-16).

The posterior apertures are small and numerous and are located around the optic nerve. They transmit the *long and the short ciliary nerves and vessels* (Fig. 6-16).

Anteriorly, the sclera is directly continuous with the cornea, the line of union being known as the *corneoscleral junction* (or sclerocorneal junction or limbus). Just posterior to this junction, and lying within the sclera, is a circularly running canal called the *sinus venosus sclerae* (*the canal of Schlemm*). On section, this canal appears oval in shape and is lined with endothelium (Figs. 6-3 and 6-12). The outer wall of the canal forms a groove in the sclera. Posterior to the canal is a projecting ridge of scleral tissue known as the *scleral spur* (Fig. 6-12). The scleral spur is triangular on section, with its apex pointing anteriorly and inward; it gives attachment to the ciliary muscle.

Structure   The sclera may be divided, for purposes of description, into three layers: 1) the episclera, 2) the scleral stroma, and 3) the lamina fusca.

Episclera   The episclera is the outermost layer and consists of loose connective tissue. It is connected to the fascial sheath of the eyeball (Tenon's capsule) by fine strands of tissue. It merges with the underlying scleral stroma. Anteriorly, the episclera has a rich blood supply from the anterior ciliary arteries, which form a plexus that extends between the extrinsic muscle insertions and the corneo-scleral junction. These vessels lie deep to the conjunctiva and normally are inconspicuous. However, in the presence of inflammation they become very red and congested (see p. 113). The episclera becomes progressively thinner toward the back of the eye.

Scleral Stroma   This consists of dense fibrous tissue intermingled with fine elastic fibers (Fig. 6-5). The individual collagen fibrils (type I and type III) vary in diameter from 28 to 280 µm, with periodicities of 80 and 21 µm. The bundles of fibrils run in whorls, loops, and arches, and, although they are approximately parallel with the surface, many pass from layer to layer seemingly at random, forming a feltlike matting of the bundles (Fig. 6-6). The irregular arrangement of the collagen fibrils is largely responsible for the opacity of the sclera, in contrast to the transparency of the cornea where the fibrils run parallel with the surface.

A few flat elongated fibroblasts are found between the collagen bundles (Fig. 6-5), together with an occasional melanocyte.

A viscoelastic structure, the sclera responds to a deforming force in a biphasic manner—a brief lengthening (elastic response) followed by a slow stretching (viscid response).

Lamina Fusca   This is the innermost layer of the sclera (Fig. 6-5). It is faintly brown, because of the presence of melanocytes, which form a thin, irregular layer. The lamina has many grooves, caused by the passage of the ciliary vessels and nerves. It is separated from the external surface of the choroid by a potential space—the *perichoroidal space*. Connecting the lamina fusca with the choroid are fine collagen fibers that provide a weak attachment between the sclera and the choroid.

Figure 6-5

Photomicrograph of a section of sclera, showing the stroma and the lamina fusca. Note the presence of elongated fibroblasts between the collagen bundles in the stroma. Note also the melanocytes in the lamina fusca. A small area of choroid packed with pigment cells is seen below. (Plastic section; H&E; × 400.)

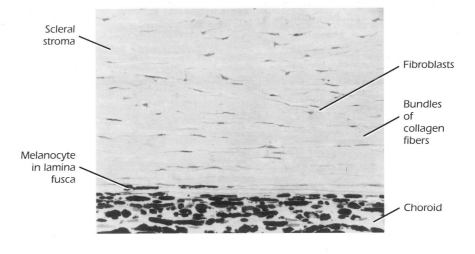

Scleral stroma

Fibroblasts

Bundles of collagen fibers

Melanocyte in lamina fusca

Choroid

Blood Supply The sclera is a relatively avascular structure. However, anterior to the insertions of the recti muscles, the *anterior ciliary arteries* form a dense *episcleral plexus*. The posterior part of the sclera receives small branches from the *long and short posterior ciliary arteries* (Fig. 6-16).

Nerve Supply The sclera is supplied by the *ciliary nerves*, which pierce the sclera around the optic nerve. The many short ciliary nerves supply the posterior portion, while the two long ciliary nerves supply the anterior region.

Functions The tough, fibrous structure of the sclera protects the intraocular contents from trauma and mechanical displacement. The firmness and strength of the sclera, together with the intraocular pressure, preserve the shape of the eyeball and maintain the exact position of the different parts of the optic system. The strength and firmness of the sclera provide a rigid insertion for the extraocular muscles.

 Clinical Notes

Changes in Scleral Color with Age and in Disease The anterior portion of the sclera is visible clinically beneath the transparent conjunctiva, as the white of the eye. In the adult the sclera has a dull white color. In children, when the sclera is thin, the pigment cells of the underlying choroid show through, giving the sclera a bluish tinge. In the elderly, the sclera may have a yellowish color due to fatty deposits.

Figure 6-6

Photomicrograph of a section of sclera, showing bundles of collagen fibers and nucleated fibroblasts. Note that many of the collagen bundles run parallel with the surface, but considerable numbers are randomly arranged to form a feltlike structure. (H&E; × 400.)

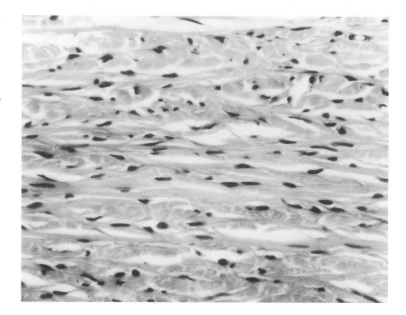

In patients with osteogenesis imperfecta, Ehlers-Danlos syndrome, and other collagen diseases that produce a defect in collagen synthesis, the sclera is abnormally thin and is blue. The blue color, as explained above, is caused by the underlying choroidal pigment cells showing through the thin sclera.

It might be noted that the yellow appearance of the eyeball in jaundice is due not to pigment in the sclera but to bilirubin in the vascular conjunctiva.

Thickness of the Sclera as a Factor in Cupped Disc, Tendon Recessions and Advancements, and Trauma   Sclera thickness varies considerably in different parts of the eyeball, the sclera being thinnest just behind the insertions of the recti muscles. In glaucoma, the raised intraocular pressure causes the lamina cribrosa to bulge outward. This is responsible for the development of the cupped disc in the chronic form of glaucoma.

In strabismus, which is commonly treated with tendon recessions or advancements, it is important to remember that the sclera is very thin (about 0.3 mm or less) where the tendons are sutured to the sclera.

A blow to the eyeball may rupture the sclera, usually at the sites of muscle insertion. Almost always this is associated with damage to the underlying choroid and retina.

Perforations of the Sclera and the Spread of Neoplasms   Wherever blood vessels and nerves pierce the sclera, the passage provides a pathway for the spread of intraocular tumors, such as melanomas, from inside the eyeball to the exterior. The most common site of extraocular extension of a tumor is along the optic nerve.

Blood Supply of the Sclera, the Development of the Ciliary Flush, and the Healing of Surgical Incisions While the blood supply to the scleral stroma is poor, the episclera has a rich arterial supply. This is particularly important from the clinical point of view, in that an episcleral plexus—formed by branches of the anterior ciliary arteries—exists beneath the conjunctiva. Normally, this plexus is inconspicuous, but in the presence of inflammation involving the cornea, iris, and ciliary body, marked vasodilatation may occur, especially in the limbal area surrounding the cornea. This pronounced vasodilatation is known as a *ciliary flush*.

The rich blood supply to the episclera results in rapid healing of surgical incisions.

Nerve Supply of the Sclera and Eye Pain The sclera receives a profuse sensory innervation. It follows, therefore, that inflammations of the sclera will cause a dull, aching pain. Since the extraocular muscles are inserted into the sclera, the pain is made worse by ocular movement.

Cornea The transparent cornea forms the anterior one-sixth of the eyeball (Fig. 6-3 and Fig. 8-23). Because its curvature is greater than over the rest of the eyeball, a slight sulcus, the *sulcus sclerae*, marks the junction of the cornea with the sclera. Seen from the front, the cornea is convex but somewhat elliptical in shape. Although the dimensions of the cornea vary considerably from one person to another, the approximate measurements are about 10.6 mm vertically but about 11.7 mm horizontally. Posteriorly, the cornea is concave and circular, measuring about 11.7 mm in diameter. The cornea is thinnest at its center, measuring about 0.5 to 0.6 mm, and thicker at the periphery, measuring about 0.7 mm.

The radius of curvature of the anterior surface of the cornea is about 7.7 mm; that of the posterior surface, 6.9 mm. However, it should be pointed out that it is frequently more curved in the vertical than in the horizontal planes (regular astigmatism).

The cornea is the main structure responsible for the refraction of light entering the eye. It separates the air, with a refractive index of 1.00, from the aqueous humor, with a refractive index of 1.33. (For further measurements, see Table 6-1.)

Structure Microscopically, the cornea consists of five layers (Fig. 6-7). From front to back, they are 1) the epithelium, 2) Bowman's layer (membrane), 3) the substantia propria, 4) Descemet's membrane, and 5) the endothelium.

Epithelium The corneal epithelium is stratified and consists of five layers of cells (Fig. 6-8). Its total thickness measures about 50 to 60 μm. The superficial cells are flattened, nucleated, nonkeratinized squamous cells, and the deepest cells are columnar. At the corneoscleral junction (limbus), the epithelium becomes thicker and may consist of 10 or more layers of cells. Here, the epithelium becomes continuous with the bulbar conjunctiva. The corneal epithelium is devoid of melanocytes except at the limbus in dark races. The greater part of the epithelium is also devoid of the immunocompetent dendritic cells, *Langerhans' cells*; however, these cells are present in the peripheral corneal epithelium.

Table 6-1   Important Measurements of the Human Cornea Used in Refractive Surgery

Thickness (µm)		Radius of curvature (mm)	
Peripheral	700	Anterior	7.7
Central	540	Posterior	6.9
Refractive index		Central radius of curvature and refractive power	
Air	1.00	Air-tear	7.7 mm = +43.6 D
Tear	1.336	Tear-cornea	7.7 mm = +5.3 D
Cornea	1.376	Cornea-aqueous	6.9 mm = −5.8 D
Aqueous	1.336	Total central refractive power = 43.1 D	

Data from Holladay JT, Waring GO III. Optics and topography of radial keratotomy. In: Waring GO III, ed. *Refractive keratotomy for myopia and astigmatism.* St. Louis: Mosby, 1992:37–144.

    Figure 6-7

Diagram showing structure of the cornea.

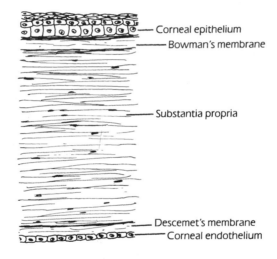

The superficial cell layer is two to three cells thick (Fig. 6-8). They are flat, have horizontal nuclei, and are attached to one another by desmosomes. Electron microscopic examination of the outer surfaces of the superficial cells (Fig. 6-9) shows microvilli and microplicae (ridges) that extend into the superficial tear film. Some of the cells appear to be lighter and have many microvilli, while other darker cells have fewer microvilli and are centrally located. It is believed that the microvilli and microplicae of these surface cells assist in retaining the tear film and thus in keeping the cells moist. As the superficial cells age, they lose their attachments to one another and are lost in the tear film.

The middle-zone cells are polyhedral in shape, with convex anterior surfaces and concave posterior surfaces (sometimes called wing cells). The nuclei are oval or round. Multiple desmosomes attach the cells to their neighbors. The lateral borders of the cells show many interdigitations, and the presence of numerous gap junctions permits free intercellular communication in this zone.

Figure 6-8

(A) Photomicrograph of a section of the cornea, showing the corneal epithelium; the clear Bowman's membrane or layer; the substantia propria; the narrow, clear Descemet's membrane; and the corneal endothelium. (H&E; × 260.)
(B) Photomicrograph of a high-power view of the corneal epithelium. The epithelium is stratified, the deepest cells are columnar, and the superficial cells are squamous and nonkeratinized. Note the clear zone, beneath the epithelium, containing Bowman's membrane or layer. (H&E; × 400.)

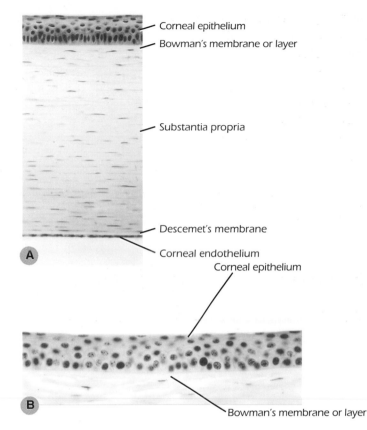

Corneal epithelium
Bowman's membrane or layer
Substantia propria
Descemet's membrane
Corneal endothelium
Corneal epithelium
Bowman's membrane or layer

The deepest basal cells are tall columnar cells that form a single layer resting on a basement membrane (Fig. 6-8). The lateral borders interdigitate with one another and are attached by desmosomes and gap junctions. Hemidesmosomes attach the basal plasma membrane to the basement membrane. The hemidesmosomes are also tethered to the stroma by *anchoring fibrils* that pass through the basement membrane and Bowman's layer. The anchoring fibrils are composed of type VII collagen, and after multiple branching in the stroma end in a complex mesh of type VI collagen fibrilis, known as *anchoring plaques*.

The basement membrane is prominent and stains positive with periodic acid–Schiff (PAS). It is strongly attached to the underlying Bowman's layer.

Running between the epithelial cells are the naked nerve endings of sensory nerve fibers, which are sensitive mainly to pain.

It has been estimated that a complete turnover of corneal surface epithelial cells takes place every 7 days. New cells are formed by mitotic division in the limbal basal cell layer. Centripetal ameboid movement of the cells occurs from the periphery of the cornea to the center. At the limbus the epithelium is thrown into radial folds (*palisades of Vogt*) that provide an increased surface area of basal cells, which is ideal for the production of new cells.

Figure 6-9

Scanning electron micrographs of the cornea. (A) Cut edge of the cornea, showing
corneal surface epithelium, Bowman's membrane or layer, and bundles of collagen
fibers in stroma. (× 455.) (B) Surface of corneal epithelial cells, showing many
microvilli. (× 2340.) (Courtesy of Fred Lightfoot.)

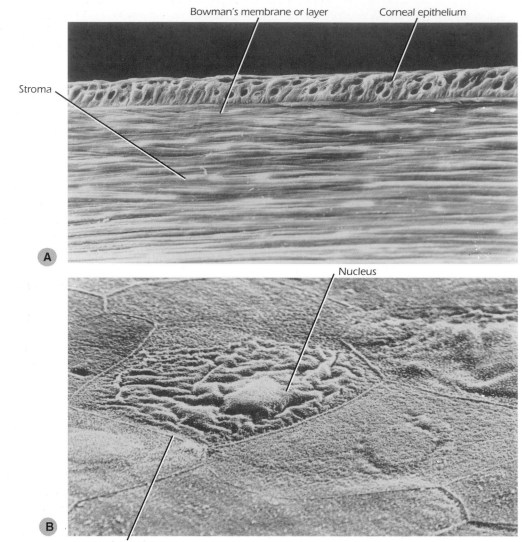

Bowman's Layer Bowman's layer lies immediately beneath the basement membrane of the corneal epithelium (Figs. 6-7 and 6-8). It measures about 8 to 12 μm in thickness. It is acellular and consists of interwoven collage fibrils embedded in intercellular substances. Electron microscopy reveals its collagen to be finer and more randomly arranged than that in the substantia propria. Bowman's membrane ends abruptly at the limbus. Its deep surface merges into the substantia propria.

Substantia Propria or Stroma This forms about 90 percent of the corneal thickness (Figs. 6-7 and 6-8). Transparent, fibrous, and compact, it consists of many lamellae of collagen fibrils that run parallel with the surface (Fig. 6-9). The parallel collagen fibrils are mainly of type I collagen, with smaller amounts of types III, V, and VI. It is estimated that there are about 200 to 250 flattened lamellae, each of which is about 2 μm thick. The direction of the collagen fibrils in any given lamella is the same, but they run at right angles to those of adjacent lamellae. The lamellae are bound together by fibrils that pass from one lamella to another.

The collagen fibrils, which tend to be larger in the posterior part of the cornea, measure between 21 and 65 nm in diameter. The collagen fibrils are embedded in glycosaminoglycans. Lying between adjacent lamellae are flattened fibroblasts with many processes. Occasional macrophages, lymphocytes, and polymorphonuclear leukocytes are also seen.

Descemet's Membrane This lies on the posterior surface of the substantia propria and is the basement membrane of the endothelium. The membrane is strong and homogeneous and measures 10 μm in thickness. It is sharply defined from the substantia propria and is thicker than the endothelium (Figs. 6-7 and 6-8). When incised, it tends to curl up in the anterior chamber and easily separates from the substantia propria and the endothelium.

Descemet's membrane is composed of fine type IV collagen fibrils arranged in a hexagonal pattern and embedded in matrix. It is PAS-positive. At the periphery of the cornea, there are small protrusions of the membrane into the anterior chamber, occurring with increasing frequency with age. These minute protrusions covered with endothelium, are called *Hassall-Henle bodies*. At the corneal margin the membrane terminates abruptly and becomes continuous with the trabecular tissue on the inner wall of the sinus venosus sclerae (see p. 151). The anterior border ring of the trabecular network is known as the *line of Schwalbe*.

Endothelium The *corneal endothelium* consists of a single layer of flattened cells (Figs. 6-7 and 6-8) that are polygonal in shape and whose plasma membranes interdigitate with one another. The cell cytoplasm contains numerous mitochondria, a prominent endoplasmic reticulum, and a Golgi apparatus, indicating that the endothelium plays an active role in the synthesis and transport of fluid. The cells cover the posterior surface of Descemet's membrane and are continuous with the endothelial cells that line the spaces of the iridocorneal angle and the anterior surface of the iris. The cells are connected by tight junctions and their free surfaces show a few microvilli. These cells play a major role in controlling the normal hydration of the cornea, both by a barrier function, limiting access of water from the aqueous humor to the corneal stroma, and by an active transport mechanism.

Blood Supply and Lymphatic Drainage The cornea is avascular and devoid of lymphatic drainage. The capillary blood vessels derived from the anterior ciliary arteries of the conjunctiva and sclera end at the circumference of the cornea. The cornea is nourished by diffusion from the aqueous humor and from the capillaries at its edge. The central part of the cornea receives oxygen indirectly from the air via oxygen dissolved in the tear film, whereas the peripheral part receives oxygen by diffusion from the anterior ciliary blood vessels.

Nerve Supply   These nerve fibers are derived from the ophthalmic division of the trigeminal nerve, mainly through the long ciliary nerves. The long ciliary nerves enter the sclera from the perichoroidal space a short distance posterior to the limbus. Here they divide up to form the *annular plexus*. Branches then pass forward in a radial pattern to enter the substantia propria of the cornea. Further division occurs, and the fibers lose their myelin sheaths. They then unite to form a *subepithelial plexus*. Fine terminal branches now pierce Bowman's membrane and pass between the epithelial cells to form the *intraepithelial plexus*. There are no specialized nerve endings. The axons are naked and devoid of a Schwann cell sheath.

Function   The cornea is the most important refractive medium in the eye. This refractive power occurs on the anterior surface of the cornea, where the refractive index of the cornea (1.38) is greatly different from that of the air. The importance of the tear film in maintaining the normal environment for the corneal epithelial cells has already been stressed (see p. 119). The transparency of the cornea results from the uniform spacing of the collagen fibrils in the substantia propria. Any increase in tissue fluid between the fibrils causes cloudiness of the cornea. The endothelial cells play a major role in limiting fluid uptake by the corneal stroma. As mentioned previously, this probably occurs as the result of both its barrier function and its active transport function.

Clinical Notes

Distortions of the Shape of the Cornea and Astigmatism   The shape of the cornea is often not a section of a perfect sphere. Commonly, it is more curved in a vertical than in a horizontal plane. This condition, in which the refracting power is not the same in all directions, is called *astigmatism*. It results in parallel rays of light not focusing at a point. The effects of astigmatism can be neutralized with the assistance of cylindrical lenses.

Central Corneal Shape and Refractive Power   The use of contact lenses and the performance of modern corneal refractive surgery has made it imperative that surgeons have a knowledge of the normal corneal shape and power. Some of the more important measurements are summarized in Table 6-1.

Surgical Anatomic Zones of the Cornea   For practical purposes the surface of the cornea can be divided into two general regions: the central optical zone and the remainder of the cornea. The central optical zone is the refractive region responsible for forming the image on the foveal part of the retina. It measures approximately 3 to 4 mm in diameter and overlies the pupil of the eye. The remainder of the cornea serves only as a mechanical support. However, this area is of optical importance in peripheral vision and when the pupil is widely dilated; it is also of vital importance for epithelial cell replacement.

Surgically four concentric anatomic zones are now recognized and are useful when performing keratotomies and excimer laser keratomileusis (photorefractive keratectomy). The diameters of these zones are summarized in Table 6-2.

Refractive Surgery　　Recently, refractive surgery has become widely used. In these procedures the corneal curvature is altered to change the focusing of the light rays on the retina. For the correction of myopia, an attempt is made to flatten the central corneal surface.

In *radial keratotomy*, a series of radial incisions are made in the peripheral part of the cornea, resulting in a flattening of the central corneal curvature. This flattening is accomplished by the induction of gaping wounds in the corneal stroma, which then gradually repairs itself.

Another example of refractive surgery is *photorefractive keratectomy*. In this procedure an excimer laser beam is used to ablate a thin area of the anterior corneal surface, thereby changing its curvature. Epithelial cells then repopulate the area overlying the damaged stroma.

More recently, a newer form of refractive surgery called *laser in situ keratomileusis (LASIK)* has been introduced. This involves the careful cutting and raising of a thin flap of corneal tissue about 160 μm in depth. The exposed stroma is then ablated by a laser beam to change the curvature of the cornea. The corneal flap is then replaced.

Aging Changes in the Cornea　　With advancing years, the cornea becomes less translucent and dustlike opacities, due to condensation in the stroma, may occur in the deeper parts of the stroma. Bowman's and Descemet's membranes also increase in thickness.

Arcus senilis appears as white arcs superiorly and inferiorly, separated from the limbus by a clear interval of nearly 1 mm. Ultimately, the arcs form a complete circle. The condition is due to an infiltration of extracellular lipid and is present in almost every person over 60 years old.

The appearance of small protrusions at the periphery of Descemet's membrane that occur in the aged has already been noted. They are known as *Hassall-Henle bodies* and usually do not interfere with vision.

Table 6-2　Summary of the Anatomic Zones of the Cornea with Their Approximate Diameters

Corneal Zone	Approximate Diameter (mm)	Characteristics
Central optical	3–4	Most spherical, symmetric; overlies pupil
Paracentral (mid)	4–7	Generally spherical but flatter than central zone
Peripheral	7–11	Cornea flattens the most here
Limbal	11–12	Abuts the scleral sulcus and the sclera

Data from Holladay JT, Waring GO III. Optics and topography of radial keratotomy. In: Waring GO III, ed. *Refractive keratotomy for myopia and astigmatism.* St. Louis: Mosby, 1992:37–144.

Effect of Trauma on the Cornea   Because a portion of the cornea is exposed between the eyelids, injuries from foreign bodies or abrasions are very common. Damage to the corneal epithelium causes considerable pain. The cornea is extremely sensitive and receives a profuse nerve supply from the long and short ciliary nerves, which are branches of the ophthalmic division of the trigeminal nerve. The naked axons are sensitive to pain and to cold.

The stratified squamous epithelium covering the anterior surface of the cornea is capable of rapid regeneration after an abrasion. Bowman's layer, which is in fact the superficial layer of the stroma, serves as a barrier to the underlying stroma. When damaged it is not reformed but is replaced by fibrous tissue. When damaged the stroma is also replaced by fibrous tissue. Descemet's membrane is the basement membrane of the endothelial cells. When injured, it can be regenerated by these cells. It is a strong membrane and resistant to trauma. It is somewhat elastic, and when torn it curls up in the anterior chamber. The cells of the endothelium are closely bound to one another and can be stripped off as a sheet.

Regeneration of Corneal Epithelial Cells   Following superficial corneal damage, the corneal epithelial cells are replaced by the centripetal movement of new cells from the periphery of the cornea to the center. The radial folds of epithelium at the limbus (*palisades of Vogt*) are ideally suited for the production of new cells.

Edema of the Cornea   The corneal epithelium and the corneal endothelium maintain the normal tissue fluid content of the corneal stroma. The junctional complexes of the epithelial cells prevent passage of tear fluid into the cornea or loss of tissue fluid into the tear fluid. The endothelium limits the uptake of aqueous humor by way of both its barrier function and its active transport mechanism. Trauma to either of these layers will result in edema of the stroma. Death of the surface cells causes edema, but the density of Bowman's layer tends to inhibit spread into the deeper stroma. Acute glaucoma can produce corneal edema by opening up the gaps between the endothelial cells. Because of the high intraocular pressure (above 60 mm Hg), the aqueous fluid is pushed through the corneal stroma, where it accumulates beneath and among the epithelial cells.

Vascularization of the Cornea Associated with Inflammations and Infections
Normally, the cornea is an avascular structure. The cornea is nourished by diffusion from the aqueous humor and from the capillaries at its edge. The central part of the cornea receives its oxygen indirectly from the atmosphere via oxygen dissolved in the tears.

Corneal inflammations and infections can result in invasion of the cornea at its circumference by new blood vessels. These bring cellular and humoral defense mechanisms closer to the site of infection. Unfortunately, the transparency is thus compromised, and if the condition persists an opacity may develop. Then new blood vessels arise from the superficial vascular plexus of the conjunctiva and the deep plexus from the anterior ciliary arteries. Normally, capillary loops from these plexuses end at the limbus. The new blood vessels may enter the cornea around the entire circumference or be confined to a segment. Later, when the cause of the new vascularization has abated, the blood vessels can atrophy and become empty, resembling ghost vessels.

Corneal Transplants   It has long been known that the cornea is an immunologically privileged site for grafting. This has been attributed to the avascularity of the cornea and the absence of the dendritic, antigen-presenting Langerhans' cells in the corneal epithelium. These cells are, however, present in the peripheral cornea.

The Limbus   The limbus (corneoscleral junction, or sclerocorneal junction) is an important landmark for the ophthalmologist (Fig. 6-10). It is an area measuring about 1.5 to 2.0 mm wide, and there is a shallow groove on its outer surface, known as the *external scleral sulcus.* On the inner surface a similar groove, called the *internal scleral sulcus,* contains the trabecular meshwork and the sinus venosus sclerae (canal of Schlemm). The posterior lip of the internal sulcus forms a projecting ridge of scleral tissue known as the *scleral spur* (Figs. 6-10, 6-11, and

 Figure 6-10

Diagram of structures seen in the anterior portion of the eyeball in the region of the corneoscleral limbus.

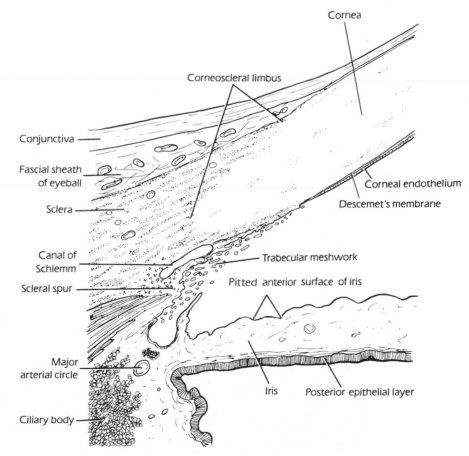

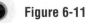

Figure 6-11

Diagram of structures present in the corneoiridial angle of the anterior chamber.

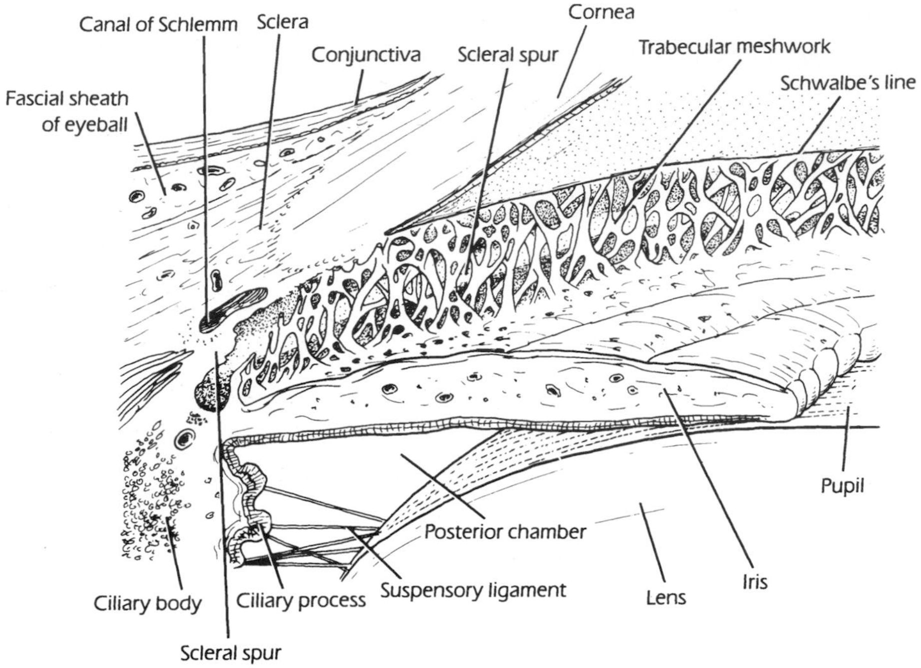

Canal of Schlemm   Sclera
Conjunctiva   Scleral spur
Cornea
Trabecular meshwork
Schwalbe's line
Fascial sheath of eyeball
Pupil
Ciliary body   Ciliary process   Suspensory ligament   Posterior chamber   Lens   Iris
Scleral spur

6-12). The scleral spur is triangular, with its apex pointing anteriorly and inward. Attached to the anterior surface of the spur is the trabecular meshwork. The posterior surface of the spur gives attachment to the ciliary muscle.

At the limbus each layer of the cornea can be traced laterally (Fig. 6-10). The corneal epithelium becomes the epithelium of the bulbar conjunctiva. Here, the epithelial cells are thrown into folds by the subepithelial connective tissue, which resembles the dermal papillae. When observed from the surface, the crests of the epithelial folds run radially into the cornea; these are known as the *palisades of Vogt*. The folds greatly increase the surface area of the basal cells, which is important for regeneration purposes (see p. 150). The connective tissue within the folds contains blood vessels and lymphatics. Bowman's layer becomes continuous with the lamina propria of the conjunctiva and the fascial sheath of the eyeball (Tenon's capsule). The substantia propria of the cornea gradually loses its uniform and orderly arrangement and becomes the sclera. Descemet's membrane ends abruptly at Schwalbe's line, and just posterior to this the trabecular meshwork begins (Fig. 6-11). This is composed of branching sheets of fenestrated connective tissue, which together form a spongelike system of passages (Fig. 6-12) that communicate with the anterior chamber.

At the limbus, the corneal endothelium is continuous laterally with the endothelium that lines the passages of the trabecular meshwork described above, and then continues to the anterior surface of the iris.

Figure 6-12

Diagram of the structures present in the corneoiridial angle of the anterior chamber, showing Schwalbe's line, the scleral spur, the trabecular meshwork, and the canal of Schlemm.

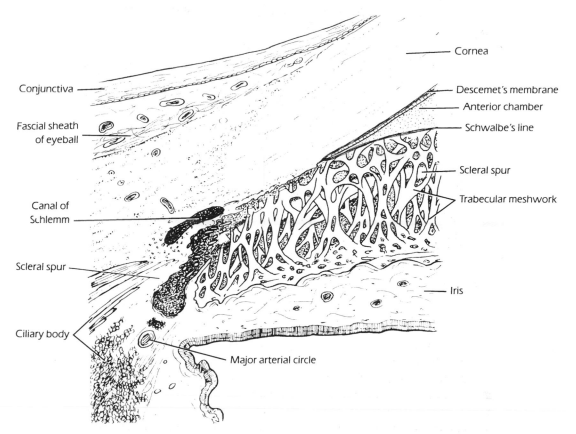

Sinus Venosus Sclerae (Canal of Schlemm) The sinus venosus sclerae is a canal lined with endothelium that runs circularly around the eyeball at the corneoscleral junction (Figs. 6-12 and 6-13). In places the canal breaks up into branches that coalesce again (Fig. 6-14). The sinus, which is oval or triangular in cross-section, lies within the internal scleral sulcus (Figs. 6-12 and 6-13). It is therefore related posteriorly to the scleral spur. The inner wall of the sinus is related to the trabecular meshwork and to the anterior chamber. There is no direct communication between the venous sinus and the passages of the trabecular meshwork or the cavity of the anterior chamber. In fact, the lumen of the venous sinus is separated from the lumen of the passages by the sinus endothelium, the connective tissue wall of the sinus, and the endothelial lining of the passages. Electron microscopic examination of the endothelial cells lining the wall of the sinus venosus sclerae shows the presence of giant vacuoles in the cytoplasm. These are now believed to play a role in the outflow of aqueous

Figure 6-13

Photomicrograph of a section through the region of the corneoscleral junction, showing the anterior chamber, the trabecular meshwork, and the canal of Schlemm. (H&E; × 400.)

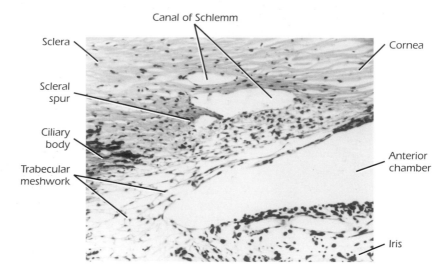

humor from the anterior chamber. Serial sections have shown that the vacuoles can expand and fuse with the apical and basal plasma membranes of the cells to form a transcellular channel. This would explain how the aqueous humor leaves the lumen of the trabecular passages to enter the lumen of the sinus venosus.

The scleral sinus is drained by 25 to 35 *collector channels*, which join the deep scleral venous plexus (Fig. 6-14). The deep scleral plexus drains via an intrascleral plexus and an episcleral plexus into the anterior ciliary veins. A few of the collector channels bypass the deep scleral venous plexus and pass directly through the sclera. These channels are known as the *aqueous veins*, because they contain clear aqueous humor and not blood. The aqueous veins drain into the conjunctival veins close to the corneoscleral junction. These very small aqueous veins can be seen in the living subject when the eye is examined with a slit lamp.

Function   Ninety percent of the outflow of aqueous humor from the anterior chamber occurs through the passageways of the trabecular meshwork, the sinus venosus sclerae, the collector channels, and the aqueous veins. The principal resistance to the flow of the aqueous through the eye is the trabecular meshwork. The pores of the meshwork become progressively smaller as the sinus venosus sclerae is approached. In most people, the trabecular meshwork offers a precisely controlled resistance to outflow, and the cells lining the passageways can, by changing their shape in response to chemicals, hormones, and neurotransmitters, regulate the flow through the meshwork within a narrow range. The flattened cells lining the passages are also capable of phagocytosing any debris in

Figure 6-14

(A) Diagram of the anterior chamber of the eye, with the greater part of the cornea removed to reveal Schwalbe's line and the extent of the trabecular meshwork. The canal of Schlemm is also shown. (B) Diagram showing the canal of Schlemm and its relationship with the veins and arteries in that region. Note that the canal is drained by the collector channels that join the deep scleral venous plexus or bypass the plexus to drain into the conjunctival veins.

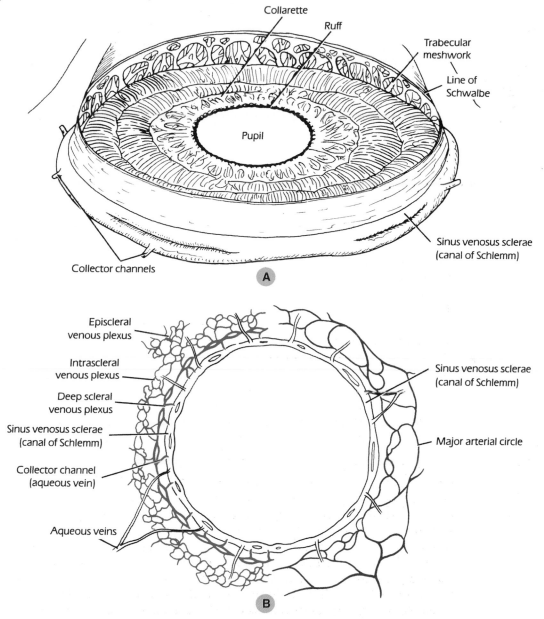

the aqueous. The trabeculae are known to thicken with age; and this thickening, combined with accumulation of debris, can severely increase the resistance to outflow and cause glaucoma.

The endothelial cells lining the sinus venosus sclerae form the final barrier to the outflow of aqueous humor. It is now generally agreed that the following mechanisms are responsible for the drainage of the aqueous:

1. *Transcellular channels formed by giant cytoplasmic vacuoles.* This means is now thought to be responsible for the passage of the greatest volume of aqueous humor. As pointed out previously, the vacuoles are first formed on the basal side of the cell. After considerable enlargement, but still remaining in contact with the basal plasma membrane, they touch and fuse with the apical plasma membrane. Thus for a period there exists a channel from one surface of the endothelial cell to the other. The aqueous now flows down a pressure gradient and enters the sinus venosus sclerae. Later, the vacuole disappears, only to be replaced by others. Some authorities believe that the cytoplasmic filaments of the endothelial cells may press on the channels, controlling the flow and even acting as one-way valves.

2. *A small flow between the endothelial cells.* This involves the passage of aqueous humor between the intercellular attachments and must be extremely small.

3. *Active transport across the endothelial cells through small pinocytotic vesicles.* This mechanism contributes very little to the total aqueous flow.

The question of whether the sinus venosus sclerae in a normal individual contains blood has been debated for years. Studies appear to show that the collector channels and aqueous veins offer very little resistance to the aqueous outflow; consequently, the sinus venosus usually contains no blood and is filled with aqueous humor flowing down a pressure gradient.

 Clinical Notes

The Anatomic Limbus and the Surgical Limbus   The limbus is an important landmark, an area measuring about 1.5 to 2.0 mm wide. It is the site where the cornea and sclera merge with each other. The anatomic limbus is defined by Schwalbe's line. The surgical limbus is defined by the beginning of the bluish area marking the transition zone between the cornea and the sclera. The surgical limbus is located slightly anterior to the anatomic limbus. The surgical limbus marks the point of entry for virtually all types of anterior segment surgery.

Having reflected the conjunctiva, the posterior border of the surgical limbus can be identified between the transparent bluish cornea and the opaque white sclera. An incision along the posterior border will pass in front of the canal of Schlemm and the anterior part of the trabecular meshwork. An incision made where the conjunctival epithelium merges with the corneal epithelium enters the anterior chamber of the eye anterior to the trabecular meshwork.

Sinus Venosus Sclerae (Canal of Schlemm) and Glaucoma   Glaucoma is one of the most common causes of blindness. In the majority of patients it is due to increased resistance to outflow of the aqueous humor through the trabecular meshwork into the sinus venosus sclerae. The resulting increase in intraocular pressure leads to atrophy of the optic nerve and defects of the visual field. In most patients the cause is unknown, but in some it follows trauma or inflammation of the eyeball. Tissue debris and inflammatory exudate block the passages of the trabecular network, preventing adequate drainage of the aqueous humor. (See also p. 154.)

Vascular Pigmented Layer

The vascular pigmented layer, or *uveal* tract*, consists, from back to front, of the choroid, the ciliary body, and the iris forming a continuous structure (Fig. 6-3).

Choroid

The choroid is a thin, soft, brown coat lining the inner surface of the sclera. It is extremely vascular. The choroid extends from the optic nerve posteriorly to the ciliary body anteriorly. It is thickest at the posterior pole (about 0.22 mm) and gradually thins anteriorly (about 0.1 mm). Its inner surface is smooth and firmly attached to the pigmented layer of the retina; its outer surface is roughened. It is firmly attached to the sclera in the region of the optic nerve and where the posterior ciliary arteries and ciliary nerves enter the eye. It is also tethered to the sclera where the vortex veins leave the eyeball.

Between the sclera and the choroid is a potential space, the *perichoroidal space*. Running across this space are thin, pigmented sheets of connective tissue called the *suprachoroid lamina*. Running in the perichoroidal space are the long and short posterior ciliary arteries and nerves. At the optic nerve the choroid becomes continuous with the pia and arachnoid.

Structure   The choroid may be divided into three layers: 1) the vessel layer, 2) the capillary layer, and 3) Bruch's membrane.

The Vessel Layer   This external layer consists of loose connective tissue containing melanocytes in which are embedded numerous large and medium-sized blood vessels (Fig. 6-15). The arteries are branches of the short posterior ciliary arteries and extend anteriorly. The veins are much larger and converge to join four of five vorticose veins that pierce the sclera to join the ophthalmic veins (Fig. 6-16).

The Capillary Layer   This intermediate layer consists of a network of wide-bore capillaries with saclike dilatations (Fig. 6-15). They are fed by arteries from the vessel layer and drained by veins into the vessel layer. The capillaries are supported by delicate connective tissue containing melanocytes. They are lined by a continuous layer of fenestrated endothelial cells. It should be noted that the density of the capillaries is greatest and the bore is widest at the macula.

Bruch's Membrane   This inner homogeneous layer measures 2 to 4 μm thick (Fig. 6-15) and consists of five different components: 1) the basement membrane of the endothelium of the capillaries of the capillary layer, 2) an outer layer of

---

*The word *uva* (Latin) means "grape." The term *uveal tract* was given to a dissection of the choroid, ciliary body, and iris, because this structure is brown and spherical, and resembles a grape, the optic nerve forming the stalk.

Figure 6-15

(A) Photomicrograph of low-power view of section through the wall of the eyeball, showing the choroid as a highly vascular, pigmented coat. (Plastic section; H&E; × 100.) (B) Photomicrograph of section through the choroid, showing the vessel layer, the capillary layer, and the region known as Bruch's membrane. (Plastic section; H&E; × 400.)

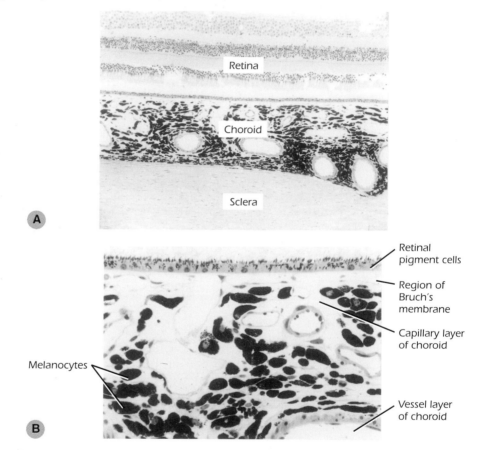

collagen fibers, 3) a meshwork of elastic fibers, 4) an inner layer of collagen fibers, and 5) the basement membrane of the pigment epithelium of the retina. The function of this membrane is not exactly known, although it is believed to play a role in the passage of tissue fluid from the choroidal capillaries to the retina.

Blood Supply   The choroid receives its blood supply mainly from the posterior ciliary arteries (Fig. 6-16). A number of recurrent branches arise from the anterior ciliary arteries. All these arteries are branches of the ophthalmic artery. The four or five vorticose veins drain the choroid and pierce the sclera to join the ophthalmic veins.

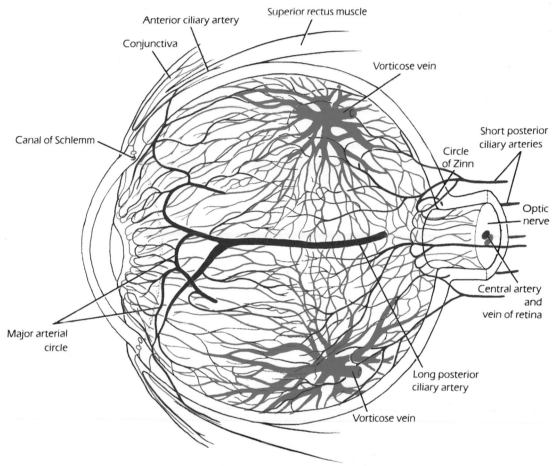

Figure 6-16

Diagram showing the arterial supply and venous drainage of the choroid, the ciliary body, and the iris.

Nerve Supply   The choroid is innervated by the long and short ciliary nerves (see Fig. 10-16). The long ciliary nerves are branches of the nasociliary nerve, a branch of the ophthalmic division of the trigeminal nerve. They carry sensory nerve fibers and sympathetic fibers. The short ciliary nerves arise from the ciliary ganglion and carry parasympathetic fibers and sympathetic fibers.

The long and short ciliary nerves pierce the sclera around the optic nerve and run forward in the perichoroidal space. Branches are given off to the choroid to form plexuses. Terminal branches reach the blood vessel walls. Experiments have shown that stimulation of the sympathetic nerves causes strong vasoconstriction of the choroidal blood vessels.

Function   The principal function of the choroid is to nourish with its blood vessels the outer layers of the retina. It also serves to conduct many blood vessels forward to the anterior regions of the eye. It is also thought that changes in the blood flow in the choroidal blood vessels may serve to produce heat exchange from the retina. It has been suggested that the blood flow in the choroidal arteries assists in regulating intraocular pressure. It might be noted that the tight junctions between the retinal pigment epithelial cells act as a barrier controlling the movement of choroidal tissue fluid into the retina. The large number of pigment cells in the choroid absorb excess light that penetrates the retina, thus preventing reflection.

Ciliary Body

The ciliary body is continuous posteriorly with the choroid and anteriorly with the peripheral margin of the iris (Figs. 6-3 and 6-12). Considered as a whole, the ciliary body is a complete ring that runs around the inside of the anterior sclera. It measures about 6 mm wide (6.5 mm on the temporal side and 5.5 mm on the nasal side) and extends forward to the scleral spur and backward to the ora serrata of the retina. On the outside of the eyeball, the ciliary body extends from a point about 1.5 mm posterior to the corneal limbus to a point 7.5 to 8.0 mm posterior to this on the temporal side and 6.5 to 7.0 mm on the nasal side. The ciliary body is triangular on cross-section, with its small base facing the anterior chamber of the eye and its anterior outer angle facing the scleral spur. Its apex extends posteriorly and laterally to become continuous with the choroid. The anterior surface or base is ridged or plicated and is called the *pars plicata* (Fig. 6-17). The posterior surface is smooth and flat and is called the *pars plana*. It is the pars plicata that surrounds the periphery of the iris and gives rise to the *ciliary processes* (Figs. 6-17, 6-18, and 6-19). In the intervals between the ciliary processes, the fibers of the zonule (suspensory ligament) of the lens pass to attach to the surface of the pars plicata (Figs. 6-19 and 6-20). The equator of the lens is situated about 0.5 mm from the ciliary processes. The posterior margin of the pars plana of the

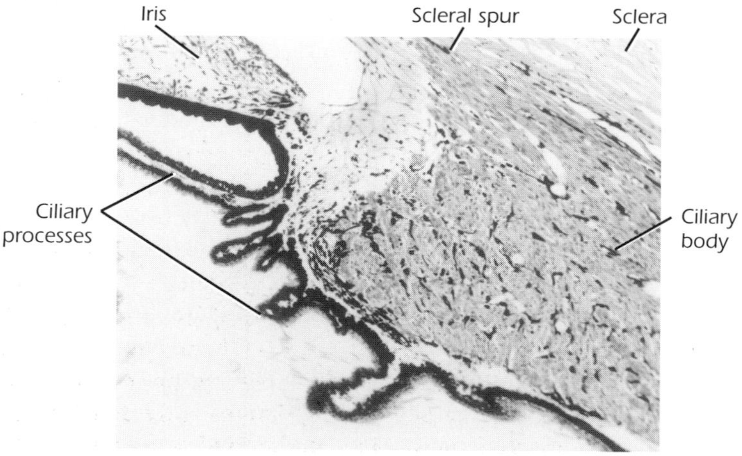

Figure 6-17

Photomicrograph of a section of the anterior portion of the eyeball, showing the sclera, the ciliary body, the ciliary processes, and the root of the iris. (H&E; × 100.)

Iris   Scleral spur   Sclera

Ciliary processes

Ciliary body

Figure 6-18

Photomicrograph of a section of two ciliary processes. Note the two layers of ciliary epithelium that cover the processes. The inner layer of cubical cells is nonpigmented and constitutes the anterior continuation of the nervous part of the retina; the deeper layer consists of cubical cells that are packed with melanin pigment and constitute the anterior continuation of the pigmented layer of the retina. (H&E; × 400.)

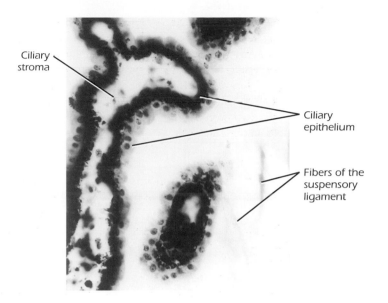

ciliary body has a scalloped edge that fits into and corresponds with the toothlike edge of the ora serrata of the neural part of the retina.

Structure   For purposes of description, the ciliary body is made up of 1) the ciliary epithelium, 2) the ciliary stroma, and 3) the ciliary muscle (Fig. 6-17).

Ciliary Epithelium   The ciliary epithelium consists of two layers of cubical cells that cover the inner surface of the ciliary body (Fig. 6-20). Embryologically, they represent the two layers of the optic cup. The nonpigmented inner layer of cells constitutes the anterior continuation of the nervous part of the retina. These cells also line the anterior chamber. The pigmented outer layer of cells constitutes the anterior continuation of the pigmented layer of the retina, the retinal pigmented epithelium. These cells rest against the stroma of the ciliary body. It is interesting to note that the basal surface of the nonpigmented cells faces the interior of the eye, while the base of the pigmented cells is directed toward the stroma. As a result, the apices of the nonpigmented and pigmented cells face each other; in places they are separated by small spaces called *ciliary channels.*

The basement membrane of the nonpigmented cells faces the posterior chamber and is continuous with the inner limiting membrane of the nervous part of the retina. The basement membrane of the pigmented cells faces the stroma and is continuous with the basement membrane of the pigmented epithelium of the retina (Fig. 6-20).

As seen by electron microscopy, the nonpigmented cells have the following characteristics. The basal and lateral plasma membranes have extensive foldings, which interdigitate with neighboring cells (Fig. 6-20). The cytoplasm contains a well-developed Golgi apparatus and extensive granular and agranular endoplasmic reticulum. Many mitochondria are present. These cells resemble other

Figure 6-19

Scanning electron micrograph of the posterior surface of the ciliary body, showing the ciliary processes and the fibers that form the suspensory ligament, or zonule. In the intervals between the ciliary processes the fibers of the ligament pass to attach to the surface of the pars plicata. (× 65.) (Courtesy of Fred Lightfoot.)

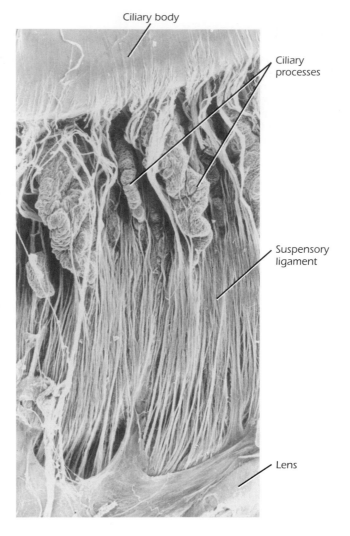

epithelial cells that are actively engaged in transporting water and ions and producing a secretion.

The pigmented cells are packed with melanosomes. The remaining scant cytoplasm contains a small Golgi apparatus and numerous mitochondria. The basal plasma membrane has marked infolding, indicating that the cells are actively involved in ion transport. The structure of the two layers of ciliary epithelium appears to suggest that both layers are involved in producing aqueous humor. The presence of numerous cell attachments suggests that the activities of the two cell layers may be coordinated.

Ciliary Stroma   The ciliary stroma (Fig. 6-21) consists of bundles of loose connective tissue, rich in blood vessels and melanocytes, containing the embedded ciliary muscle. The connective tissue extends into the ciliary processes, forming a connective tissue core.

Figure 6-20

(A) Diagram showing the two layers of cubical cells forming the ciliary epithelium. Note that the basal surface of the nonpigmented cells faces the interior of the eye (posterior chamber); the base of the pigmented cells is directed toward the stroma of the ciliary body. (B) Diagram showing the posterior surface of the ciliary body, the ciliary processes, and the fibers of the suspensory ligament. The right half of the lens has been omitted to show the pupil and the posterior surface of the iris.

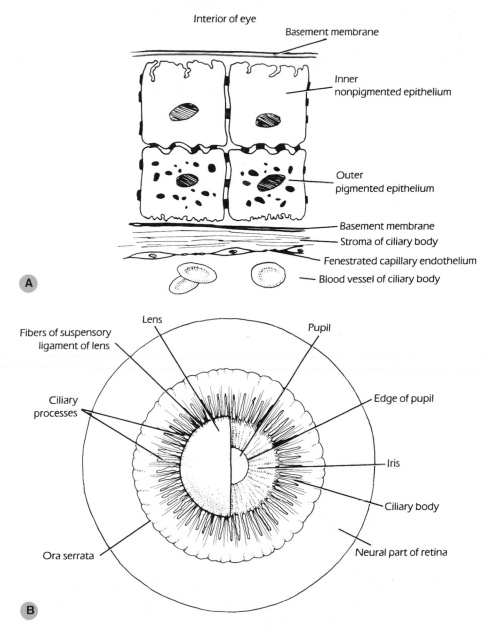

Figure 6-21

Photomicrograph of a section of the ciliary body, showing a feltwork of smooth muscle fibers and connective tissue. Note the presence of many melanocytes and blood vessels. (H&E; × 200.)

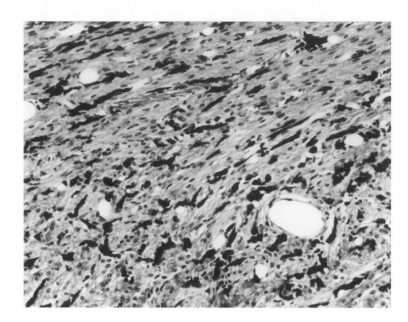

The blood vessels consist of the ciliary arteries, veins, and capillary networks. At the base or peripheral edge of the iris is the major arterial circle, formed mainly by branches of the long posterior ciliary arteries (Fig. 6-28). The endothelium of the capillaries that lie close to the ciliary epithelium is fenestrated.

Ciliary Muscle   The ciliary muscle forms the bulk of the substance of the ciliary body and consists of smooth muscle fibers (Fig. 6-21). The muscle fibers may be divided into three main groups; most of the fibers are attached to the scleral spur (Fig. 6-22). These groups are as follows: 1) The *longitudinal or meridional fibers*—the most external and closest to the sclera—pass posteriorly into the stroma of the choroid. 2) The *oblique or radial fibers* run from the first layer to the third layer, and radiate out from the scleral spur. 3) The *circular fibers*, the most internal, run around the eyeball like a sphincter. They lie close to the peripheral edge of the lens.

It is the contraction of the ciliary muscle, especially the longitudinal and the circular fibers, that pulls the ciliary body forward in accommodation. This forward movement is responsible for relieving the tension in the suspensory ligament, making the elastic lens more convex and thereby increasing the refractive power of the lens.

The ciliary muscle is innervated by the postganglionic parasympathetic fibers derived from the oculomotor nerve. The nerve fibers reach the muscle via the short ciliary nerves.

Functions   The ciliary body is concerned with the suspension of the lens and with the process of accommodation (see p. 202). The anterior surface of the ciliary processes produces the aqueous humor (see p. 194). The posterior surface faces the vitreous body and probably secretes glycosaminoglycans into the body (see p. 204).

Figure 6-22

Diagram showing the arrangement of the smooth muscle fibers in the ciliary body. Note the relationship of the ciliary body to the iris, the anterior chamber, the canal of Schlemm, and the corneoscleral limbus.

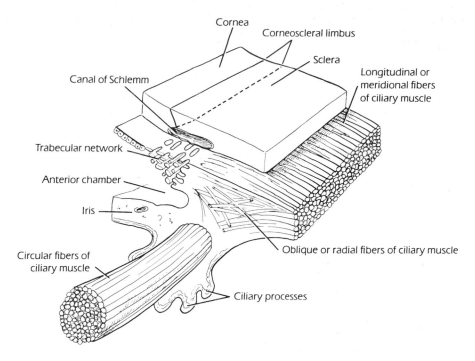

Iris

The iris is a thin, contractile, pigmented diaphragm with a central aperture, the *pupil* (Fig. 6-3 and Fig. 8-23). It is suspended in the aqueous humor between the cornea and the lens. The periphery of the iris, which is attached to the anterior surface of the ciliary body, is called the *ciliary margin*, or root of the iris. The pupil is surrounded by the *pupillary margin* of the iris. The iris, measuring about 12 mm in diameter, is thickest about 2 mm from the pupillary margin and is thinnest at the ciliary margin.

The anterior surface of the lens is convex and presses lightly against the iris, causing it to bulge anteriorly. The pupil varies in diameter from 1 to 8 mm, and in about 25 percent of normal subjects the pupils differ slightly in size. The iris divides the space between the lens and the cornea into an anterior and a posterior chamber. The aqueous humor, formed by the ciliary processes in the posterior chamber, circulates through the pupil into the anterior chamber and finally exits into the sinus venosus sclerae at the iridocorneal angle.

The color of the iris varies from light blue to dark brown; the color may vary from one eye to another in the same person and in different parts of the same iris. The color of the iris is produced by the pigment in the melanocytes. The blue iris has less pigment in the melanocytes compared with the brown iris. The blue color results from the absorption of light, with long wavelengths and the reflection of the shorter blue waves that are seen by the observer. In whites at birth, the iris is usually blue, later becoming darker as more melanin accumulates in the superficial melanocytes. In blacks at birth, the melanocytes throughout the iris contain more melanin. In an albino person the melanocytes are devoid of pigment, so that the hemoglobin in the blood vessels of the iris and retina show as a reddish glow.

Anterior Surface   The anterior surface of the iris is divided into a central *pupillary zone* and a peripheral *ciliary zone* (Fig. 6-23). The line of demarcation is formed by a circular ridge, the *collarette*, which lies about 2 mm from the pupillary margin. The collarette forms a wavy line, and here the iris is thickest.

The anterior surface of the iris is devoid of epithelium and has a velvety appearance. It shows a series of radial streaks caused by trabeculae or bands of connective tissue that enclose oval-shaped crypts (Fuch's crypts). The trabeculae are most pronounced in the region of the collarette. The crypts communicate with the tissue spaces of the iris. In the ciliary region there are long radial ridges produced by the underlying blood vessels. These are branches of the major arterial circle located in the ciliary body (Fig. 6-28). At the collarette they anastomose to form an incomplete minor vascular circle of the iris.

Near the outer part of the ciliary region are a number of concentric furrows, which become deeper when the pupil dilates. They are recognized as dark lines and are known as *contraction furrows* (Fig. 6-23). These are merely caused by the folding of the iris as the pupil dilates.

At the pupillary margin, the pigmented posterior epithelium extends anteriorly around the edge of the pupil for a short distance. The epithelium has radial folds, which give its boundary a crenated appearance, sometimes called the *ruff* (Figs. 6-23 and 6-24). When the pigmented epithelium of the iris extends around the pupil margin anteriorly to an excessive degree, it is called *ectropion uvae* and can be an important sign of abnormal traction on the iris tissues, induced by tumor or other significant pathologic processes. The pupil is never fixed and is constantly changing in size in response to the sphincter and dilator pupillae muscles.

Posterior Surface   The posterior surface of the iris is black and shows a number of radial contraction folds, which are most prominent in the pupillary region (Fig. 6-23). Circular folds are also present at the periphery.

Structure   Microscopically, the iris consists of two layers: 1) the stroma, situated anteriorly and derived from mesenchyme, and 2) two epithelial layers located posteriorly and derived from the neural ectoderm (Fig. 6-24).

Stromal Layer   The stroma of the iris consists of highly vascular connective tissue containing collagen fibers, fibroblasts, melanocytes, and matrix. The stroma also contains nerve fibers, the smooth muscle of the sphincter pupillae, and the myoepithelial cells of the dilator pupillae.

Figure 6-23

(A) Diagram showing the features seen on the anterior surface of the iris. The pupillary zone extends from the pupil to the collarette, and the ciliary zone extends from the collarette to the peripheral edge of the iris, where it joins the ciliary body. (B) Diagram showing the features on the black posterior surface of the iris. Note the radial contraction folds, which are most prominent in the pupillary region.

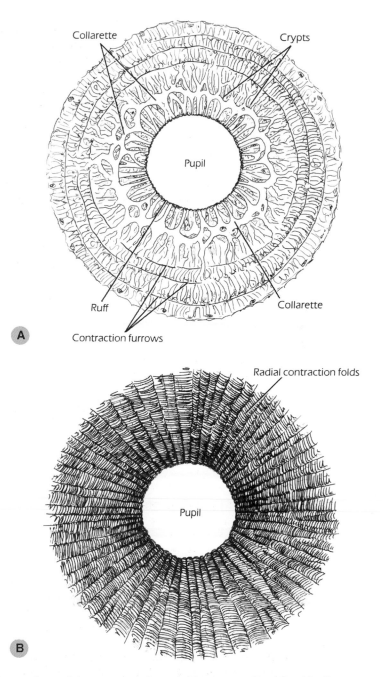

The anterior surface of the stroma is bare, with no covering of epithelium (Fig. 6-24). Here, there is a compact, dense arrangement of fibroblasts, melanocytes, and collagen fibers (Fig. 6-25). Numerous crypts (Fuch's crypts) are present, communicating with the tissue spaces of the stroma and with the anterior chamber. The aqueous humor thus has direct communication with the tissue spaces of the iris.

Figure 6-24

(A) Photomicrograph of a section of iris close to the pupillary margin. Note the formation of the ruff from the pigmented posterior epithelium (H&E; × 400.) (B) Photomicrograph of a section of iris, showing the general structure. Note the absence of epithelium on the anterior surface, the presence of numerous pigmented melanocytes in the stroma, and the posterior epithelial cells packed with melanin. (H&E; × 200.)

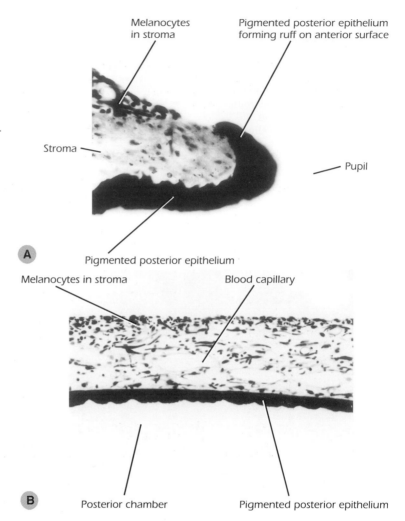

The collagen fibrils have a diameter of about 60 nm, and a periodicity of 50 to 60 nm. They are loosely arranged, the spaces between them being filled with fluid rich in mucopolysaccharides. There are no elastic fibers.

The fibroblasts have numerous branching processes and at the periphery blend with those of the trabecular meshwork at the iridocorneal angle. The melanocytes also show numerous branching dendritic processes, and the cytoplasm contains varying numbers of melanosomes. Mast cells, macrophages, and lymphocytes are also present in the stroma.

The *sphincter pupillae muscle* is located in the pupillary zone of the iris (Fig. 6-26). It forms a ring of smooth muscle fibers around the pupil, measuring about 1 mm wide. The bundles of smooth muscle cells are separated by connective

Figure 6-25

Scanning electron micrograph of the anterior surface of the iris. (A) The surface to be covered by an incomplete layer of fibroblasts (arrows). (× 3850.) (B) In the intervals between the fibroblasts are melanocytes containing large numbers of melanin granules (arrows). (× 4375.) (Courtesy of Fred Lightfoot.)

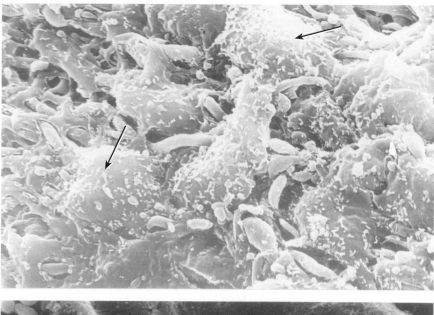

A

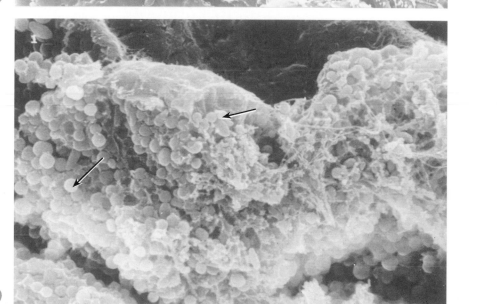

B

Figure 6-26

(A) Diagram showing the arrangement of the fibers of the dilator pupillae and the sphincter pupillae of the iris. (B) Diagram showing the two posterior epithelial layers of the iris. Note that the two cells are apposed to each other apex to apex, and that the basal process of the anterior cell forms the myoepithelium of the dilator pupillae.

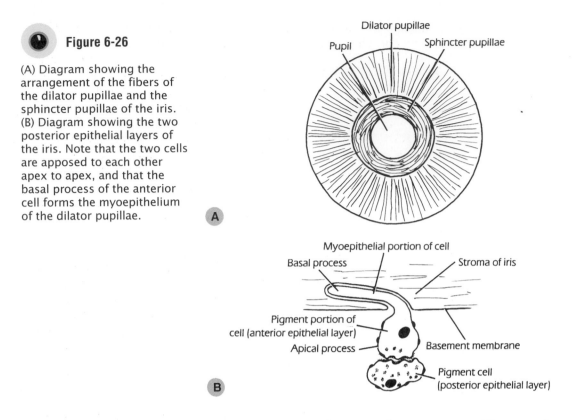

tissue that contains blood vessels and motor and sensory nerves. Electron microscopy shows that within the muscle bundles, groups of smooth muscle cells, six to eight in number, are connected to each other by gap junctions. Nerve fibers usually end on one muscle cell situated at the periphery of each muscle group. When the sphincter pupillae contracts, the pupil constricts. The nerve supply of the sphincter pupillae is from the parasympathetic postganglionic fibers in the short ciliary nerves. They are derived from the oculomotor nerve.

The *dilator pupillae muscle* is a thin layer of myoepithelium that extends from the iris root as far as the sphincter pupillae (Fig. 6-26). The myoepithelial cells are derived from the anterior layer of the iris pigment epithelium that covers the posterior surface of the iris (Fig. 6-26). The apical processes form the pigment cells, while the basal processes form the muscle fibers. The muscle processes are fusiform in shape and measure about 4 μm thick and 60 μm long. The myofilaments are present throughout the cells but are more concentrated in the muscular processes. The muscular processes are joined by gap junctions and are surrounded by a basement membrane. Nonmyelinated nerve fibers terminate close to the plasma membrane. When the dilator pupillae contracts, the pupil enlarges. The nerve supply of the dilator pupillae is from the postganglionic fibers of the superior cervical sympathetic ganglion via the long ciliary nerves.

It is interesting to note that both the sphincter pupillae muscle fibers and the myoepithelial cells of the dilator pupillae are derived from the external layer of the optic cup.

Epithelial Layers　　There are two posterior epithelial layers, one called anterior and the other posterior. The two epithelial layers consist of cells that are derived embryologically from the neuroectoderm of the two layers of the optic vesicle. The cells of the two layers are apposed to each other apex to apex; between these lies a potential space that can, under certain circumstances, fill with fluid and become a real space, forming an iris cyst. The anterior (epithelial) layer lies in contact with the stroma of the iris (Fig. 6-26) and is closely associated with the muscular processes of the dilator pupillae (see above). The anterior layer contains relatively few melanin granules that are found in the apical cytoplasm. This anterior layer is continuous with the outer pigmented layer of the ciliary epithelium.

The posterior (epithelial) layer is bathed with aqueous humor and faces the posterior chamber. The cells are larger than those of the anterior layer and are cuboidal in shape. They are packed with melanin granules. This layer is continuous with the inner nonpigmented layer of the ciliary epithelium.

The apical plasma membranes of both epithelial layers have numerous microvilli that project into small intercellular spaces. The lateral plasma membranes of adjacent cells of both layers are connected by tight junctions and desmosomes. Scanning electron micrographs of the posterior surface of the posterior epithelial layer show longitudinal furrows and pits and, at the periphery, circumferential folds. Transmission electron micrographs of the basal plasma membrane show numerous infoldings and a basement membrane.

Pupil Movements

Miosis (Contraction)　　The sphincter pupillae constricts the pupil in bright light and during accommodation. This occurs in response to parasympathetic nerve activity.

Mydriasis (Dilation)　　The dilator pupillae dilates the pupil in low-intensity light and during excitement or fear. This occurs in response to sympathetic nerve activity.

Blood Supply　　The arterial supply of the iris is provided by radial vessels that lie in the iris stroma (Fig. 6-27). The arteries arise from the *major arterial circle* located in the stroma of the ciliary body. The major arterial circle is formed from the two long posterior ciliary arteries and the seven anterior ciliary arteries.

The radial arteries converge in a spiral pattern toward the pupillary margin and form the radial ridges seen on the anterior surface of the iris. The spiral pattern of the arteries permits adaptation to the movement of the iris as the pupil dilates or constricts. On reaching the collarette, the arteries anastomose to form an incomplete *minor arterial circle* of the iris (Fig. 6-28).

The veins follow the arteries and form a corresponding minor venous circle. The radial veins do not drain into a major venous circle but converge and drain into the vorticose veins.

The endothelial lining of all the blood vessels of the iris, including the capillaries, is nonfenestrated and there are tight junctions between the endothelial

Figure 6-27

(A) Diagram summarizing the arterial and venous drainage of the eyeball. (B) Diagram summarizing the arterial and venous drainage of the iris.

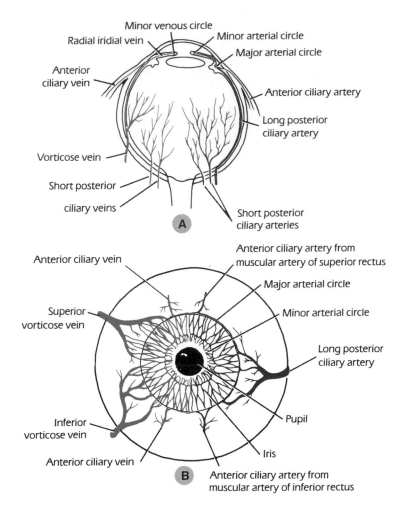

cells. This is of great significance since it makes them less permeable. When the anterior chamber and the iris are subjected to an inflammatory process, the vessels in the iris leak protein and other large molecules. This is easily seen on slit-lamp examination of the anterior chamber, because protein in the aqueous changes its optical properties. The endothelium is surrounded by a thick basement membrane. In the arteries and veins there is no elastic lamina, and the smooth muscle fibers are few in number. The tunica adventitia is well developed. Electron microscopy shows the presence of numerous tubular bodies (Weibel-Palade bodies) in the cytoplasm of the capillary endothelial cells. Their significance is not understood, but they are believed to bud off from the Golgi apparatus.

Nerve Supply   The iris receives its sensory and autonomic nerve supply from the long and short ciliary nerves. The long ciliary nerves are branches of the

Figure 6-28

Diagram showing the arterial supply and venous drainage of the anterior portion of the eyeball. The vortex vein, which is normally present at the equator, has been included for completeness.

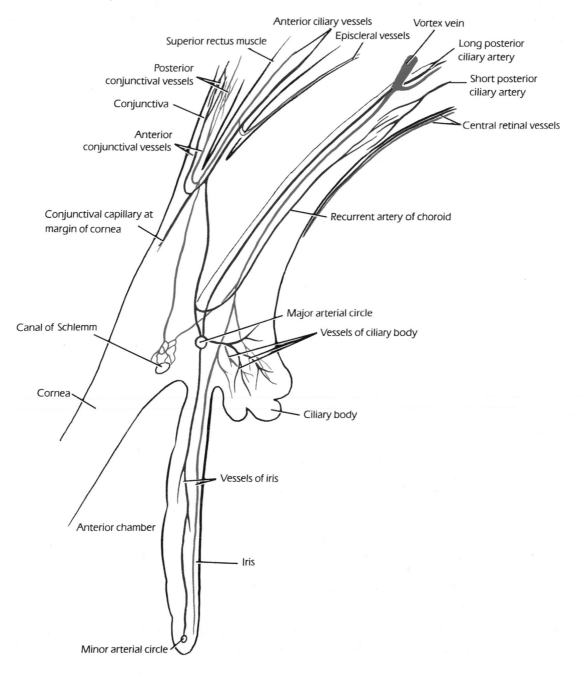

nasociliary branch of the ophthalmic division of the trigeminal nerve. They contain sensory fibers that ascend in the trigeminal nerve. The long ciliary nerves also contain postganglionic sympathetic fibers from the superior cervical sympathetic ganglion. These fibers innervate the dilator pupillae and are vaso-motor to the blood vessels.

The short ciliary nerves arise from the ciliary ganglion and contain postgan-glionic parasympathetic nerve fibers. This pathway originates in the Edinger-Westphal nucleus of the oculomotor nerve. The parasympathetic innervates the sphincter pupillae. A few sympathetic fibers also travel in the short ciliary nerves.

Function   The ability to dilate and constrict the pupil permits the iris to control the amount of light entering the eye and impinging on the retina. Thus, with poor illumination the pupil is dilated by the dilator pupillae and with excessively bright light the pupil is constricted by the constrictor pupillae. However, it should be pointed out that the actual contribution that the pupil makes in controlling light entry is fairly small and represents only a tenfold change in the amount of light, that is, one log unit. This represents a small part of the six log units to which the retina can actually remain effectively sensitive. During accommodation for near vision, the pupil also constricts, thus restricting the incoming light to the center part of the lens, so that spherical aberration is diminished.

Clinical Notes

The iris, ciliary body, and choroid together form the middle coat of the eyeball, which is known as the *uveal tract.*

Circulatory Metastases   The uveal tract is highly vascular, receiving its main blood supply from the posterior ciliary arteries and minor contributions anteriorly from the anterior ciliary arteries. Because of its extreme vascularity, it is com-monly involved in other general systemic diseases and may be a site for circula-tory metastases.

Lesions of the Choroid and Atrophy and Destruction of the Retina Because the uveal tract provides nourishment for the outer part of the retina, a lesion of the choroid may interfere with nutrition to the adjacent retina and cause atrophy and de-struction of the retina.

Age Changes in the Choroid   In the aged the choroid may show signs of atrophy and depigmentation. At the periphery of the fundus, the red glow may have a patchy appearance. Bruch's membrane may show evidence of thickening from small yellow dots, referred to as *drusen,* scattered about the central area. The choroidal blood vessels commonly show evidence of sclerosis after the age of 60 years.

Malignant Melanoma of the Uveal Tract   These arise from the melanocytes of the choroid, ciliary body, and iris. They are the most common malignant intra-ocular tumors.

Ciliary Body and Iris in Inflammations   Inflammations of the ciliary body and iris are associated with a deep, boring pain in the eye and with a ciliary injection. A ciliary injection is a dilatation of the anterior ciliary arteries that supplies these structures.

The iris, ciliary body, and anterior part of the choroid share a common blood supply and are together often involved in an inflammatory process.

Iris Adhesions The close anatomic relationship between the iris and the lens may result in the production of adhesions between these structures following iritis. Such adhesions, or *posterior synechiae*, may cause a small, irregular pupil that does not constrict to light. These posterior adhesions occur in contradistinction to adhesions of the iris to the endothelium and trabecular meshwork, which are called *anterior synechiae*. If the entire pupillary margin is stuck to the lens, a pupillary block glaucoma can occur.

The Pars Plana of the Ciliary Body and Surgery The pars plana is surgically an important anatomic structure. Because of its relative avascularity and position anterior to the retina, incisions through the sclera and choroid into the vitreous should be made at this point to avoid hemorrhagic complications and retinal detachments.

Nervous Layer—The Retina

The nervous coat, or retina, is the internal layer of the eyeball (Fig. 6-3). This layer is where the optical image is formed by the eye's optical system. Here, photochemical transduction occurs so that nerve impulses are created and transmitted along visual pathways to the brain for higher cortical processing. The retina is a thin, transparent membrane having a purplish-red color in living subjects. Its thickness varies from 0.56 mm near the optic disc to 0.1 mm at the ora serrata. It is thinnest at the center of the fovea. The retina is continuous with the optic nerve posteriorly, and it extends forward to become the epithelium of the ciliary body and the iris. The outer surface of the retina is in contact with Bruch's membrane of the choroid; the inner surface is in contact with the vitreous body. The retina is firmly attached at the margins of the optic disc and at its anterior termination at the ora serrata. It should be remembered that the retina extends more anteriorly on the medial side, so that the ora serrata lies closer to the limbus on that side (Fig. 6-29). An approximate landmark on the outside of the eyeball is the point of insertion of the medial rectus muscle medially and the lateral rectus muscle laterally.

The retina consists of an outer pigmented layer and an inner neurosensory layer, which are embryologically derived from neuroectoderm. The outer layer is derived from the outer layer of the optic cup; the inner layer, from the inner layer of the optic cup. The posterior, receptive part of the retina extends forward from the optic nerve to a point just posterior to the ciliary body. Here the nervous tissues of the retina end and its anterior edge forms the wavy ring, called the *ora serrata* (Fig. 6-29). The anterior, nonreceptive part of the retina at the ora serrata becomes continuous with the pigmented and nonpigmented columnar cell layers of the ciliary body and its processes. At the iris, both layers of cells continue on to its posterior surface, and they both become pigmented.

Figure 6-29

Diagram of a horizontal section of the right eyeball at the level of the optic nerve. The vitreous body has been removed to reveal the extent of the neural retina.

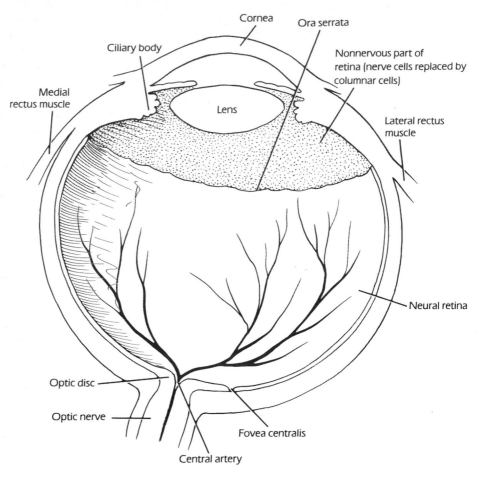

At the center of the posterior part of the retina is an oval, yellowish area, the *macula lutea*, which is the retinal area for the most distinct vision. It has a central depression, the *fovea centralis* (Fig. 6-29).

The optic nerve leaves the retina about 3 mm to the medial side of the macula lutea at the *optic disc* (Fig. 6-29). The optic disc is slightly depressed at its center, where it is pierced by the *central retinal artery and vein*. At the optic disc, there is a complete absence of *rods* and *cones;* thus, it is insensitive to light and is referred to as the *blind spot.* On ophthalmoscopic examination, the optic disc is seen to be pale pink, much paler than the surrounding retina.

Pigmented Layer of the Retina

The retinal pigment epithelium (often abbreviated RPE) consists of a single layer of cells that extends forward from the margin of the optic nerve to the ora serrata anteriorly; here it continues forward with the continuation of the nervous layer as the pigmented ciliary epithelium (Figs. 6-30, 6-31, and 6-32). The cells are narrow and tall in the posterior polar region and become flattened near the ora serrata. On tangential section, the cells are hexagonal. The basal end of each cell is much infolded and rests on a basement membrane, which forms part of Bruch's membrane of the choroid. The apical ends of the cell show multiple microvilli measuring 5 to 7 µm long (Figs. 6-32 and 6-33). These project between and surround the outer segments of the rods and cones, and there are no specialized attachments between them (Fig. 6-34). The microvilli are embedded in glycosaminoglycans, which may act as an adhesive binding the pigment layer to the neural layer. The adjacent cell membranes are bound together in the basal region by the zonula adherens, which encircles the cell, and in the apical region by the zonula occludens, which also surrounds the cell and practically obliterates the intercellular space. These tight junctions are very important in maintaining the isolation of the retina from the systemic circulation (see p. 286).

The cell nuclei occupy the basal part of the cytoplasm and there are numerous round or ovoid melanin granules that extend into the microvilli. There are a well-developed granular and agranular endoplasmic reticulum and a Golgi apparatus. Lysosomes are present in large numbers, together with residual bodies, or phagosomes. It is now known that the apical microvilli continuously erode the outer ends of the rods. The pigment cells then phagocytose the debris, which includes the lamellar structures found in the outer processes of the photoreceptor cells. Lysosomes play an active role in breaking down the contents of the phagosomes and lipofuscin granules are the final products of this process.

Functions   The pigment cells have numerous functions, including the absorption of light, participation in the turnover of the outer segments of the photoreceptors,

 Figure 6-30

Photomicrograph of a section of the eyeball, showing the retina and the choroid. (H&E; × 130.)

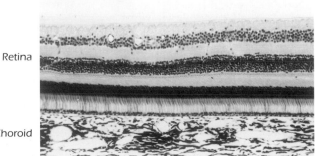

Retina

Choroid

Figure 6-31

Photomicrograph of a section of the retina, showing the different layers. Identify layers 1, 2, 4, 6, and 8. The numbers refer to layers shown diagrammatically in Figure 6-32. (H&E; × 400.)

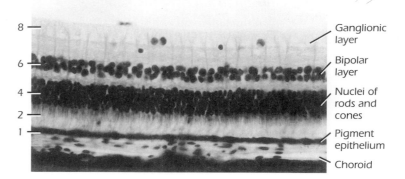

Figure 6-32

(A) The 10 layers of the retina, as seen in an ordinary histologic section. (B) Diagram showing the arrrangement of the nerve cells. Note that the cell processes of the supporting cells of Müller form the outer and inner limiting membranes.

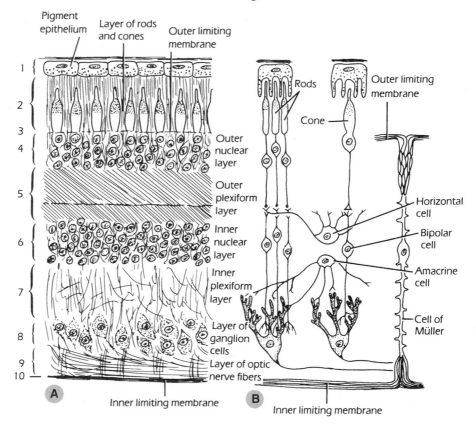

Figure 6-33

Diagrams showing in detail the structure of (A) a rod and a cone, and (B) a pigment cell. Note the relationship of the pigment cell to the outer segments of the rods. (C) Outer segment of a rod. (D) Outer segment of a cone.

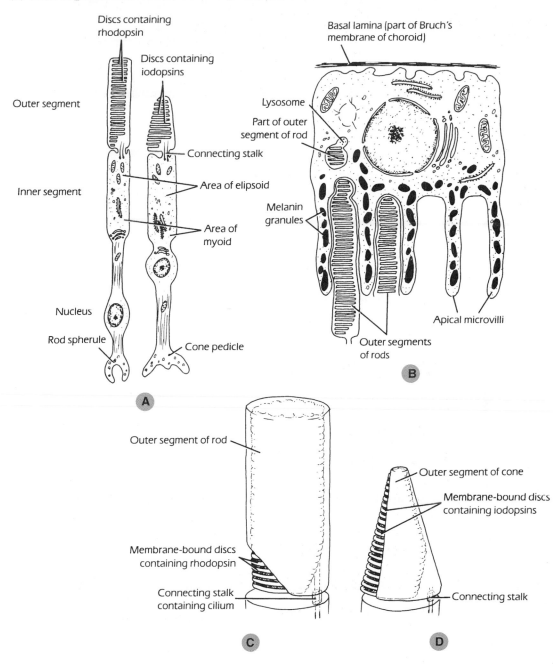

Figure 6-34

Electron micrograph of a section of pigment epithelial cells of the retina, showing the microvilli at the apical ends of the cells (arrows) projecting between the outer segments of the rods. (× 14,000.) (Courtesy of Dr. T. Kuwabara.)

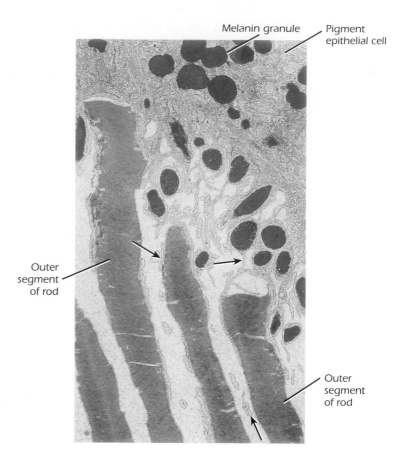

and the formation of rhodopsin and iodopsin by storing and releasing vitamin A, which is a precursor of the photosensitive pigments. These cells may also have a secretory function.

The pigment cells absorb light by an antireflection mechanism that prevents the return of light into the photoreceptive layer of the neural retina, with the resulting loss of image sharpness.

The pigmented epithelium, which is developed from the outer layer of the optic cup, and the rods and cones, which are developed from the inner layer of the optic cup, are separated by a potential space that constitutes the remains of the cavity of the optic vesicle. Although the layers are very close together, they can become separated, a condition known as *detached retina* (see p. 191).

Clinical Notes

Blood-Retina Barrier   The pigment epithelial cells are joined to each other by tight junctions that completely encircle the cells. This arrangement forms a barrier that limits the flow of ions and prevents diffusion of large toxic molecules from the choroid capillaries to the photoreceptors of the neural retina.

Albinism   In oculocutaneous and ocular albinism, there is a lack of melanin pigment in the pigment cells of the retina and the uvea. On clinical examination of the eye* one can see through the iris (a condition called transillumination of the iris) and visualize the ciliary processes and the lens, and the pupil is red. The fundus is light red, and the retinal and choroidal vessels can be seen against the white sclera. The number of pigment cells present is normal, but the melanin pigment is deficient.

Neural Retina

Structure   The neural retina is embryologically derived from the inner layer of the optic cup. It consists of three main groups of neurons: 1) the photoreceptors, 2) the bipolar cells, and 3) the ganglion cells. It also possesses other important neurons, the horizontal cells and the amacrine cells, that modulate their activity. Supporting cells are also present.

The photoreceptors are similar to sensory receptors elsewhere in the body. The bipolar cells are similar to the neurons in the posterior root ganglia and form the first-order neurons. The ganglion cells are similar to the relay neurons found in the spinal cord and brain stem and form the second-order neurons. The axons of the ganglion cells become myelinated after they have passed through the lamina cribrosa and entered the substance of the optic nerve. The myelin sheaths of these axons are formed from oligodendrocytes rather than Schwann cells, because the optic nerve is comparable to a tract within the central nervous system. The optic nerves and the optic tracts conduct their impulses to the lateral geniculate body (see p. 389), where most of the axons terminate by synapsing with nerve cells. The nerve cells of the lateral geniculate body form the third-order neurons, and their axons terminate in the visual cortex. Thus, the number of neurons involved in conducting light impulses from the retina to the visual cortex is the same as that found in other sensory pathways.

Photoreceptors   There are two types of photoreceptors, the rods and the cones (Figs. 6-31 and 6-32). The rods are mainly responsible for vision in dim light and produce images consisting of varying shades of black and white, while the cones are adapted to bright light and can resolve fine details and color vision. The total number of the rods in the retina has been estimated to be about 110 to 125 million and of the cones, 6.3 to 6.8 million. The density of the rods and cones varies in different parts of the retina. The rods are absent at the fovea, rising rapidly in numbers toward the periphery and then slowly diminishing at the extreme periphery of the retina; it is estimated that about 30,000 rods per square millimeter are present at the extreme periphery. The cones, on the other hand, are most dense at the fovea and the numbers decrease at the periphery. It is interesting that the number of rods and cones is much greater than the number of ganglion cells. (There are approximately 1 million ganglion cells in each retina and about 100 photoreceptor cells per ganglion cell.) It follows that large numbers of rod and cones activate a single axon in the optic nerve.

Both the rods and cones are long, narrow cells whose names describe the shape of their free ends. The outer ends of the cells interdigitate with the pigment

*In approximately 10 percent of the population, a slight degree of transillumination of the iris is possible and it is a normal finding.

epithelium and are referred to as the *outer segments. Connecting stalks* join the outer segments to the *inner segments.*

The *rod cells* are slender cells about 100 to 120 µm long (Figs. 6-32 and 6-33). The outer segment is the true photoreceptor of the cell and contains the photosensitive pigment rhodopsin. Electron microscopic examination shows that the outer segment contains 600 to 1000 transversely arranged membrane-bound lamellae, or discs, stacked on one another like a pile of coins (Fig. 6-34). The rhodopsin molecules are located within the membrane of the discs. Each disc measures approximately 2 µm in diameter and about 14 nm thick (Fig. 6-35).

There is clear evidence that the discs are formed at the base of the outer segment and are then pushed up to the free end of the outer segment. When the discs reach the tip of the segment, the free end and the contained discs are phagocytosed by the cells of the pigment epithelium. This sloughing of the discs of the rods does not occur in a continuous fashion, but, rather, in a 24-hour cycle, wherein most of the discs are shed at once in the early morning.

The connecting stalk, which is eccentrically placed, contains a modified cilium (Fig. 6-35). The cilium possesses the usual nine doublet microtubules but does not have a central pair. It originates in a basal body found in the inner

Figure 6-35

Electron micrograph of a portion of the outer and inner segments of a rod, showing the transversely arranged membrane-bound discs stacked one on another. The connecting stalk contains a modified cilium, which originates in a basal body in the inner segment. (× 45,000.) (Courtesy of Dr. T. Kuwabara.)

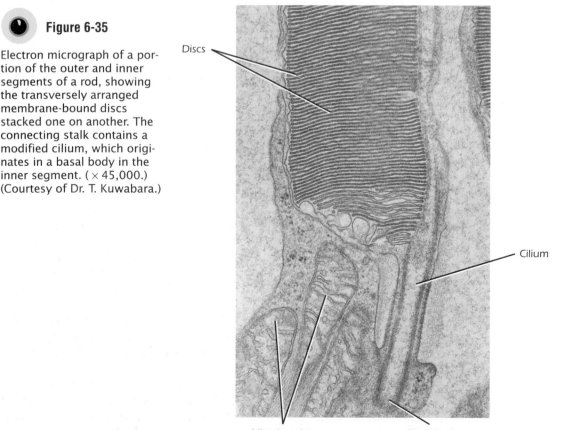

Discs

Cilium

Mitochondria   Basal body

Figure 6-36

Electron micrograph of a portion of the outer segment of a cone. Note that the membranes of the transversely arranged discs are continuous with the outer plasma membrane (arrow). (× 56,000.) (Courtesy of Dr. T. Kuwabara.)

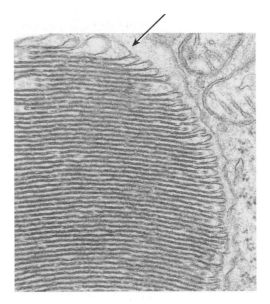

segment. Developmental studies of the outer segments of the rods show that in fact they are modified cilia.

The inner segment consists of two areas, the *ellipsoid*, situated next to the connecting stalk, and the *myoid*, located toward the vitreous (Fig. 6-33). The ellipsoid contains the basal body, with numerous mitochondria, and the myoid contains the granular and agranular endoplasmic reticulum, free ribosomes, and a Golgi apparatus.

The remainder of the rod cell is made up of the *outer fiber*, the *cell body*, the *inner fiber*, and the *spherule* (Fig. 6-33). The rod outer fiber, about 1 μm wide, joins the inner segment to the cell body. The rod inner fiber contains numerous microtubules and connects the cell body to a pear-shaped spherule. The rod spherule contains many presynaptic vesicles and it synapses with the dendrites of the bipolar cells.

The *cone cells* are also long, slender cells, measuring about 65 to 75 μm in length (Figs. 6-32 and 6-33). They have a structure similar to that of the rods, with an outer segment, a connecting stalk, and an inner segment. The outer segment is conical, considerably wider than a rod at its base, and tapering down to a rounded tip. The membranes of the transversely arranged discs are continuous with the outer plasma membrane (Figs. 6-33 and 6-36); thus the laminae of the discs, unlike those of the rods, are continuous with the extracellular space. The tips of the cones are not phagocytosed by the pigment cells. Several photochemicals are found in the cones; they are similar in composition to rhodopsin and are known as *iodopsins*. As in the rods, the photosensitive pigments are incorporated into the disc membrane.

The cone outer segment is connected to the inner segment by an eccentrically placed modified cilium (Fig. 6-33). The structure of the inner cone segment resembles that of the inner segment of the rod. The inner cone segment merges with the body, which contains a large, pale-staining nucleus. The body of the cone is connected by the inner fiber to the expanded end, called the *cone pedicle*. This synapses with the dendrites of the bipolar cells.

Bipolar Cells   The bipolar cells have a radial orientation. One or more dendrites of the bipolar cells pass outward to synapse with the photoreceptor cell terminals (Fig. 6-32). The single axon is directed inward to synapse with ganglion cells and amacrine cells. Several types of bipolar cells have been identified on the basis of their synaptic connections. *Rod bipolar cells* connect several rod cells to one to four ganglion cells. *Flat or diffuse bipolar cells* connect many cone cells with many ganglion cells. *Midget bipolar cells* connect a single cone cell with a single midget ganglion cell. The latter arrangement provides a direct pathway from the cone to a single optic nerve fiber.

Ganglion Cells   The ganglion cells are so named because they resemble cells found in nervous ganglia. They are situated in the inner part of the retina (Fig. 6-31). The ganglion cells are the second neurons in the visual pathway. They vary in diameter from 10 to 30 µm. Most of them are small (midget ganglion cells), but a small number are large. In most of the retina the ganglion cells form a single layer. However, the number of layers increases from the periphery of the retina to the macula, where there may be as many as 10 layers. They decrease again toward the fovea, where they are absent.

The ganglion cells are multipolar cells and their dendrites synapse with the axons of bipolar cells and amacrine cells (Fig. 6-32). The midget ganglion cells are linked by single midget bipolar neurons to a single cone cell.

The ganglion cells have nonmyelinated axons that make a right-angled turn when they reach the inner surface of the retina. The axons then converge at the exit of the optic nerve at the optic disc. The optic nerve fibers pass through the sclera at a site known as the *lamina cribrosa* (Fig. 6-38); it is the weakest part of the sclera. After piercing the lamina, the nerve fibers become myelinated, the myelin sheath being formed from oligodendrocytes. In some individuals the ganglion cell axons are partially myelinated, usually in areas near the optic disc; such areas are non-seeing and will produce a blind spot (see p. 403).

Other Important Nerve Cells   In addition to the rod and cone cells, bipolar cells, and ganglion cells, there are two types of neurons called horizontal and amacrine cells.

The *horizontal cells* are situated close to the terminal expansions of the rods and cones (Fig. 6-32). The cells are multipolar and have one long and several short processes, which run horizontally parallel with the retinal surface. The long process may be as long as 1 mm. The cytoplasm contains an organelle made up of tubular membranes covered by many ribosomes (called Kolmer's crystalloid). The horizontal cells associated with the cones have short processes that have synaptic junctions with seven cone pedicles. The horizontal cells associated with the rods have short processes that synapse with 10 to 12 rod spherules. The long processes make contact with rods and cones some distance away and with bipolar cells. The horizontal cells respond to the neurotransmitter liberated by the rods and cones following excitation by light. They are then believed to liberate an inhibitory transmitter, gamma-aminobutyric acid (GABA), that inhibits the activity of the bipolar cells some distance away, thus sharpening contrast and increasing spatial resolution. It is also possible that the horizontal cells integrate visual stimuli.

Amacrine cells were so named because it was believed that they had no axons. They can be recognized by their large cell bodies, with abundant cytoplasm and lobulated indented nuclei. They are situated close to the ganglion cells and their long processes radiate widely and synapse with one another and with the dendrites of the ganglion cells and the axonal endings of the bipolar cells (Fig. 6-32). The amacrine cells are stimulated by the bipolar cells, which in turn excite the ganglion cells. The long horizontal pathways ensure that laterally placed ganglion cells are excited. They also appear to serve as modulators of photoreceptor signals. Different types of amacrine cells have now been identified according to their neurotransmitter content.

Supporting Cells   Because the neural retina develops from the optic cup, which is an outgrowth of the central nervous system, it is not surprising that the supporting cells are similar to neuroglial cells. One of these runs radially and is called the *Müller cell* (Fig. 6-32). It is long, narrow, and pale-staining, with long processes extending from it through almost the whole thickness of the neural retina. Subsidiary branches extend out horizontally, surrounding and supporting the nerve cells. Müller cells thus fill in most of the space of the neural retina not occupied by the neurons.

Toward the outer surface of the neural retina, electron microscopy has shown that there exists a row of zonulae adherentes between the photoreceptor cells and the radial processes of the Müller cells. This forms a dense-staining line seen by light microscopy and traditionally (but erroneously) called the *outer limiting membrane* (Fig. 6-32). Tufts of microvilli project from the ends of the Müller cells in the spaces between the inner segments of the rods and cones.

At the vitreous surface of the neural retina the Müller cell processes have expanded terminations covered by a basement membrane. The combination of the terminations and the basement membrane forms the so-called *inner limiting membrane* recognized by light microscopy.

Other processes of the Müller cells make extensive contacts with the walls of blood capillaries. These interesting glial-like cells probably play an important role in supporting the neurons of the retina; possibly they also assist in nourishing the retinal neurons. They may be responsible for the uptake of neurotransmitter substances and electrical insulation of receptors and neurons.

Other glial-like cells, called retinal astrocytes, perivascular glial cells, and microglial cells, have also been described. The retinal microglial cells have a phagocytic function and probably have immunologic functions.

Layers   Traditionally, based on light microscopic findings, the whole retina was said to be composed of 10 layers (Fig. 6-32). These are, from outside inward, as follows:

1. The pigment epithelium	6. The inner nuclear layer
2. The rods and cones	7. The inner plexiform layer
3. The external limiting membrane	8. The ganglion cells
4. The outer nuclear layer	9. The nerve fiber layer
5. The outer plexiform layer	10. The internal limiting membrane

Once the retina was examined with the electron microscope, it was found that no real layers exist. In this account, the different functional components of the retina have been described. However, should the reader wish to identify the composition of the various "layers," he or she ought to consult Fig. 6-32. Note that the outer nuclear layer consists of the nuclei of the rod and cone cells. The outer plexiform layer is made up of the synapses between the terminal processes of the rod and cone cells, the bipolar cells, and the horizontal cells. The inner nuclear layer consists of the nuclei of the bipolar cells, the horizontal cells, the amacrine cells, and the Müller cells. The inner plexiform layer is made up of the synaptic connections between the bipolar, amacrine, and ganglion cells. The ganglion cell layer consists of the nuclei of the ganglion cells. The nerve fiber layer consists of the axons of the ganglion cells that are converging toward the optic disc. The external and internal limiting membranes have been described previously.

Specialized Areas of the Neural Retina

Macula Lutea and Fovea Centralis   As stated previously, the macula lutea is an oval, yellowish area at the center of the posterior part of the retina. It measures about 5 mm in diameter and lies about 3 mm to the lateral side of the optic disc. The yellow coloration of the macula is caused by a yellow carotenoid pigment, *xanthophyll,* which is present in the retinal layers from the outer nuclear layer inward.

The fovea centralis is a depressed area in the center of the macula lutea (Fig. 6-37). It measures about 1.5 mm in diameter. The sides of the depression are called the *clivus*; the floor of the depression, the *foveola*. The depressed area is formed by the nerve cells and fibers of the inner layers of the retina being displaced peripherally, leaving only the photoreceptors in the center. This arrangement permits incoming light to have greater access to the photoreceptors than elsewhere, and this greater accessibility explains in part why this central depressed area has the most distinct vision. There are no blood vessels overlying the fovea and no rod cells in the floor of the fovea. It is here that there is the highest concentration of cones (147,000 per square millimeter). The closeness of packing of the photoreceptors and therefore the angle each subtends ultimately limit the visual acuity obtainable by the retina, and, therefore, the eye.

Optic Disc   The optic disc lies about 3 mm medially to the macula lutea (Fig. 6-38). It is pale pink or almost white and much paler than the surrounding retina. It measures about 1.5 mm in diameter. The edge of the disc is slightly raised, while the central part has a slight depression. It is in this depression that the central retinal vessels enter and leave the eye.

Figure 6-37

Photomicrograph of a section of the retina, showing the fovea centralis. Note there are no blood vessels and no red cells in the floor of the fovea. (H&E; × 200.)

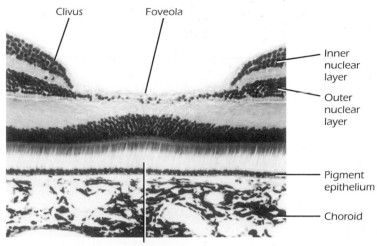

Clivus

Foveola

Inner nuclear layer

Outer nuclear layer

Pigment epithelium

Choroid

Cones

 Figure 6-38

Photomicrograph of a section through the optic disc and the commencement of the optic nerve. The arrow indicates the site of the lamina cribrosa. (H&E; × 52.)

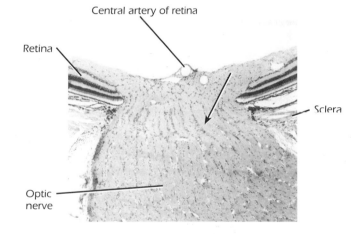

Central artery of retina

Retina

Sclera

Optic nerve

It is at the optic disc that the optic nerve fibers exit the eye by piercing the sclera. This area of the sclera is known as the *lamina cribrosa*. It is a relatively weak area and can be made to bulge out by a rise in pressure inside the eyeball. A rise in cerebrospinal fluid pressure in the meningeal sheath that surrounds the optic nerve may cause the optic disc to bulge into the eyeball. It is believed that the external pressure on the optic nerve impedes the axon flow of its fibers and this causes the optic disc to swell. Posterior to the optic disc, the nerve fibers are myelinated, whereas anterior to the disc they are nonmyelinated. At the optic disc, there is a complete absence of *rods* and *cones*; thus, it is insensitive to light and is referred to as the *blind spot*.

Ora Serrata   The ora serrata is the scalloped anterior margin of the retina. Here the nervous tissues of the retina end (Fig. 6-39). The anterior, nonreceptive part

Figure 6-39

(A) Photomicrograph of a section of the anterior part of the retina, showing the ora serrata. (H&E; × 200.) (B) Photomicrograph of a section of the anterior nonreceptive part of the retina. Note that it consists of a single layer of pigment epithelium, with a deeper layer of nonpigmented columnar epithelium. (H&E; × 400.)

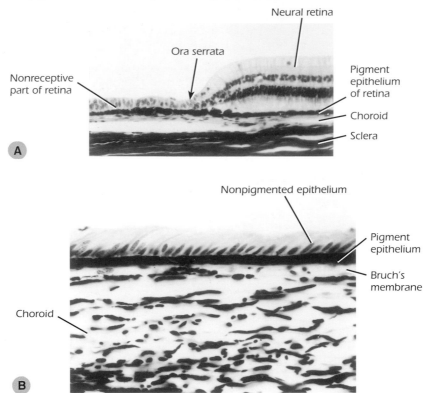

of the retina extends forward from the ora serrata over the ciliary body to the posterior surface of the iris; it consists of a single layer of pigment cells with a deeper layer of nonpigmented columnar epithelium. Recall that on the posterior surface of the iris both layers of cells are pigmented. The ora serrata is about 8.5 mm from the limbus; nasally, it is 1 mm closer to the root of the iris than on the temporal side.

Blood Supply   The blood supply of the retina is from two sources. 1) The outer laminae, including the rods and cones and outer nuclear layer, are supplied by the choroidal capillaries; the vessels do not enter these laminae, but tissue fluid exudes between these cells. 2) The inner laminae are supplied by the central artery and vein. The retinal arteries are anatomic end arteries, and there are no arteriovenous anastomoses. It should be emphasized that the integrity of the retina depends on both of these circulations, neither of which alone is sufficient.

The *choroidal vessels* are described on pages 281 and 282.

Figure 6-40

Diagram showing the arterial supply and venous drainage of the optic disc and optic nerve.

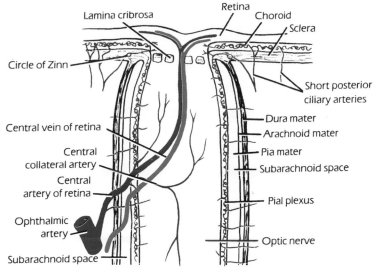

The *central retinal artery* is the first branch of the ophthalmic artery. It measures about 0.3 mm in diameter and runs forward adherent to the dural sheath of the optic nerve. It enters the inferior and medial side of the optic nerve about 12 mm posterior to the eyeball. To do so, it first pierces the dura and arachnoid, from both of which it obtains a covering. It then bends forward within the subarachnoid space (Fig. 6-40). Within a short distance it turns at a right angle and enters the optic nerve by piercing the pia mater. Here again, the artery acquires a sheath derived from the pia mater. On reaching the center of the optic nerve, the artery bends anteriorly, and then, surrounded by a sympathetic plexus and accompanied by the central vein, pierces the lamina cribrosa to enter the eyeball. At this location the posterior ciliary arteries form an anastomotic circle in the sclera around the optic nerve. Small branches from this circle penetrate the choroid to supply the optic disc and the adjacent retina. A number of very small anastomoses occur between the branches of the posterior ciliary arteries and the central retinal artery. Occasionally a larger connection, known as the *cilioretinal artery*, exists between the two arterial systems.

The central artery now divides into two equal superior and inferior branches (Fig. 6-41). After a few millimeters these branches divide dichotomously into superior and inferior nasal and temporal branches. This last division takes place either inside the optic nerve or on the surface of the optic disc. The branches of the central artery and vein emerge from the center of the disc, usually toward the nasal side. The four arteries now supply a quadrant of the retina; there is no overlap, and there is no anastomosis between branches within a quadrant. The nasal branches run a relatively straight course toward the ora serrata, but the temporal branches arch above and below the fovea centralis and then pass to the ora.

Figure 6-41

Left ocular fundus as seen through an ophthalmoscope.

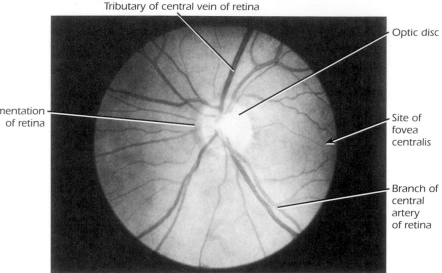

The arterial branches run in the nerve fiber layer close to the internal limiting membrane. It will be remembered that this membrane is the basement membrane of the Müller cells together with their expanded terminations. The membrane is extremely thin and transparent, and this accounts for the fact that the retinal blood vessels can be easily seen with the ophthalmoscope.

The arterioles are distributed throughout the different layers of the neural retina, reaching as far as the internal nuclear layer. There are no arteriolar anastomoses. In structure they resemble arterioles found elsewhere, but the internal elastic lamina is absent and smooth muscle cells occur in the tunica adventitia. The arterioles give rise to a diffuse capillary network whose walls are lined with nonfenestrated endothelial cells. Outside the endothelium are numerous pericytes beneath the endothelial basement membrane. The retinal capillaries form superficial and deep nets but do not extend outside the inner nuclear layer.

The capillary networks are most concentrated in the macula but are absent from the fovea centralis. This capillary free zone, called the *foveal vascular zone*, is approximately 500 μm in diameter. In diabetes mellitus, the diameter of this avascular zone becomes enlarged. At the periphery of the retina the capillaries are less numerous and at the ora serrata they are absent. The arteries of the retina are innervated by sympathetic postganglionic fibers and possibly receive some parasympathetic nerve fibers.

The retina is protected from circulating molecules of large size by the presence of the nonfenestrated endothelium of the capillaries and, as mentioned previously, by the tight junctions at the site of the retinal pigment epithelium.

These two barriers prevent anything except small molecules from entering the milieu of the photoreceptors.

The *central vein of the retina* is formed by tributaries that accompany the arteries (Figs. 6-40 and 6-41). The diameter of the vein is about one-third to one-fourth larger than that of the corresponding artery. The pattern of the veins, although similar, is not identical to that of the arteries. It should be noted that the arteries tend to lie superficial (i.e., toward the vitreal surface) to the veins and thus cross superficial to the veins. The venules arise from the capillary networks and join one another to form the larger superficial retinal veins.

The central vein of the retina leaves the eyeball through the lamina cribrosa accompanied by the central artery. The vein lies on the lateral side of the artery in the optic nerve. The vein crosses the subarachnoid space and has a longer course in the space than the artery (Fig. 6-40). The vein pierces the dural sheath farther from the eyeball than the artery and drains directly into the cavernous sinus or the superior ophthalmic vein.

Blood-Retina Barrier   As in the brain, the neural retina is protected from large molecular toxic substances by a barrier. The outer third of the neural retina is protected by the zonulae occludentes that close off the spaces between the pigment epithelial cells of the pigment layer of the retina. The remainder of the retina that is supplied by the central artery is protected by the zonulae occludentes that close off the spaces between the nonfenestrated endothelial cells of the retinal capillaries.

Lymphatic Drainage   There are no lymphatic vessels in the retina.

Clinical Notes

Detachment of the Retina   The neural retina is firmly attached to the underlying pigment epithelium at the optic disc and the ora serrata. Elsewhere the attachment is weak, and this is especially so in the region just posterior to the ora serrata. It is often erroneously stated that the attachment is particularly weak at the macula. This is not accurate, but unfortunately, for reasons not known, subretinal fluid tends to accumulate in this area.

Three factors normally keep the two parts of the retina in apposition: 1) the negative pressure created by the absorption of fluid between the two parts of the retina; 2) the presence of viscous mucopolysaccharides between the microvilli of the pigment cells and the photoreceptor cells; and 3) it is believed, an electrostatic force existing between the two parts of the retina, causing them to adhere.

The neural retina is susceptible to pathologic separation from the underlying pigment epithelium. This may follow trauma to the eyeball or degenerative changes in the neural retina. Vitreous traction on the retina, or the presence of a hole or a tear, allows accumulation of fluid between the pigment epithelium and the neural retina, causing the layers to be separated or detached. Such a separation represents a reopening of the lumen of the embryonic optic vesicle.

Significance of Blood Supply of the Retina   The outer plexiform layer of the sensory retina divides the neural retina into two halves. The inner vitreal half receives its blood supply from the central retinal artery. The outer half contains no blood vessels and is supplied by the choroid capillaries derived from the ciliary vasculature.

Outer Retinal Degeneration Following Retinal Detachment   Simple retinal detachment causes the separation of the neural retina from the underlying choroidal vascular supply and produces outer retinal degeneration.

Central Retinal Artery Occlusion and Retinal Degeneration   Complete or partial central artery occlusions most commonly occur at the level of the lamina cribrosa just before the artery enters the retina. Here, the central artery has the structure of a medium-sized artery and is subject to atherosclerosis. Once the central artery divides into its four major fundus vessels, these have the structure of an arteriole. Here the arterioles cross internal to the venules, with both vessels enclosed in a common connective tissue sheath. Disease changes in the arteriolar wall can be seen with the ophthalmoscope as a nicking or narrowing of the venous blood column.

In complete central artery occlusion there is a sudden onset of unilateral blindness. In branch arteriole occlusion there is partial loss of sight corresponding to the sector supplied by the arteriole. It has been estimated that total arterial occlusion lasting about $1^1/_2$ hours will produce irreversible retinal degeneration. The changes begin in the inner vitreal half of the retina and are seen clinically as a white discoloration of the fundus. Because normally the vitreal half of the retina is absent from the fovea centralis and the outer half of the foveal retina is nourished by the underlying capillaries of the chorion, this part is unaffected by central artery occlusion and remains as a rounded red area surrounded by a grayish-white discolored retina.

Optic Nerve

The optic nerve for convenience of description may be divided into an orbital part and an intracranial part.

Structure

Orbital Part   The nerve fibers of the optic nerve are the axons of the cells in the ganglionic layer of the retina. They converge on the optic disc and exit from the eye through the lamina cribrosa (Fig. 6-38). The fibers of the optic nerve are nonmyelinated within the eyeball; posterior to the disc, the nerve fibers are myelinated, but the sheaths are formed from oligodendrocytes rather than Schwann cells. This can be explained on the basis that the optic nerve is comparable to a tract within the central nervous system, in that developmentally the optic nerves and the retinae are parts of the brain.

About 1,200,000 myelinated axons make up the optic nerve, the great majority 1 µm in diameter. About 8 percent are larger, measuring from 2 to 10 µm in diameter.

The optic nerve is about 4 cm long and runs backward and medially through the posterior part of the orbital cavity. It then passes through the optic canal in the lesser wing of the sphenoid bone into the cranial cavity and joins the optic chiasma. The optic nerve is surrounded by three meningeal sheaths, which are continuous with those surrounding the brain—the thick, fibrous dura; the thin, delicate arachnoid; and the vascular pia (see Fig. 12-3). At the eyeball all three layers fuse with the sclera. At the optic canal the sheaths are continuous with the corresponding coverings of the brain, and the dural sheath becomes continuous with the meningeal layer of the dura.

The pia mater closely invests the optic nerve, sending into its substance septa that support the nerve fibers and the central artery and vein of the retina (see Fig. 12-3). The subarachnoid space around the brain continues forward as a tubular extension around the optic nerve to the back of the eyeball. As pointed out previously, if the cerebrospinal fluid pressure should rise abnormally, the lamina cribrosa would bulge inward, producing a convex disc as seen through the ophthalmoscope.

The central artery and vein cross the subarachnoid space about 12 mm posterior to the eyeball to enter the optic nerve (Fig. 6-40). Here the vein may be compressed in disorders of raised cerebrospinal fluid pressure, producing retinal venous engorgement and papilledema.

Intracranial Part   The intracranial part of the optic nerve is described in Chapter 13, page 384.

Blood Supply

In the orbital cavity the optic nerve receives arterial branches from the posterior ciliary arteries and the central artery of the retina (Fig. 6-40). The axons on the surface of the optic disc receive their arterial supply from branches of the central artery of the retina. These vessels are reinforced by branches from the partial arterial circle of Haller-Zinn, which is derived from the short posterior ciliary arteries behind the lamina cribrosa.

The venous drainage of the optic nerve is into the central vein of the retina.

Clinical Notes

Structure of the Optic Nerve and Regeneration

The optic nerve may be regarded as an anterior extension of the white matter of the brain. It is made up of approximately one million axons, which arise from the ganglion cells of the neural retina and pass to the lateral geniculate body. Here, they are relayed to the visual cortex. While in the retina the axons are unmyelinated and transparent; on passing through the lamina cribrosa, they become myelinated and white. Because the optic nerve does not possess Schwann cells, it is unable to regenerate.

Meningitis and Optic Perineuritis

The optic nerve, like the brain, is covered by three layers of meninges and is surrounded by an extension of the subarachnoid space. Inflammations of the meninges of the brain can thus spread to those around the optic nerve, causing a perineuritis.

Meningeal Sheath of the Optic Nerve and Cerebrospinal Fluid Pressure

A rise in cerebrospinal fluid pressure can extend to the back of the eyeball, causing a bulging of the optic disc and papilledema. It should be remembered that the optic disc (lamina cribrosa) shows a normal posterior bowing, which should not be confused with a pathologic bowing secondary to glaucoma.

Optic Nerve Head (Optic Disc) and Papilledema

The optic disc, unlike the surrounding retina, does not possess the cells of Müller; these cells hold the nerve fibers together. For this reason, the optic disc easily swells in individuals with papilledema, leaving the surrounding retina flat.

Crescent of Choroid or Sclera at Optic Disc

Sometimes the retina does not quite reach the edge of the optic disc. This leaves a crescent of pigmented choroid that can be easily seen with the ophthalmoscope. In some persons the choroid and the retina do not reach the optic disc and a white scleral crescent can then be seen.

Chambers of the Eyeball

The eye contains two chambers: the anterior chamber and the posterior chamber.

Anterior Chamber

This chamber of the eyeball is a small cavity lying behind the cornea and in front of the iris (Fig. 6-3). It is filled with aqueous humor. Its volume is about 0.2 mL. It measures about 3 mm anteroposteriorly in its central portion.

At the peripheral margin of the anterior chamber is the corner between the cornea, sclera, ciliary body, and iris; this is called the *angle*. It is here that the trabecular meshwork (Fig. 6-42) is located, with its channels for the drainage of the aqueous humor (see p. 152).

It should be noted that the anterior chamber is bounded in front by the cornea and a small area of the sclera. Posteriorly, the chamber is bounded by the anterior surface of the iris, a small area of the anterior surface of the lens exposed by the pupil, and a part of the ciliary body (Fig. 6-42).

Posterior Chamber

This chamber of the eyeball is a small, slitlike cavity. Its volume is about 0.06 mL. The posterior chamber is filled with aqueous humor and communicates through the pupil with the anterior chamber. The posterior chamber (Fig. 6-42) is bounded anteriorly by the iris, peripherally by the ciliary processes, and posteriorly by the lens and the zonule (suspensory ligament).

Aqueous Humor

The aqueous humor is a clear fluid that fills the anterior and posterior chambers of the eyeball (Fig. 6-42). The volume of aqueous in the anterior and posterior chambers is about 0.2 mL.

Formation, Circulation, and Drainage   Constantly in motion, the aqueous is formed by the ciliary processes of the ciliary body in the posterior chamber. This occurs mainly as the result of active transport by the nonpigmented cells of the ciliary epithelia. The process takes place against a concentration gradient and

● **Figure 6-42**

Diagram of the anterior portion of the eye, showing the origin, circulation, and drainage of the aqueous humor.

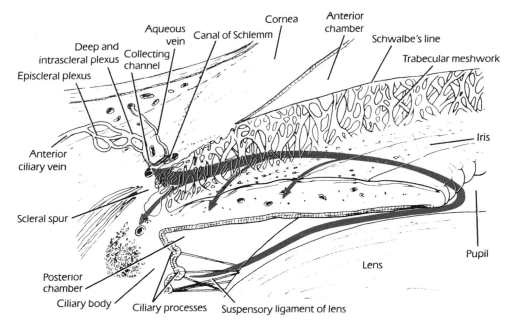

requires cellular energy in the form of adenosine triphosphate. Ultrafiltration of fluid from the capillaries in the ciliary processes across the ciliary epithelia has long been thought to contribute to its formation. However, experimentation has revealed that the hydrostatic forces across the ciliary epithelia favor reabsorption of aqueous into the ciliary processes rather than diffusion out of the processes. The rate of formation of aqueous humor is about 1 to 2 μL per minute. The entire volume of aqueous is replaced every 1 to 2 hours, or about 1 percent per minute.

The aqueous humor flows between the suspensory ligaments of the lens and then through the pupil into the anterior chamber (Fig. 6-42). Ninety percent of the outflow occurs through the passageways of the trabecular meshwork, the sinus venosus sclerae, the collector channels, and the aqueous veins (for details, see p. 154). The remaining 10 percent of the outflow probably occurs through the anterior surface of the ciliary body, where it enters the extracellular spaces and diffuses into the suprachoroidal space to enter the vortical veins. Some of the flow may take place through the scleral fenestra into the vortical veins and some may be absorbed into the choroidal veins and then into the vortical veins. Very small amounts of aqueous may enter the blood vessels of the iris or diffuse through the vitreous to enter the blood vessels of the retina and optic nerve. Diffusion through the cornea is another possible route. It should be emphasized that these accessory drainage pathways are of minimal importance in the normal individual.

Functions   The aqueous humor supplies the metabolic needs of the avascular lens and the cornea. The aqueous contains glucose, amino acids, and high concentrations of ascorbic acid; it also contains dissolved gases. By means of its pressure it supports the wall of the eyeball and maintains its optical shape.

Intraocular Pressure

The normal intraocular pressure is about 10 to 20 mm Hg. This varies slightly with each heartbeat and with respiration. Three chief factors are responsible for maintaining a normal intraocular pressure: 1) the rate of formation of aqueous humor by the cells of the ciliary processes, 2) the rate of drainage of aqueous humor through the trabecular meshwork, and 3) the pressure in the episcleral veins into which the sinus venosus sclerae (canal of Schlemm) drains.

Although many factors can modify the intraocular pressure, normally the pressure varies only momentarily. Fortunately, the structures resisting the pressure, namely, the elasticity of the cornea and the sclera, remain constant.

Clinical Notes

Blood–Aqueous Humor Barrier and Inflammation   The blood–aqueous humor barrier is formed by the zonula occludens of the nonpigmented ciliary epithelium. This barrier can become disrupted by the inflammatory process. The nonfenestrated capillary endothelial cells in the surrounding tissues can also become leaky.

Influence of Age and Disease on Aqueous Drainage   Two areas of resistance to the circulation of aqueous humor normally exist: 1) where the anterior surface of the lens is in contact with the iris, and 2) where the aqueous leaves the anterior chamber to enter the veins.

The iris-lens resistance may increase because of such factors as age, diabetes mellitus, miotics, posterior synechiae, and increased aqueous viscosity caused by hemorrhage or inflammation. The drainage of aqueous from the anterior chamber into the venous system can be inhibited by such factors as age changes in the trabecular meshwork, with thickening of the columns; melanin debris blocking the passages through the meshwork; or corticosteroid administration closing the outflow channels by alteration of acid mucopolysaccharide content of the meshwork.

Glaucoma   In this disease of the eye, the intraocular pressure becomes pathologically high and can lead to blindness. It was briefly discussed earlier in this chapter. The cause of the condition is an obstruction to the aqueous drainage from the anterior chamber.

There are two main forms of glaucoma: *open-angle* and *closed-angle.* In open-angle glaucoma the relationship between the iris root, the trabecular meshwork, and the cornea is normal. However, the drainage resistance is increased as the result of a block in the juxtacanalicular trabecular tissue. This may be caused by a degenerative condition in which the collagen content of the trabecular fibers becomes progressively increased and thus the columns expand and the pores of the meshwork are narrowed. Hemorrhage or macrophage blockage of the passageways can also cause this form of glaucoma.

In closed-angle glaucoma, the iris root is displaced forward, blocking the trabecular meshwork and obstructing the outflow. Many causes can be responsible, including inflammation of the iris, trauma, and hemorrhage.

Refractive Media of the Eye

The refractive media of the eye consist of the cornea, the aqueous humor, the lens, and the vitreous body. The cornea and the aqueous humor have been described.

Lens

The lens is a transparent, biconvex structure situated behind the iris and the pupil and in front of the vitreous body (Fig. 6-3). The convexity of its anterior surface is less than that of its posterior surface (Fig. 6-43). The center points on its anterior and posterior surfaces are referred to as the *anterior and posterior poles*, respectively; a line joining the poles forms the *axis of the lens*; the marginal circumference of the lens is called the *equator*. In the adult the lens measures approximately 10 mm in diameter and 4 mm thick. The equator of the lens is encircled by the ciliary processes of the ciliary body and lies 0.5 mm from them. The lens, which has considerable flexibility, is kept in position by the suspensory ligaments.

The dioptric power of the entire eye is about 58 diopters, with the cornea responsible for most of this refractive ability. The lens contributes only about 15 diopters to the total power. The importance of the lens is that it can change its dioptric power, allowing distant and near objects to be focused on the retina. The range of dioptric power is reduced with age, being about 8 diopters by the age of 40 and only 1 to 2 diopters by age 60. The lens has a refractive index of about 1.36 in the periphery and 1.4 in the inner zone.

The lens continues to grow throughout life, measuring about 6.5 mm in diameter at birth and 10.00 mm in the adult. It also increases in thickness, the thickness possibly reaching 5 mm in the aged.

Structure

The lens is made up of three parts: 1) an elastic capsule, 2) a lens epithelium, which is confined to the anterior surface of the lens, and 3) the lens fibers.

The *capsule* of the lens is an elastic basement membrane that envelops the entire lens (Fig. 6-43). It is thickest on the anterior and posterior surfaces close to the equator, measuring about 20 µm, and thinnest at the posterior pole, measuring about 3 µm. The inner surface of the anterior part of the capsule is in direct contact with the lens epithelium, while posteriorly it contacts the superficial lens fiber cells. The thick basement membrane is formed by the lens epithelium anteriorly and by the superficial lens fibers posteriorly.

Under the light microscope (Figs. 6-44 through 6-47) the capsule has a homogeneous appearance, but with the electron microscope it is seen to consist of 40 lamellae. Each lamella resembles a unit basal lamina and measures about 40 nm. It consists of type IV collagen fibrils embedded in a matrix of glycoproteins and sulfated glycosaminoglycan. According to researchers, the elastic capsule can be stretched up to about 60 percent of its circumference without tearing.

Figure 6-43

(A) Diagram of the lens in equatorial view. (B) Diagram of the lens capsule, showing its areas of thickening. (C) Diagram of a section of adult lens, showing the various lens nuclei within the lens cortex.

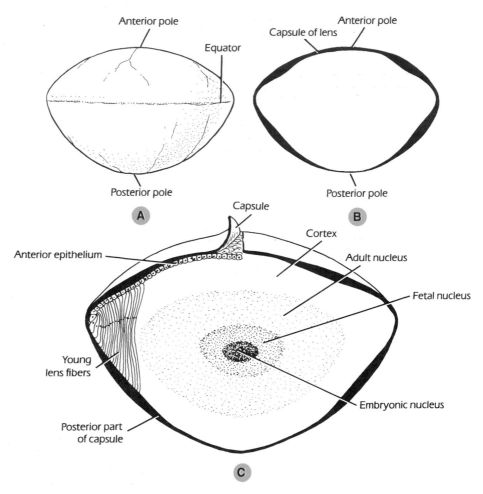

Inserted into the region of the equator are the zonular fibers that connect the lens to the ciliary processes.

The lens capsule serves as a diffusion barrier and is freely permeable to low-molecular-weight compounds but restricts the movement of large colloidal particles. The chief function of the capsule is to mold the shape of the lens in response to the pull of the zonular fibers during accommodation.

The *lens epithelium* is cuboidal and lies beneath the capsule (Fig. 6-45). It is found only on the anterior surface of the lens (Fig. 6-46). At the equator, these cells elongate and form columnar cells, which become arranged in meridional rows

Figure 6-44

(A) Diagram showing the formation of lens fibers from the anterior lens epithelium in the germinal zone at the equator. Note the forward movement of the lens nuclei to form the lens bow. (B) Diagram showing the formation of complicated suture patterns, as more and more lens fibers are produced throughout life.

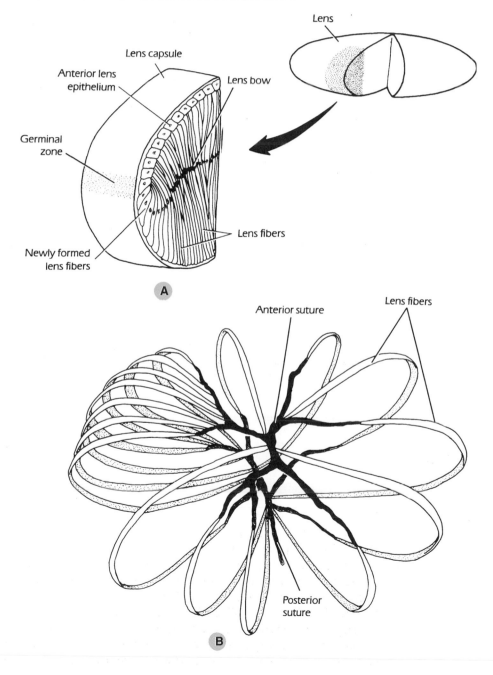

Figure 6-45

Photomicrograph of a section of the anterior portion of the lens, showing the clear capsule and the underlying lens epithelium. The lens fibers that constitute the main mass of the lens are also shown. (H&E; × 500.)

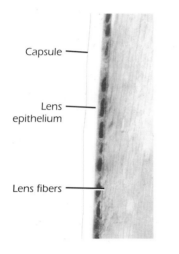

Capsule —

Lens epithelium —

Lens fibers —

 Figure 6-46

Photomicrograph of a section of the posterior portion of the lens, showing the clear capsule and the lens fibers. (H&E; × 1000.)

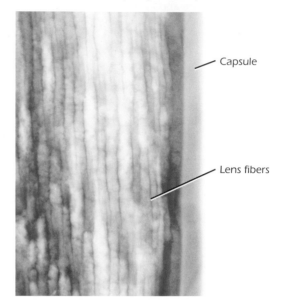

Capsule

Lens fibers

 Figure 6-47

Photomicrograph of a section of the lens close to the equator, showing the anterior lens epithelium and the nuclei of the lens epithelial cells. As the lens epithelial cells elongate, the nuclei disappear and the cells become lens fibers. (H&E; × 800.)

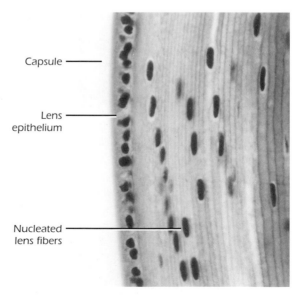

Capsule —

Lens epithelium —

Nucleated lens fibers —

(Fig. 6-47). It is at the equator that the lens epithelial cells become transformed into lens fibers. At the equator lens mitotic activity is at a maximum.

The function of the lens epithelium is mainly twofold. The cells located at the equator are actively dividing and differentiating into lens cell fibers. The remaining, more centrally placed cells are involved in the transport of substances from the aqueous humor to the lens interior, and in the secretion of the capsular material.

The lens *fibers* constitute the main mass of the lens (Fig. 6-46). The fibers are formed by the multiplication and differentiation of the lens epithelial cells at the equator. The lens cell elongates and turns meridionally (Figs. 6-44 and 6-47). As the basal part of the cell elongates, the process moves along the internal surface of the capsule in a posterior direction. As the apical part of the cell elongates, it slips beneath the internal surface of adjacent lens cells. To begin with, the nucleus remains intact, but later it fragments and disappears. This process continues (and does so throughout life); preceding generations of cells are repeatedly pushed into the lens substance. As the cell progressively elongates anteriorly, the nucleus moves anteriorly, so that it takes up a position anterior to the nuclei of the more superficial cells. This anterior movement of the nuclei as the fibers pass deeper produces the nuclear pattern known as the *lens bow* (Fig. 6-44).

Each elongated lens cell is now called a lens fiber. It is a hexagonal prism in cross-section and very long, measuring about 10 mm. The fibers run meridionally from the posterior to the anterior lens surface; they are U-shaped. The earliest formed fibers are those in the center or *nucleus* of the lens; the later fibers form the outer or *cortex* of the lens. In this manner a lens cut on section has a laminated appearance.

It will be remembered that in the fetus (see p. 9) the ends of opposing lens fibers in the same layer abut in a manner producing patterns known as *sutures*. The anterior suture is an erect Y shape, and the posterior is an inverted Y. As the lens increases in size, the lens fibers are unable to stretch the anteroposterior distance, so that progressively more complicated suture patterns are formed (Fig. 6-44).

As the result of this continuous production of lens fibers from the embryonic stage and the progressive internalizing of the fibers, some writers refer to the earliest fiber mass in the center of the lens as the *embryonic nucleus* (Fig. 6-43). This is followed by the *fetal nucleus* with its Y-shaped sutures. Those fibers that are formed after birth constitute the earliest part of the fiber mass known as the *adult nucleus*. The size of the embryonic and fetal nuclei remains constant, while that of the adult nucleus is always increasing. The area surrounding the adult nucleus, containing the recently formed nucleated fibers, is referred to as the *lens cortex* (Fig. 6-43).

The lens fibers have a few small vesicles, microfilaments, microtubules, and an occasional mitochondrion in their cytoplasm. The fibers are tightly packed, there being very little intercellular space. The lens fibers are held together by the interlocking of their adjacent plasma membranes. In some places this takes the form of a tongue-and-groove or ball-and-socket type of interdigitation. It is interesting to note that the interdigitations are less complicated in the superficial zones of the lens, and this may permit molding of the lens shape during accommodation. In addition, the lens fibers exhibit numerous gap junctions—which may explain how deep lens fibers can survive some distance from the surface, and away from a source of nourishment.

During development, the lens fiber cells lose their nuclei and the cytoplasmic organelles become specialized for the production of lens proteins, known as *crystallins*. The crystallins are of at least two types, alpha and beta, and they constitute up to 60 percent of the lens fiber mass. The high refractive index of the lens is due to the crystallins. The differing concentrations of the crystallins in different parts of the lens produce regional differences in the refractive index. This probably compensates for the spherical and chromatic aberrations that might exist if the concentrations of the crystallins were uniform throughout the lens.

The close relationship that exists between the lens epithelial cells and the lens fibers, as seen by the interdigitation of the plasma membranes and the existence of numerous gap junctions, makes the lens a syncytium. This would explain why, from a physiologic point of view, the lens acts like a single cell.

Suspension

The lens is held in position by a series of delicate, radially arranged fibers (Figs. 6-19 and 6-20), collectively known as the *suspensory ligament of the lens*, or *zonule*. The zonule fibers arise from the epithelium of the ciliary processes and run toward the equator of the lens. The fibers fuse to form about 140 bundles. The larger bundles are straight and reach the lens capsule in front of the lens. Together they form the *anterior zonular sheet*.

The smaller fibers curve backward and are attached to the posterior surface of the lens to form the *posterior zonular sheet*. As the zonular fibers reach the lens, they break up into fine fibers that become embedded in the outer part of the lens capsule.

When the eye is at rest, the elastic lens capsule is under tension, causing the lens constantly to endeavor to assume a globular rather than a discoid shape. The equatorial region, or circumference, of the lens is attached to the ciliary processes of the ciliary body by the zonule, as previously noted. The pull of the radiating fibers of the zonule tends to keep the elastic lens flattened, permitting the eye to focus on distant objects.

Accommodation

To accommodate the eye for close objects, the ciliary muscle contracts. The meridional fibers pull the choroid and ciliary body forward, and the circular fibers, acting as a sphincter, move the ciliary body inward. This relieves the tension on the radiating fibers of the zonule. This process allows the elastic lens to assume a more nearly globular shape. At the same time, the sphincter pupillae muscle contracts, so that the pupil becomes smaller and only the light rays going through the thickest, central part of the lens impinge on the retina.

With advancing age, the lens becomes denser and less elastic, and, as a result, the ability to accommodate is lessened (presbyopia).

Clinical Notes   **Age Changes In the Lens**   The lens continues to grow throughout life and does not discard any of its cells. These are continually added to the central portion of the lens as lens fibers, so that the central portion of the lens becomes less pliable and more compact. The lens capsule also increases in thickness with age. It has been estimated that the lens in a subject aged 65 years is one-third larger than that in a 25-year-old subject.

With increasing age, the central portion or nucleus becomes sclerosed and yellowish. The increasing refractive index of the nucleus compensates for the flattening of the lens. The increased density eventually reduces visual acuity. It is important, however, not to confuse this increased density with the onset of cataract.

Cataract   In this condition the lens becomes opaque. Senile cataract is the most common form, and must be distinguished from various degrees of nuclear sclerosis, noted above. The cause of senile cataract is not known. It is characterized by the accumulation of metabolic products within the lens fibers and by a disturbance between the osmotic balance of the lens and the aqueous humor. Other forms of cataract are congenital, those associated with other intraocular diseases, those occurring following ocular trauma, and those associated with systemic diseases, such as diabetes mellitus and scleroderma.

Cataract Surgery   The most commonly performed type of cataract surgery is referred to as *phacoemulsification*. In this procedure, the dense nucleus of the lens is broken up (emulsified) by an ultrasound instrument and the pieces are removed by vacuum.

There are various methods for breaking up the lens, including dividing it into pieces, each of which is then broken up and phacoemulsified; the debris is then vacuumed through the opening in the anterior wall of the lens capsule. Another technique is called "phaco chop" or "stop and chop." In this procedure, the lamellar structure of the lens nucleus is taken advantage of by exerting pressure with a small cleaving instrument, either from the front of the lens or combined with pressure from the back of the lens. By this means the lens is split along its normal fracture lines into smaller pieces, which can then be safely emulsified.

Lens Capsule and Cataract Surgery   Because much of the current cataract surgery is done within the lens capsule and intraocular lenses are inserted within it, a knowledge of the consistency of the capsule, its normal dimensions, and its ability to stretch to accept the intraocular lens is very important clinically.

The resilient nature of the capsule allows a circular piece of the anterior wall to be carefully removed (*capsulorrhexis*). If this procedure is carried out without tearing the capsule (curvilinear continuous capsulorrhexis), it can be safely dilated during the introduction of an intraocular lens.

In the adult, after removal of the lens substance, the capsule collapses and its total diameter increases to approximately 9.5 to 10.5 mm. Following the implantation of a posterior-chamber intraocular lens, the capsule assumes an oval shape with an uneven stretch around its circumference. According to researchers who experimented with human lenses using short- and long-term fixation of post-mortem eyes, the introduction of a lens into the capsule stretches the equator from approximately 10.5 mm to 11.9 mm and the maximum diameter never exceeds 12.0 mm. Furthermore, with the capsule remaining intact and not tearing, it is not possible to stretch the equatorial diameter more than 12.0 mm. Thus, it is feasible to introduce an intraocular lens with a diameter of 12.0 mm into an intact lens capsule by capsulorrhexis and still have stable fixation.

Defects of Refraction

Hypermetropia (Farsightedness)   In this condition, either the eyeball is too short anteroposteriorly or the lens of the eye is not strong enough to bend the light rays sufficiently (Fig. 6-48). In either case, parallel light rays entering the eye cannot come into sharp focus on the retina, and the image falls behind the retina. In order to see a distant object clearly, the hypermetropic, or farsighted, person increases the strength of the lens of the eye by accommodation. Only then can the image be focused on the retina. Such an individual thus is unable to focus on a near object, and hence is called hypermetropic, or farsighted. This condition can be corrected by placing a convex lens in front of the eye, as in the use of eyeglasses (Fig. 6-48).

Myopia (Nearsightedness)   In this condition, the eyeball is too long antero-posteriorly, or, rarely, the lens of the eye is too strong (Fig. 6-48). In either case, parallel light rays entering the eye cannot come into sharp focus in the retina, and the image falls in front of the retina. Such an individual is unable to see a distant object clearly. If the individual moves close to the object, however, the image eventually comes into sharp focus on the retina. The person is myopic, or nearsighted. This condition can be corrected by placing a concave lens in front of the eye in order to diverge the light rays (Fig. 6-48).

Presbyopia   With increasing age, the lens loses its elasticity. As a result, the individual is unable to accommodate for near vision because the lens cannot assume a spherical shape. In order for an older person to see both near and distant objects clearly, bifocal glasses frequently are necessary. The upper part of the lens permits focusing on distant objects, and the lower part of the lens, which is stronger, makes it possible to focus on near objects, such as reading material.

Vitreous Body

The vitreous body fills the eyeball behind the lens (Fig. 6-49). It thus occupies about four-fifths of the eyeball and lies between the lens and the retina. Anteriorly, the vitreous body has a saucer-shaped depression for the lens called the *hyaloid fossa*. The vitreous is a transparent gel having a more dense cortex and a more liquid center.

The cortex of the vitreous is attached at several points around its circumference to neighboring structures. In the region of the pars plana of the ciliary body and the adjacent ora serrata is an attachment that is known as the *vitreous base*. The vitreous is also attached to the neural part of the retina, especially at the margin of the optic disc. Behind the lens, the vitreous is attached to the lens along the periphery of the hyaloid fossa; this attachment is particularly firm in the young and weakens with age.

A narrow channel 1 to 2 mm wide runs forward from the optic disc to the posterior pole of the lens. Its course is usually somewhat curved. This channel is

Figure 6-48

(A) Optics of a simple camera; (B) optics of the eye; (C) parallel light rays focusing behind the retina in hypermetropia; (D) correction of hypermetropia with a convex lens; (E) parallel light rays focusing in front of the retina in myopia; (F) correction of myopia with a concave lens.

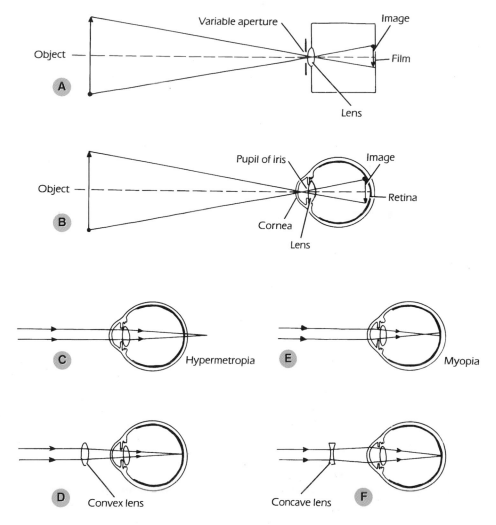

called the *hyaloid canal* and during fetal life it contains the hyaloid artery. The hyaloid artery is a branch of the central artery of the retina, and in the developing eyes it nourishes the lens. The hyaloid artery disappears about 6 weeks before birth, and the canal becomes filled with liquid.

The vitreous is a colorless, transparent gel consisting of 98 percent water. It has a refractive index of 1.33, which is nearly the same as that of aqueous humor. Chemically, the vitreous contains large quantities of hyaluronic acid, amino

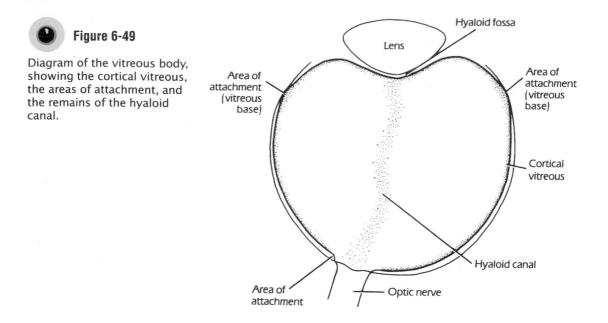

Figure 6-49

Diagram of the vitreous body, showing the cortical vitreous, the areas of attachment, and the remains of the hyaloid canal.

acids, soluble proteins, salts, and ascorbic acid. It possesses an organized network of fine collagen fibrils that form a scaffolding, which can be seen under polarized light. The fine-diameter fibrils are mainly of type II collagen. The cortex of the vitreous contains more collagen than the central region.

Occasional cells called *hyalocytes* that resemble mononuclear phagocytes are present in the cortex; in addition to phagocytosis they are thought to form collagen and to synthesize sodium hyaluronate. A few fibroblasts are also present and they may be involved with collagen synthesis.

Dark-field slit-lamp illumination of the eye has revealed that within the adult human vitreous there are fine parallel fibers coursing in an anteroposterior direction. The fibers are mainly concentrated in the cortex and arise from the vitreous base anteriorly and pass posteriorly. The fibers seen near the hyaloid canal undulate. They are continuous and do not branch and are inserted into the cortex posteriorly. Electron microscopic studies have concluded that the fibrils seen with the slit lamp must in fact be composed of collagen fibrils.

In the past it was customary to state that the vitreous body was bounded by anterior and posterior hyaloid membranes. Electron microscopic examinations have shown these so-called membranes to be merely increased densities of the fiber network at the periphery of the cortex. Such a network blends with the basement membrane of the Müller cells of the retina and the basement membrane of the ciliary epithelial cells.

Age Changes

At adolescence, the vitreous begins to undergo a physical change. There is a decrease in the volume of the gel and an increase in the liquid volume. This process of liquefaction begins in the central vitreous and progresses with age.

The underlying mechanism for vitreous liquefaction is not known but it is thought to be due to an alteration in the hyaluronic acid–collagen interaction. The importance of the liquefaction of the vitreous in relation to retinal detachment is referred to below.

Functions

The vitreous body transmits light and contributes slightly to the dioptric power of the eye. It supports the posterior surface of the lens and assists in holding the neural part of the retina against the pigmented part of the retina. The vitreous probably plays an important role in retinal metabolism by serving as a repository for chemical substances and influencing the movements of solutes and solvents.

Clinical Notes

Detachment of the Vitreous

The vitreous is a hydrogel with an internal scaffolding of collagen fibrils. The cortical region of the vitreous is denser due to the denser collagen network. The network is attached to the retina at the ora serrata and the optic disc. Elsewhere the attachment to the retina is weak, and in pathologic conditions the vitreous is easily detached.

Accumulation of Fluid in the Retrolenticular Space

The hyaloid fossa (patellar fossa) on the anterior surface of the vitreous for the lens shows a potential space between the vitreous and the lens, called the *retrolenticular space*. Blood or exudates can accumulate in this space in pathologic conditions.

Senile Changes in the Vitreous

In the aged the vitreous tends to undergo degeneration and liquefaction. This process may lead to vitreous detachment and predispose to retinal detachment.

CHAPTER 6
Clinical Problems

Answers on Page 210.

1 A 16-year-old boy was making a pipe bomb in his basement when it suddenly exploded. On examination in the emergency room, it was found that his right eye had been severely damaged, with perforation and prolapse of intraocular tissue. Because of the extensive prolapse of the retina and the poor prognosis for recovery of vision in that eye, the ophthalmologist decided to enucleate the eye. What anatomic structure in the orbit is preserved to form a socket for the prosthesis? Following the operation, will the globe be able to move naturally by the extraocular muscles? What is meant by the terms *suspensory ligaments* and *check ligaments*?

2 Discussing the operations to correct strabismus with a fourth-year medical student, an ophthalmologist was asked whether the superior and inferior recti or the oblique muscles are ever operated on for the condition. The ophthalmologist replied that, although the medial and lateral recti are the commonest muscles to be shortened or lengthened in this condition, sometimes it may be necessary to operate on the other muscles. However, the fascial relationships for the inferior rectus and the inferior oblique muscles make the operation difficult. What is the name of the fascia that is closely related to the inferior rectus and the inferior oblique muscles?

In reattachment of the tendons of the recti to the eyeball in operations for the correction of strabismus, is the sclera thick or thin in this situation?

3 When performing surgical incisions into the sclera, does the surgeon have to worry about wound healing in a relatively avascular structure?

4 A 45-year-old man is walking along a street when he passes some workers digging a hole in the road. A gust of wind blows some dirt into the air, and suddenly the man experiences an acute, stabbing pain in his left eye. Although he blinks his eyes vigorously for several minutes, the pain persists. Because of the severity of the pain and excessive lacrimation, the man immediately goes to the emergency room of a local hospital. On examination of the cornea with a slit lamp, the ophthalmologist can identify a small abraded area where the corneal epithelium is missing. Does the cornea heal quickly? Describe the structure and function of the cornea. How does the cornea receive its nourishment? Is the cornea resistant to most infections?

5 An 80-year-old woman visited her ophthalmologist for a routine check-up. What changes normally occur in the cornea with age? What is arcus senilis? What are Hassall-Henle bodies?

6 If a surgical incision is made between the transparent bluish cornea and the white sclera at the limbus, where will the knife enter the eyeball relative to the canal of Schlemm?

7 Define the uveal tract and describe its blood supply. What part does the uveal tract play in the nourishment of the retina?

8 An inflammation of the ciliary body and iris may give rise to a so-called ciliary injection. Describe the arteries that give rise to the ciliary injection.

9 What is meant by the terms *blood-retina barrier* and *blood–aqueous humor barrier*?

10 Describe the normal ophthalmoscopic appearances of a) the macula, b) the optic disc, and c) the retinal arteries and veins.

11 An 88-year-old man suddenly experiences complete blindness of his right eye. The diagnosis is central retinal artery occlusion. Describe the blood supply of the neural retina.

12 The optic nerve is said to be an outward extension of the white matter of the brain. Explain that statement. What part do the coverings of the optic nerve play in the production of papilledema in patients with raised intracranial pressure?

13 Describe in detail the formation, circulation, and drainage of the aqueous humor. Where do areas of resistance to the drainage normally occur? What is the difference between open-angled and closed-angled glaucoma?

14 Name the different refractive media of the eye. Give the approximate normal dioptric power of each structure.

15 Explain in detail the mechanisms involved in accommodating the eye. Describe the histologic structure of the lens. Explain how the lens structure changes with age. Define the embryonic nucleus, the fetal nucleus, and the adult nucleus of the lens.

16 Describe the structure of the vitreous and explain where it is strongly attached to the neural retina. What senile changes normally occur in the vitreous, and how may these predispose to retinal detachment?

17 What factors are responsible for keeping the neural and pigmented layers of the retina in apposition?

18 Explain why an individual suffering from hypermetropia needs convex lenses, whereas a myopic individual requires concave lenses.

19 Explain the problem of presbyopia. What is structurally responsible for the lens losing its elasticity in old age?

20 Describe the structure of the iris. What is responsible for its color? What is the innervation of the sphincter and dilator pupillae muscles?

CHAPTER 6
Answers to Clinical Problems

1 The fascial sheath of the eyeball (fascial bulbi, Tenon's capsule) is preserved to form a socket for the prosthesis. Because the extraocular muscles have fascial sleeves that are continuous with the sheath of the eyeball, the socket will move when the muscles contract.

The suspensory ligament is a hammock-like thickening of the inferior part of the fascial sheath of the eyeball. It is attached by means of the medial and lateral check ligaments to the lacrimal and zygomatic bones.

The medial and lateral check ligaments are expansions of the tubular sheaths of the medial and lateral recti muscles. They are strong and are attached, as noted above, to the lacrimal and zygomatic bones (see p. 133). Since these expansions may limit the actions of these muscles on the eyeball, they are called medial and lateral check ligaments.

2 The portion of the fascial sheath of the eyeball that is closely related to the inferior rectus and the inferior oblique muscles is thickened inferiorly to form the suspensory ligament, as noted previously. This thickened ligament receives contributions from the fascia covering the inferior rectus and the inferior oblique muscles as they cross each other below the eyeball. The presence of these fascial septa sometimes makes the freeing up of these two muscles difficult surgically.

The sclera varies in thickness in different parts of the eyeball. It is particularly thin in the region where the recti tendons are attached (about 0.3 mm or less).

3 No, the surgeon does not have to worry. Even though the blood supply to the scleral stroma is poor, the episclera or outer layer of the sclera has a rich blood supply from the anterior and the posterior ciliary arteries. This excellent blood supply ensures that rapid healing occurs.

4 Abrasions of the cornea heal quickly unless complicated by infection. The cornea consists of five layers: 1) the corneal epithelium, 2) Bowman's membrane, 3) the substantia propria, 4) Descemet's membrane, and 5) the endothelium. The structure of the cornea is described on page 143.

The cornea is the most important refractive medium of the eye. The refractive power occurs on the anterior surface of the cornea, where the refractive index is 1.38.

The cornea receives its nourishment by diffusion from the aqueous humor and from the capillaries at its edge. The central part of the cornea receives its oxygen directly from the air, whereas the peripheral part receives its oxygen by diffusion from the anterior ciliary blood vessels at the corneal margin.

The cornea is very resistant to infection. It is sensitive, however, to gonococcus, *Chlamydia trachomatis*, herpes simplex, and herpes zoster.

5 The following structural changes commonly take place in the cornea with age: 1) The cornea becomes less translucent, and dustlike opacities, due to condensation in the stroma, may occur in the deeper parts of the stroma; 2) Bowman's and Descemet's membranes increase in thickness; and 3) Hassall-Henle bodies appear at the periphery of Descemet's membrane (see p. 147).

Arcus senilis consists of white arcs that appear superiorly and inferiorly in the cornea and ultimately form a complete circle.

There is left a clear interval of 1 mm between the arcs and the limbus. The condition is due to an infiltration of extracellular lipid in the corneal stroma.

Hassall-Henle bodies occur in the aged as small protrusions at the periphery of Descemet's membrane (for details, see p. 147).

6 A surgical incision made along the posterior border of the cornea will enter the anterior chamber in front of the canal of Schlemm.

7 The uveal tract, or vascular pigmented coat, consists from back to front, of the choroid, the ciliary body, and the iris.

The profuse blood supply of the uveal tract is derived from the anterior ciliary arteries and from the long and short posterior ciliary arteries. All these arteries are branches of the ophthalmic artery. A major arterial circle located in the stroma of the ciliary body is formed from the two long posterior ciliary arteries and the seven anterior ciliary arteries. Radial branches arise from the major arterial circle to converge toward the pupillary margin of the iris. Here, they anastomose to form an incomplete minor arterial circle.

The pigmented layer of the retina and the outer laminae of the neural retina, including the rods and cones and the outer nuclear layer, are supplied by the choroidal capillaries. The vessels do not enter these laminae, but tissue fluid exudes between the cells. It should be remembered that the inner laminae of the neural retina are supplied by the central artery of the retina.

8 Ciliary injection is a clinical condition in which the blood vessels of the deep episcleral pericorneal plexus (see p. 113) become dilated. The plexus is fed by branches of the anterior ciliary arteries. In the normal eye the plexus can only just be seen. Inflammation involving the ciliary body and iris can cause ciliary injection.

9 Blood-retina barrier. The pigment epithelial cells of the retina are joined to each other by zonulae occludentes or tight junctions, which completely encircle the cells. This arrangement forms a barrier that limits the flow of ions and prevents the diffusion of large toxic molecules from the choroid capillaries to the photoreceptors of the neural retina. The remainder of the retina that is supplied by the central artery is protected by the zonulae occludentes that close off the spaces between the endothelial cells of the capillaries.

The blood–aqueous humor barrier is formed by the zonula occludens that exists between the nonpigmented ciliary epithelial cells. They encircle the cells, closing off the intercellular space. It should be pointed out that the above barriers may be disrupted by inflammatory processes.

10 The macula lutea is an oval, yellowish area at the center of the posterior part of the retina. It measures about 4.5 mm in diameter and lies about 3 mm to the lateral side of the optic disc. The macula lutea shows a central depression called the fovea centralis.

The optic disc is a round, pale pink area that lies about 3 mm medial to the macula lutea. It measures about 1.5 mm in diameter. The edge of the disc is slightly raised, while the central part has a slight depression, from which emerge the central retinal vessels. Sometimes the retina does not quite reach the edge of the optic disc, and this leaves a crescent of pigmented choroid around the disc.

The branches of the central retinal arteries and veins can easily be studied with the ophthalmoscope. The arteries tend to lie superficial, i.e., toward the vitreal surface, of the veins and thus cross superficial to the veins. The diameter of the veins is about one-third to one-fourth larger than that of the corresponding artery. The branches of the central retinal artery are described on page 189.

Although the tributaries of the central vein of the retina accompany the arteries, the pattern is not identical to that of the arteries.

11 The blood supply of the neural retina is from two sources. 1) The outer laminae, including the rods and cones and the outer nuclear layer, are supplied from the choroidal capillaries. 2) The inner laminae are supplied by the central artery of the retina (see p. 189).

The retinal arteries are anatomic end arteries and there are no arteriovenous anastomoses. The integrity of the retina depends on both of the above circulations, neither of which alone is sufficient.

12 The optic nerve may be regarded as an outward extension of the white matter of the brain. The eye develops as a diverticulum from the lateral aspect of the forebrain (see Chap. 1) and the optic vesicle and optic stalk are formed. Later, the optic vesicle becomes the optic cup. The inner layer of the cup gives rise to the ganglion cells of the neural retina, which send axons into the optic stalk. The cells of the optic stalk differentiate into supporting cells so that oligodendrocytes are formed. The oligodendrocytes are responsible for the myelination of the optic nerve axons, as they are responsible for myelination of the axons in the white matter of the brain. Thus, the development and structure of the optic nerve are very similar to those of the white matter of the central nervous system. Moreover, the optic nerve reacts to injury in the same manner as white matter, in that it does not regenerate.

The optic nerve is surrounded by the three meninges of the brain, which extend forward in the orbit to fuse with the sclera at the back of the eyeball. There is thus a tubular extension of the subarachnoid space to the lamina cribrosa. Crossing the space to enter the optic nerve are the thin-walled central retinal vein and the thick-walled central artery. A rise in cerebrospinal fluid pressure will compress the vein, causing edema of the retina and engorgement of the veins. In addition, the axon flow of the optic nerve fibers will be impeded by external pressure on the optic nerve and will cause the optic disc to bulge into the eye. By this mechanism the signs of papilledema are established.

13 A detailed description of the formation, circulation, and drainage of the aqueous humor is given on page 194. The areas offering resistance to the circulation are 1) where the lens is in contact with the posterior surface of the iris, and 2) where the aqueous leaves the anterior chamber to enter the veins. For details, see page 195. In open-angle glaucoma, the relationship between the iris root, the trabecular meshwork, and the cornea is normal. The block in the circulation is occurring in the drainage system (see p. 196).

In closed-angle glaucoma, the iris root is displaced forward and blocks the trabecular meshwork, thus obstructing the outflow (see p. 196).

14 The refractive media of the eye consist of the cornea, the aqueous humor, the lens, and the vitreous body. The dioptric power of the entire eye is about 58 diopters. The lens contributes only about 15 diopters, and most of the remainder is provided by the cornea.

15 Accommodation of the eye is described in detail on page 202. For the structure of the lens, see page 197.

The lens continues to grow throughout life, and the central portion becomes less pliable and more compact. The lens eventually becomes yellowish and the increased density eventually reduces visual acuity. The lens capsule also increases in thickness with age.

The term *embryonic nucleus* refers to the earliest fibers found in the center of the lens during embryonic development. Later, as new additional fibers are formed, and the development of Y-shaped sutures occurs, the nucleus is referred to as the *fetal nucleus.* After birth, when additional lens fibers are added, the central mass is referred to as the *adult nucleus.*

16 The structure of the vitreous is described on page 204. The vitreous body is strongly attached to the retina at the pars plana of the ciliary body, the ora serrata, and the optic disc. In the aged, the vitreous tends to undergo degeneration and liquefaction, and this may lead to vitreous detachment and thus predispose the patient to retinal detachment.

17 Three factors normally keep the neural and pigmented layers of the retina in apposition: 1) the negative pressure created by the absorption of fluid between the two parts of the retina, 2) the presence of viscous mucopolysaccharides between the microvilli of the pigment cells and the photoreceptor cells, and 3) the presence of an electrostatic force between the two parts of the retina that causes them to adhere.

18 The anatomy and light physics associated with hypermetropia and myopia are discussed on page 204.

19 Presbyopia is discussed on page 204. The continuous production of new lens fibers throughout life, and the fact that none are discarded, results in the central part of the lens becoming more compact and less pliable. The lens capsule also increases in thickness, but its rigidity is not the cause of presbyopia.

20 The structure of the iris is described on page 166. The melanin pigment granules in the melanocytes are responsible for its color. The effect of melanin pigment on the absorption of light of different wavelengths is discussed on page 165.

The sphincter pupillae is innervated by parasympathetic postganglionic fibers from the ciliary ganglion. This pathway originates in the Edinger-Westphal nucleus of the oculomotor nerve. The dilator pupillae is innervated by postganglionic sympathetic fibers from the superior cervical sympathetic ganglion.

The Anatomy of the Eyeball as Seen with the Ophthalmoscope, Slit Lamp, and Gonioscope

CHAPTER OUTLINE

The Direct Ophthalmoscope ·

The ophthalmoscope permits an observer to view another person's fundus with clarity. The retina of the patient's eye is illuminated with a bright source of light (Fig. 7-1). Light rays from the illuminated spot on the retina pass through the lens system of the patient's eye and emerge parallel with each other. These parallel rays then pass through the lens system of the observer's eye and come to focus on the observer's retina.

If the refractive powers of the patient's or the observer's eyes are abnormal, it is necessary to correct this refractive error. The ophthalmoscope has a series of about 20 lenses mounted on a turret that can be rotated until a lens of appropriate strength has been placed between the patient's and the observer's eyes.

The patient should fix his eye on a distant object. The view of the fundus is magnified 16 times and is erect. A satisfactory examination of the disc and posterior pole of the fundus can usually be made through an undilated pupil, provided that there are no opacities in the aqueous, lens, or vitreous. A better examination of the peripheral fundus can be performed through a dilated pupil. The examination is best undertaken in a darkened room.

Red Reflex

On looking through the ophthalmoscope, holding it about 1 foot away from the patient, the examiner notes that the fundus has a red appearance (Fig. 7-2). The fundus shows red because the light is being reflected back from the blood in the choroidal blood vessels, the intervening retina being transparent. Absence of the red reflex means either there is an opacity in the refractive media or the retina is not against the choroid. The possible opacities include a cataract, a vitreous hemorrhage, and a detached retina.

Figure 7-1

The optical system of the direct ophthalmoscope.

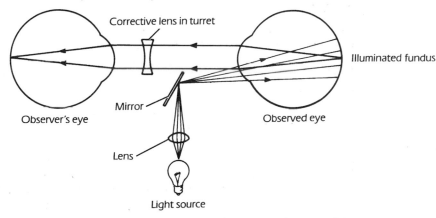

Figure 7-2

Left ocular fundus.

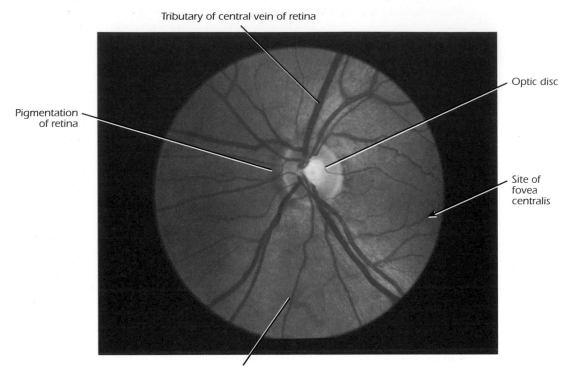

Tributary of central vein of retina

Optic disc

Pigmentation of retina

Site of fovea centralis

Branch of central artery of retina

Examination of the Normal Fundus

For this examination to be carried out successfully, the observer's eye and the ophthalmoscope must be placed as close as possible to the patient's eye. Preferably, both the examiner and the patient should be sitting. Without pupillary dilatation only about 15 percent of the fundus can be seen. With full dilation, about 50 percent of the fundus can be viewed, but the area between the equator and the ora serrata cannot be seen. In the descriptions given below we shall assume that the patient's pupil is widely dilated.

Optic Disc

This structure is circular or vertically oval with a vertical orientation (Fig. 7-2). The color is pink, with the temporal side slightly lighter than the nasal side. The disc measures about 1.5 mm in diameter and can be used as the unit of measurement. The center of the disc has a pale, almost white depression called the *physiologic cup.* The edge of the disc is usually flat and sharply defined, but the temporal edge is usually more distinct than the nasal edge. In some individuals, where the retina does not quite reach the margin of the disc, an arc or concentric ring of choroidal pigment may be visible. A common clinical observation in myopia is the presence of a white crescent on the temporal side of the disc, because the retina and choroid do not quite reach the disc on that side. Sometimes both the sclera and choroid are visible as arcs or rings around the optic disc.

The physiologic cup may have grayish areas in its base produced by the lamina cribrosa. Sometimes the bottom of the cup cannot be visualized. The location of the cup relative to the disc varies; the cup may be central or to one side, but normally it is completely surrounded by a rim of disc tissue.

The bright red central artery of the retina becomes visible on the disc surface emerging from the optic cup. Here, it divides into its superior and inferior branches. The arteries do not normally pulsate. The darker red main tributaries of the central vein of the retina pass into the cup and unite in the cup or deeper out of sight within the optic nerve.

Retinal Arteries and Veins

The arteries are bright red; the veins, darker red (Fig. 7-2). The arteries are smaller than the veins in about a 3 : 4 ratio. The arteries have thicker walls, which reflect the light as a shiny central reflex stripe. The walls of the arteries and the veins are transparent, so that the examiner observes a moving column of blood. The arteries usually cross the veins on their superficial or vitreal surface, and normally the arteries do not compress or nick the veins at the site of crossing. The branching of the vessels is variable.

Macula

The macular area lies about 2 disc diameters (2 d) on the temporal side of the optic disc (Fig. 7-2). It is darker than the surrounding retina. The superior and inferior temporal blood vessels arch above and below the macular area and no blood vessels are visible in the center of the macula. The center of the macula shows a small, dark red area called the *fovea centralis*. A small *white yellow light reflex* can be detected at the center of the fovea, caused by the reflection of the ophthalmoscope light from the concavity of the fovea.

Periphery of the Fundus

With the patient's pupil widely dilated, the peripheral fundus can be seen up to the equator. The patient has to be instructed to move the eyeball in the appropriate direction so that each quadrant of the retina can be brought into view.

Clinical Notes

Color of the Fundus

The color of the fundus depends on the melanin content of the retinal pigment epithelium, the melanin content of the melanocytes in the choroidal stroma, and the hemoglobin in the choroidal and retinal vasculature. The melanin contribution to the color parallels the complexion of the patient's skin and hair, the fundus being darker in black races and lighter in whites.

Macula

In some whites the macula is difficult to see, whereas in brunets and blacks it is easily located as a dark area. The fovea centralis also varies in appearance, and this depends on its depth. In a shallow fovea and with increasing age the foveal reflex is absent.

Retinal Vasculature

The blood vessels show wide variations in appearance. One of the common variations is the presence of arteries that run from the temporal aspect of the disc to the macular area. These cilioretinal vessels originate from the circle of Zinn, which is formed around the optic nerve in the sclera from the short posterior ciliary arteries. They are anastomoses between the ciliary arteries, that is, the choroidal circulation, and that of the retina.

Embryonic Remnant of the Hyaloid Artery

When present, this structure is seen as a small tuft of connective tissue arising from the nasal side of the optic disc and projecting forward into the vitreous. Although it may give the edge of the disc a blurred appearance, it does not interfere with vision.

Myelination of the Optic Nerve Fibers

Normally, the optic nerve fibers are not myelinated until they reach the lamina cribrosa (see p. 403) as they exit from the eyeball. Occasionally some of the fibers start their myelination early and are seen as white feathery patches near the optic disc.

Drusen

Drusen, small round hyaline bodies formed on Bruch's membrane of the choroid, may be seen. They can occur as yellow lesions anywhere in the fundus and may be associated with aging. Large, confluent drusen in the macula may predispose the patient to age-related macular degeneration.

The Slit Lamp

The slit lamp consists of two parts, a low-power binocular microscope mounted horizontally and an illumination system (Figs. 7-3 and 7-4). The illumination system consists of a bright source of light, a condenser lens, a narrow variable slit, and a projecting lens. The aperture of the slit serves as the object and provides an illuminated image in the observed eye. The image can be viewed by the microscope from either side of the narrow beam of light. The purpose of the slit lamp is to permit the observer to examine the transparent media of the eye, that is, the cornea, the aqueous humor, the lens, and the vitreous. The narrow beam provides an optical section of the transparent structures, which can be distinguished from one another by their differences in optical density. The result, a unique

Figure 7-3

The optical system of the slit-lamp biomicroscope.

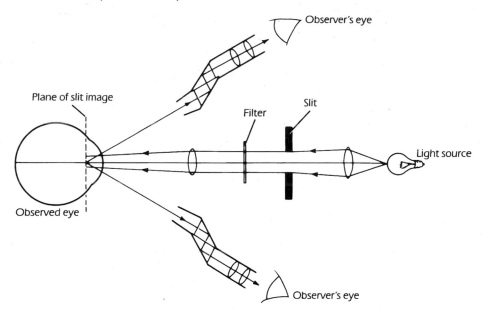

Figure 7-4

The slit-lamp biomicroscope in use.

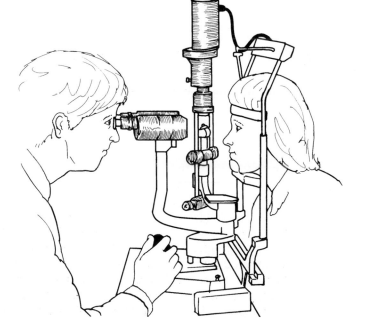

histologic section of living tissue, brought Gullstrand, the inventor of the slit lamp, the Nobel Prize in 1911.

The examiner and patient are seated on either side of the slit lamp, the patient steadying his head by placing his chin on a chin rest and his forehead against a support (Fig. 7-4). The examiner then views the eye through the binocular microscope. The examiner may alter the depth of focus so that the tissue that is of interest comes clearly into view. This is accomplished by moving the microscope in or out with a hand control. The examiner usually views first the eyelids and conjunctiva, followed by the cornea, anterior chamber, iris and pupil, lens, and anterior part of the vitreous body.

Eyelid Margin

With the slit-lamp beam widened to a full circle to illuminate the front of the eye, the eyelid margins are examined, with note made of the anterior and posterior borders. The anterior rounded border shows the eyelashes projecting in two or three rows (see Fig. 8-23). There should be no scaling, as seen in squamous blepharitis. The posterior border is sharp and resting against the eyeball. The examiner must observe the small orifices of the tarsal glands just in front of the lid margin, and the lacrimal papilla, in the center of which is the punctum lacrimale. The tear fluid can be seen as a lake nasally draining into the inferior punctum. On the medial side of the papilla there are no eyelashes and no tarsal glands; here the lid margins are rounded, with no sharp anterior or posterior borders.

Conjunctiva

Palpebral Conjunctiva

This structure is seen by everting the eyelids (see Fig. 8-23). It is a thin, transparent mucous membrane lining the inner surface of the eyelid. Within the conjunctiva can be seen a fine, subepithelial vascular network with large vessels running at right angles to the lid margin; these are branches of the palpebral (tarsal) arches (see p. 101). Within the tarsal plates the yellowish ducts of the tarsal (meibomian) glands are easily seen.

Bulbar Conjunctiva

This structure is examined by holding the lids open and asking the patient to look to the right, to the left, up, and down. Here, again, the conjunctiva is seen as a thin, transparent mucous membrane, only loosely adherent to the underlying bulbar fascia and the sclera. It is most tightly adherent to the sclera as a narrow band at the corneoscleral limbus. A superficial, bright red system of anastomosing vessels can be easily identified in the conjunctiva. These vessels move with the conjunctiva and can be made to constrict on instillation of 2.5 percent Neosynephrine. More careful examination reveals a deeply placed reddish-blue episcleral network of vessels. These vessels do not move with the conjunctiva.

A delicate, vertical fold of conjunctiva, the *plica semilunaris*, separates the bulbar conjunctiva from the *lacrimal caruncle* at the medial canthus (see Fig. 8-23).

Cornea

When the slit-lamp beam passes through the cornea, it is possible to recognize the anterior and posterior surfaces and the corneal stroma (Fig. 7-5). The anterior surface corresponds to the corneal epithelium; the posterior surface corresponds to the endothelium. The corneal stroma reflects some light and has a milky, reticular appearance. If the microscope is angled slightly, the light can be seen reflecting from the anterior and posterior surfaces. The anterior epithelium is smooth and translucent, and on it the examiner can make out mucus in the precorneal tear film. The posterior endothelial cells are yellowish in color and hexagonal in shape. Bowman's and Descemet's membranes are normally invisible, although in the aged the Hassall-Henle bodies of Descemet's membrane may be recognized as dark areas near the limbus.

Figure 7-5

The structure of the cornea and lens as seen with a slit-lamp biomicroscope. (A) The slit beam of light entering the eye. (B) The lens of an adult. (C) The cornea. Note that the slit beam of light produces a narrow section of the anterior segment of the eye, which throws the different anatomic components into relief.

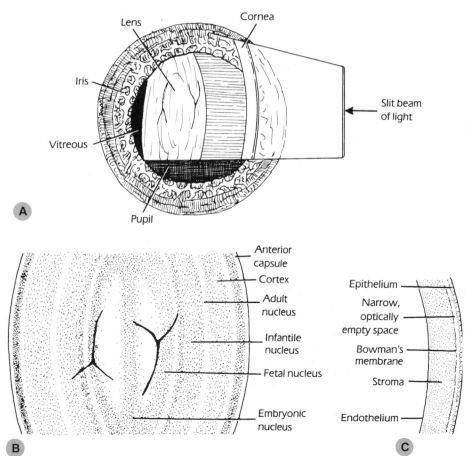

At the limbus, vascular loops that are derived from the conjunctiva and sclera can be made out at the edge of the transparent area. It is difficult to distinguish veins from arteries except by fluorescein angiography. The corneal nerves can be recognized as straight, whitish filaments with acute bifurcations in the anterior and middle layers of the cornea. They are most easily identified at the limbus, where they are larger and still possess their myelin sheath.

Aqueous Humor

Normally, the anterior chamber filled with aqueous appears optically empty and black (Fig. 7-5). If the slit beam is narrowed to a fine pencil of light, a very faint relucence can be made out along the course of the light.

Lens

When the slit-lamp beam passes through the lens, the anterior and posterior surfaces reflect light brightly (Fig. 7-5). The interior of the lens is made up of a number of discontinuity zones, some of which are brighter than others. In the adult, the lens usually has ten such bands. In the center of the lens the fetal nucleus can be identified as two planoconvex lenses with a central dark interval. This dark interval is the area of the lens that has the least optical density.

Anterior and posterior to the fetal nucleus are the anterior Y-shaped suture and the posterior inverted–Y–shaped suture (Fig. 7-5). If the beam is moved from the fetal nucleus into the adult nucleus, the sutures become increasingly branched and complicated.

The remains of the *hyaloid artery* can occasionally be recognized as a spiral structure attached to the lens near its posterior pole.

Vitreous Body

Without additional aids, the slit lamp can be used to visualize only the anterior third of the vitreous. Immediately posterior to the lens is a narrow black band, the so-called posterior lenticular space, which is devoid of structure. The cortex of the vitreous cannot be identified. Delicate, thin, wavy folds with a milky appearance can be identified within the vitreous. These filmy folds appear to be suspended in a black, optically empty space. The folds represent the fibrils present within the vitreous. In the vitreous of aged subjects, other condensations can be seen; these are thought to represent areas of degeneration. Floaters and liquefaction of the vitreous gel are particularly common in myopia.

Clinical Notes

Eyelid Margin and Conjunctiva

Notes on the clinical relevance of the anatomy of these tissues have been discussed elsewhere (see p. 105).

Figure 7-6

(A) Diagram showing that structures present in the corneoiridial angle cannot be viewed directly from outside the eye because of the opaque sclera or the internal reflection at the corneal aqueous interface. (B) Diagram showing how a gonio-prism cancels out the refractive power of the cornea, permitting structures in the corneoiridial angle to be viewed from outside the eye.

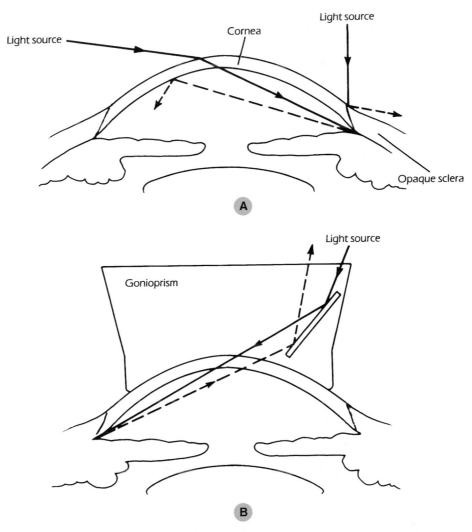

Corneal and Lens Diseases

The development of opacities and other local pathologic lesions in these structures can easily be recognized by using the slit lamp. Remains of the pupillary membrane can sometimes be seen as delicate, star-shaped pigment dots on the anterior surface of the lens capsule near the center. More commonly, grayish threads of remnants originate from the iris collarette.

Anterior Chamber Diseases

Normally, the anterior chamber filled with aqueous humor appears optically empty and black. The presence of inflammatory cells or increased protein content of the aqueous secondary to intraocular inflammation results in the narrow slit-lamp beam becoming visible, and the normal aqueous flare is accentuated. The intensity of the flare may be measured by a subjective rating of trace to 4+ by the observer.

Vitreous Body Diseases

Inflammatory cells in the vitreous may become visible by using the narrow beam of the slit lamp as paraxially as possible.

Gonioscopy

The angle of the anterior chamber of the eye cannot be seen by direct inspection because of the anteriorly advanced opaque sclera and the corneoscleral limbus (Fig. 7-6). Also, light rays arising from the angle undergo total internal reflection on reaching the curved surface of the cornea. The use of a special contact lens, a source of focal illumination, and a microscope or slit lamp makes the angle accessible. The contact lens eliminates the corneal curve and allows light to be reflected from the angle. Gonioscopy may be performed with the patient seated or recumbent.

Figure 7-7

The angle of the anterior chamber as seen with a gonioscope.

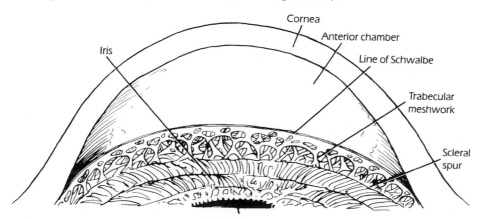

Figure 7-8

(A) Normal gonioscopic view of the eye. (B) Enlargement of an area of trabecular meshwork showing evenly spaced laser burns (arrows) in a patient with open-angle glaucoma. Laser trabeculoplasty is used in patients with open-angle glaucoma that is uncontrolled with medical treatment. The procedure successfully lowers the intraocular pressure by improving the aqueous outflow.

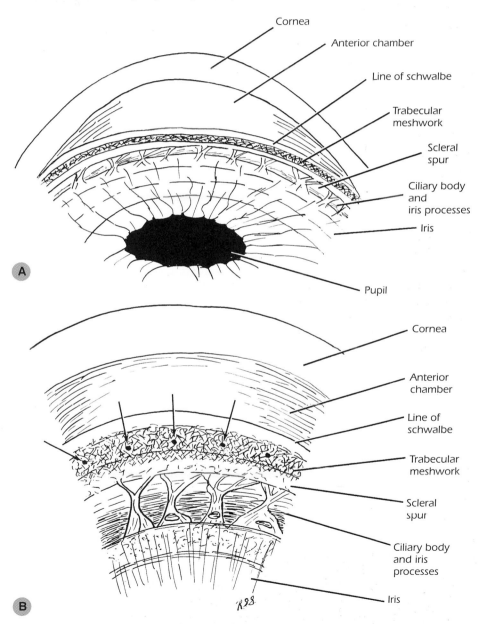

Cornea

Anterior chamber

Line of schwalbe

Trabecular meshwork

Scleral spur

Ciliary body and iris processes

Iris

Pupil

A

Cornea

Anterior chamber

Line of schwalbe

Trabecular meshwork

Scleral spur

Ciliary body and iris processes

Iris

B

Anterior Chamber Angle Examination

The angle formed by the root of the iris, the anterior border of the ciliary body, the trabecular meshwork, and the cornea can be studied (Fig. 7-7). Evaluation of the angle width (distance between the iris root and the trabecular meshwork) is important in distinguishing among open-angle, narrow-angle, angle closure, and secondary angle closure glaucoma (Fig. 7-8). The gonioscope is also useful in detecting intraocular foreign bodies lodged in the recess of the angle and in studying iris tumors and other chamber abnormalities.

In addition, with the pupil widely dilated, the gonioscope will allow the observer to view the equator of the lens, the zonule and the ciliary processes, and even the peripheral retina.

CHAPTER 7
Clinical Problems

Answers on Page 229.

1 A 10-year-old boy was having a routine eye examination. When examining the patient with an ophthalmoscope, the ophthalmologist had difficulty focusing on the child's retina. It was only when the lens turret was rotated until a lens having a −4-diopters power was in position that the fundus could be brought into focus. Can you explain this phenomenon if we assume that the patient and the examiner have emmetropic eyes?

2 A 45-year-old woman suffering from extreme nearsightedness notices some flashes of light before her left eye. Her immediate reaction is that a thunderstorm is about to take place and that she has observed flashes of lightning. There is no storm, however, and during the next few days the flashes of light recur. She also begins to notice small specks floating across her vision in the left eye, and on occasion thinks she sees what she describes as a curtain floating down within her left eye. On examination by an ophthalmologist it is noted that there is an absence of the normal red reflex. What is the possible diagnosis?

3 A 30-year-old man was having his fundi examined by means of an ophthalmoscope. The student examiner was experiencing difficulty distinguishing between retinal arteries and veins. What are the normal visible differences between retinal arteries and veins?

4 While examining a patient, an ophthalmologist asks a fourth-year student what the approximate size of the optic disc is. Is this a purely academic question? Can the information be practically useful?

5 What is the physiologic cup? How may this cup be distinguished from a pathologic cup seen in patients with glaucoma?

6 Careful examination of the fundus of a 53-year-old woman showed the presence of small arteries running from the temporal side of the optic disc to the macular area in the right eye. Examination of the left fundus did not show these vessels. What are these vessels? Are they a normal finding?

7 What is the cause of the small white light reflex found at the center of the fovea centralis when one views the fundus with an ophthalmoscope?

8 When the examiner uses the direct ophthalmoscope with the patient's pupil widely dilated, how much of the peripheral fundus can be visualized?

9 A 36-year-old woman was examined with a slit lamp. In the anterior chamber of her right eye some small white spots were visualized. Her history indicated that she had recently had an inflammation inside her right eye. What is the normal slit-lamp appearance of the anterior chamber? What is responsible for the white spots seen in this patient?

10 Describe the appearances of the cornea as seen with a slit lamp. Identify the layers of different optical density that can be visualized. What is meant by the term *optical section*?

11 What parts of the lens can be seen with a slit lamp?

12 How much of the vitreous body can be studied with the slit lamp?

13 Describe how a gonioscope can overcome the anatomic and optical obstacles to studying the angle of the anterior chamber.

CHAPTER 7
Answers to Clinical Problems

1 In young patients and examiners alike it is normal, when the examiner's eye and the patient's are brought close together, for the accommodation reflex to occur. This can easily result in an increase in strength of the lens in the patient's and the examiner's eye of +2 diopters each. Thus, to correct for this, the ophthalmoscope has to be adjusted so that a lens of −4 diopters is in position.

2 Myopia may cause the vitreous to pull on the retina secondary to the elongated shape of the eyeball. The lightning flashes seen by this patient result from the retina's being pulled on by the vitreous body. The curtain seen by the patient results from the accumulation of fluid between the two layers of the retina. Loss of the red reflex means that there is something opaque interposed between the lighted ophthalmoscope and the blood vessels of the choroid. In this patient, the retina was detached and not in contact with the choroid.

3 The arteries are bright red, and the veins are darker red or bluish. The arteries are smaller than the veins, in about a 3:4 ratio. The arteries have a shiny central reflex stripe that is absent from the veins. The arteries usually cross the veins on their superficial or vitreal surface.

4 The optic disc is approximately 1.5 mm in diameter. The size of the optic disc can be used practically as a unit of measure to estimate the size of patches or other lesions on the patient's retina.

5 The physiologic cup is the pale, almost white depression seen in the center of the optic disc. The cup observed in advanced glaucoma is larger in diameter and is deeper. Further, in glaucoma the ratio of the horizontal diameter of the optic cup to that of the optic disc increases (greater than 0.5). It should be pointed out that sometimes it is quite difficult to distinguish between a normal physiologic cup and a pathologic cup. Moreover, increased cupping is not an early sign of glaucoma.

6 These arteries, running directly from the temporal aspect of the optic disc to the macular area, exemplify the normal variation of the retinal vasculature. Called cilioretinal vessels, they originate from the circle of Zinn, which is formed around the optic nerve in the sclera from the short posterior ciliary arteries.

7 The small white light reflex at the center of the fovea centralis is produced by the reflection of the ophthalmoscope light from the concavity of the fovea.

8 With the pupil widely dilated, the peripheral fundus can be seen with the direct ophthalmoscope up to the equator. The patient must be instructed to move the eyeball in the appropriate direction so that each quadrant of the retina can be brought into view.

9 Normally, the anterior chamber is filled with a clear aqueous humor, which on slit-lamp examination appears optically empty and black. In this patient, the white spots were caused by aggregations of inflammatory cells floating in the aqueous.

10 The anterior epithelial surface of the cornea, the milky reticular appearance of the corneal stroma, and the posterior endothelial surface can be visualized easily. In the aged, the Hassall-Henle bodies of Descemet's membrane are recognized as dark areas near the limbus.

Optical section is the term used to describe the tissues illuminated by the narrow beam of light. An optical section is comparable to a histologic section cut by a microtome.

11 The anterior and posterior surfaces of the lens can be seen as bright reflected surfaces when the lens is viewed with the slit lamp. The interior of the lens in an adult shows about ten bands, some of which are brighter than others. In the center of the lens, the fetal nucleus can be identified as two planoconvex lenses with a central dark interval. Details concerning the sutures may be found on pages 201 and 202.

12 Without additional lenses, the slit lamp can visualize only the anterior third of the vitreous body.

13 The sclera and the corneoscleral limbus obstruct direct inspection of the anterior chamber. A further difficulty is that light arising from the angle undergoes total internal reflection on reaching the curved surface of the cornea. A gonioscopic contact lens applied to the cornea permits visualization of the angle.

Movements of the Eyeball and the Extraocular Muscles

CHAPTER OUTLINE

Support of the Eyeball During Eye Movements ·

The eyeball is surrounded within the orbital cavity by orbital fat. It has been suggested that the numerous connective tissue septa, running radially through the orbital fat from the fascia of the eyeball to the orbital walls, provide an important suspensory system. In addition, the suspensory ligament, with its attachment to the lateral and medial walls of the orbit by means of the check ligaments, provides further support (Fig. 8-1). The tone of the extraocular muscles almost certainly plays a role in anchoring and supporting the eyeball when the head assumes different positions.

Position of the Eyeball ·

The primary position of the eyeball means the position when the eye is directed straight ahead. *The secondary positions of the eyeball* means those positions when the eye is directed upward, downward, laterally, or medially. *The tertiary positions of the eyeball* mean those positions when the eye is directed in an oblique position (i.e., upward and downward, medially and laterally).

Terms Used in Describing Eye Movements ·

The center of the cornea or the center of the pupil is used as the anatomic "anterior pole" of the eye. All movement of the eye is then related to the direction of movement of the anterior pole as it rotates on any one of the three axes of Fick (transverse, vertical, or sagittal). The terminology then becomes as follows: *Elevation* is the rotation of the eye upward; *depression* is the rotation of the eye downward; *abduction* is the rotation of the eye laterally; and *adduction* is the rotation of the eye medially (Fig. 8-2).

Rotatory movements of the eyeball use the upper rim of the cornea (or pupil) as the marker. This point is sometimes referred to as the 12 o'clock position, or meridian. The terms *inward rotation, medial rotation*, and *intorsion* all mean the rotation of the eye medially. The terms *external rotation, lateral rotation*, and *extorsion* mean the rotation of the eye laterally (Fig. 8-2).

Duction is the term sometimes used for the movement of one eyeball from one position to another. Thus, one can have a list of ductions—*supraduction*

Figure 8-1

(A) Horizontal section of the right orbit, showing the fascial sheath of the eyeball, the fascial sheaths of the rectus muscles, and the medial and lateral check ligaments. (B) Coronal section of the right orbit, showing the relationship of the fascial sheath of the eyeball to the tendons of the extrinsic muscles—in particular the superior rectus, the levator palpebrae superioris, the inferior rectus, and the inferior oblique. The black line representing the suspensory ligament has been excessively thickened to emphasize its presence.

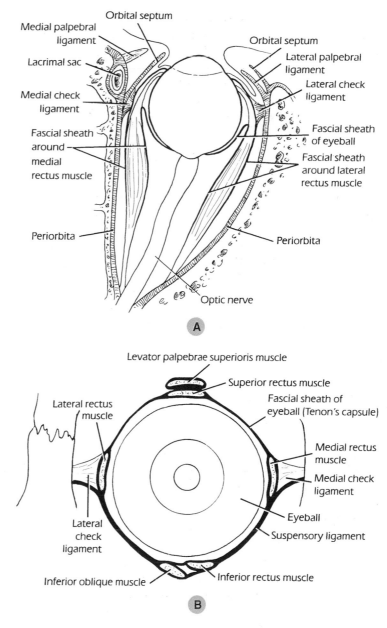

(elevation), *infraduction* (depression), *abduction* (lateral movement), *adduction* (medial movement), *incycloduction* (intorsion), and *excycloduction* (extorsion).

Axes of Rotation of the Eyeball

The movements of the eyeball may be considered as occurring around three imaginary primary axes, which pass through the center of rotation and are situated at right angles to one another (Fig. 8-3). The *vertical axis* (of Fick) passes

Figure 8-2

Diagrams illustrating the different eye movements: (A) elevation; (B) depression; (C) abduction; (D) adduction; (E) extorsion, external rotation, or lateral rotation; (F) intorsion, inward rotation, or medial rotation.

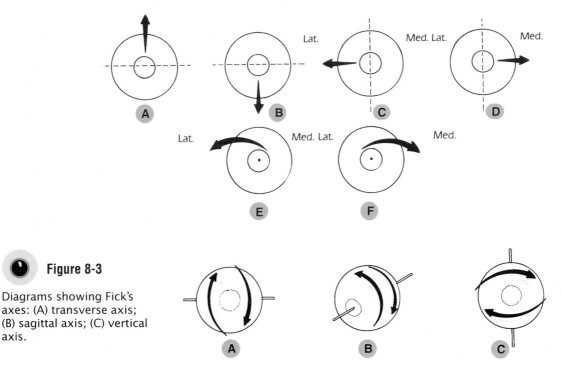

 Figure 8-3

Diagrams showing Fick's axes: (A) transverse axis; (B) sagittal axis; (C) vertical axis.

through the globe, so that the eye rotates laterally (abduction) or medially (adduction). The *transverse axis* (of Fick) passes horizontally from medial to lateral through the globe, so that the eye rotates upward (elvation) or downward (depression). The *sagittal axis* (of Fick) passes in an anteroposterior direction and corresponds to the line of vision. Inward and external rotation of the eyeball occurs around this axis.

Muscles Producing Movement of the Eyeball

The six voluntary extraocular muscles of the orbit that produce eye movements are the superior, inferior, medial, and lateral rectus muscles and the superior and inferior oblique muscles.

General Structure of the Voluntary Extraocular Muscles

Light Microscopic Structure

Skeletal muscle fibers are extremely long, cylindrical, multinucleated cells measuring many millimeters in length and from 10 to 100 μm in diameter. Each fiber is surrounded by an extracellular layer of polysaccharides, which form a basal lamina. The fibers are bound together by connective tissue to form a muscle. A tough connective tissue sheath, the *epimysium*, surrounds the whole muscle (Fig. 8-9). From the epimysium, connective tissue septa pass into the muscle mass, binding together groups of muscle cells. This connective tissue is referred to as the *perimysium*. Each muscle fiber in turn is surrounded by a delicate connective tissue envelope, the *endomysium* (Figs. 8-4 and 8-9).

The plasma membrane of skeletal muscle fibers (cells) is called *sarcolemma*, and the cytoplasm is referred to as *sarcoplasm*. The multiple nuclei of the muscle cells are found at the periphery of the cells, just beneath the plasma membrane (Figs. 8-4 and 8-5). Most of the sarcoplasm is occupied by longitudinally running *myofibrils*, which measure about 1 μm in diameter and give the fibers a longitudinally striated appearance. The myofibrils show a pattern of repeating

 Figure 8-4

Photomicrograph of a longitudinal section of one of the extraocular skeletal muscles, showing typical cross-banding and numerous peripherally located nuclei. Note the presence of abundant delicate connective tissue forming the endomysium. (H&E; × 400.)

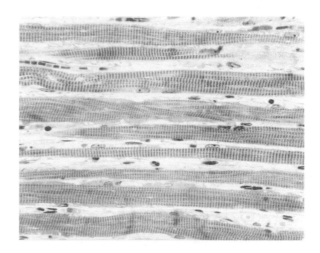

 Figure 8-5

Photomicrograph of a transverse section of one of the extraocular skeletal muscles, showing many muscle fibers with peripherally located nuclei (arrows). The muscle fibers are separated from one another by an abundance of loose connective tissue, the endomysium. Note that the endomysium contains many nerve fibers. (Plastic section; H&E; × 200.)

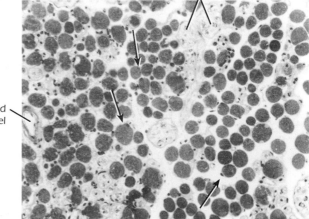

Bundles of nerve fibers

Blood vessel

Figure 8-6

Photomicrograph of a longitudinal section of skeletal muscle, showing A and I bands. (Iron hematoxylin stain; × 1200.)

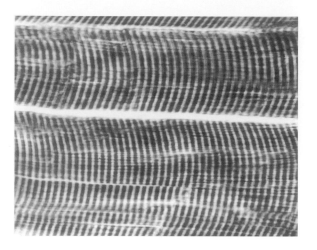

cross-bands (Figs. 8-4 and 8-6). Because these cross-bands are in close register, they give rise to the cross-striations of the whole muscle fiber.

When examined with the light microscope, each cross-striation can be seen to be made up of a dark band called the *A band* and a light band called the *I band* (Fig. 8-6). A transverse line, the *Z line*, bisects each I band. The *H bands* form the middle region of the A band. The area between two Z lines on a single myofibril is called a *sarcomere*.

Electron Microscopic Structure

The basic contractile unit of the muscle fiber is the sarcomere. With the electron microscope, the sarcomere of each myofibril is seen to be made up of two types of longitudinally running filaments (Figs. 8-7 and 8-8). The thick filament (10 nm), composed of the protein *myosin*, occupies the A band. The thin filaments (5 nm), composed of the protein *actin*, are attached to the Z line and occupy the I band. The actin filaments also extend into the adjacent A bands, where they lie between the thick myosin filaments. When a muscle contracts, the thick and thin filaments slide past one another and pull the Z lines closer together, so that the myofibril and the muscle fibers shorten. The thick myosin filaments have lateral projections that attach to the thin actin filaments and bring about the movement of the actin filaments (Fig. 8-9).

The cross-bridging between the myosin and actin filaments is the basis of the contractile process. The physical events correspond to a series of chemical events. The hydrolysis of adenosine triphosphate (ATP) to adenosine diphosphate (ADP) by ATPase in the lateral projections of the myosin filaments provides the energy. The extensive sliding movements between the myosin and actin filaments result from the repeated cycles of attachment and detachment of the cross-bridges. Since the cross-bridging occurs asynchronously when a muscle contracts, the result is a continuous rather than a jerky pull. The force of contraction appears to depend on the number of cross-bridges formed at any one time; that is, the greatest force occurs when there are the maximal number of cross-bridges between the myofilaments and when there is a maximum overlap between the myosin and actin filaments (see p. 245).

Figure 8-7

Electron micrograph of a longitudinal section of skeletal muscle, showing a single sarcomere, an A band, an I band, and a Z line. (× 13,800.) (Courtesy of Fred Lightfoot.)

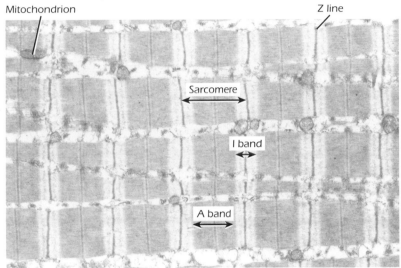

The sarcolemma, which is the plasmolemma of muscle cells, is invaginated at the A-I junction to form the *T system* of tubules. Each T tubule extends transversely into the sarcoplasm, and the cavity of each tubule is continuous with the exterior (Fig. 8-10). Another system of tubules, known as the *sarcoplasmic reticulum*, exists in the sarcoplasm. These tubules, which are the smooth endoplasmic reticulum of muscle cells, run longitudinally and do not communicate with the exterior of the muscle cell (Fig. 8-10). At the point where the T tubules lie close to the endoplasmic reticulum, the T tubules exhibit a triad consisting of a central tubule flanked on either side by two terminal cisternae. The cisternae are filled with a dense granular material containing *calsequestrin*, a protein having a high affinity for calcium. The T tubules and the sarcoplasmic reticulum play an important role in muscle contraction (see p. 245).

Skeletal muscle cells also contain the usual cell organelles and inclusions. Glycogen is found throughout the sarcoplasm, as is the oxygen-binding protein *myoglobin*.

Specific Structure of the Extraocular Muscles

The muscle fibers are arranged longitudinally, each fiber running most of the length of the muscle. In cross-section the muscle fibers are not packed closely together, and each fiber is round or oval (Figs. 8-4 and 8-5). The smaller-diameter fibers (5–15 μm) tend to occupy the periphery of the muscle, while the larger fibers (10–40 μm), which form the bulk of the muscle, occupy the center. The

Figure 8-8

Electron micrograph of a longitudinal section of skeletal muscle, showing five myofibrils that have been labeled to show the various cross-bands. (× 48,750.) (Courtesy of Fred Lightfoot.)

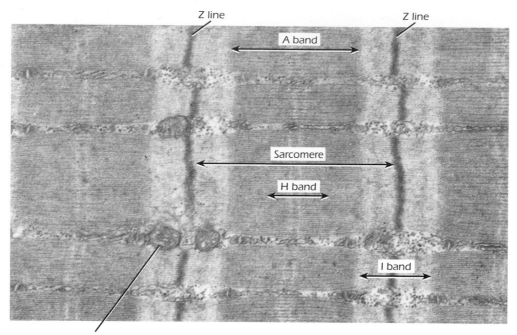

connective tissue surrounding the extraocular muscles is more delicate than that around ordinary skeletal muscle, and it contains many nerve fibers and elastic fibers. Moreover, the muscle has greater vascularity than voluntary muscles found elsewhere.

As the result of many morphologic studies done with both the light and the electron microscopes, efforts have been made to classify the different types of muscle fibers. Differences in details of innervation and physiologic response have also been used in the classification process. At least two forms of muscle fiber have been recognized: a thin (9–11 µm), slow-contracting type, and a thick (11–15 µm), fast-contracting or twitch type of fiber. The slow-contracting fibers have grapelike motor endings; the fast-contracting fibers have classic motor end-plates.

For the first 2 cm from its origin, each extraocular muscle has a thin transparent sheath. The remainder of the muscle is surrounded with a thick, opaque connective tissue sheath that is continuous with the fascial sheath of the eyeball.

Tendon of Insertion

The tendons consist of parallel running bundles of collagen fibers supported by elastic fibers. The tendon collagen fibers enter the superficial layers of the sclera and mingle with the collagen fibers so that they are no longer recognizable. The

Figure 8-9

Diagram showing the structure of skeletal muscle. Note the organization of the muscle fibers, the myofibrils, and the muscle filaments. Observe that a sarcomere, with its A, I, and H bands, extends between Z lines.

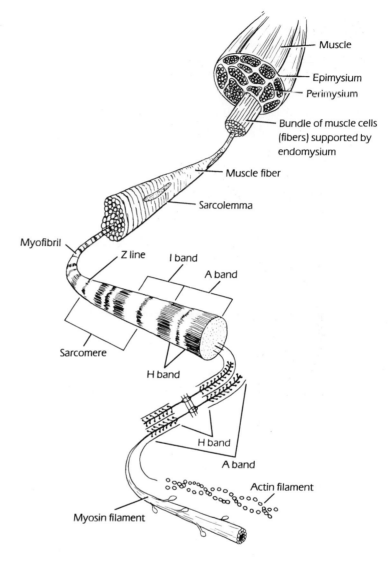

elastic fibers of the tendon cease abruptly at the point of insertion. Occasionally, slips of the tendon leave the main tendon and are attached to the sclera farther back on the globe.

Motor Innervation of the Extraocular Muscles

The motor nerve reaches the extraocular muscle in the region of the muscle's middle and posterior thirds. It breaks up into numerous branches, which run both distally and proximally between the muscle fibers (Fig. 8-11). Two types of myoneural junctions are present. The common form of motor end-plate that is found on skeletal muscles elsewhere is present in the singly innervated muscle fiber (Fig. 8-11). The second type, shaped like a bunch of grapes, is found on the multiple innervated muscle fibers. The motor fibers entering the motor

Figure 8-10

(A) Longitudinal section of skeletal muscle, showing the organization of sarcomeres. (B) Longitudinal section of skeletal muscle, showing the pathway taken by an action potential that causes the release of calcium ions from the sarcoplasmic reticulum; the calcium ions are taken up again by the calcium pump. (C) Sliding movements of the actin filaments as a myofibril contracts.

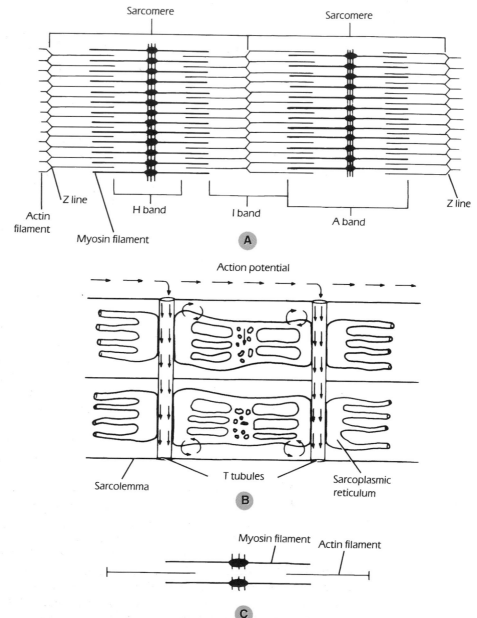

Figure 8-11

(A) Photomicrograph of several muscle fibers, showing four motor end-plates. Note the myelinated axons passing to each end-plate. (× 400.)
(B) Photomicrograph of two muscle fibers, showing two motor end-plates. Note the terminal branching of the axon as it enters the end-plate. (× 400.)

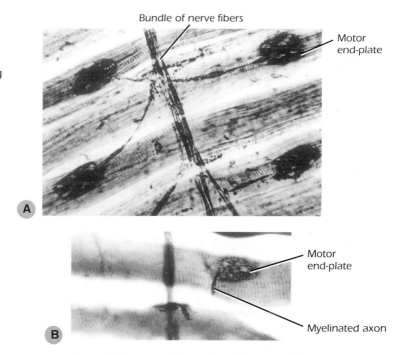

Bundle of nerve fibers

Motor end-plate

A

Motor end-plate

Myelinated axon

B

end-plate are always myelinated; the grapelike endings have smaller nerves, which are myelinated or nonmyelinated.

Myoneural Junctions in Skeletal Muscle

As each large alpha myelinated fiber enters a skeletal muscle, it branches many times. A single branch then terminates on a muscle fiber at a site referred to as a *neuromuscular junction* or *motor end-plate* (Figs. 8-11 and 8-12). On reaching the muscle fiber, the nerve loses its myelin sheath and breaks up into a number of subsidiary branches. Each branch ends as a naked axon and forms the *neural element* of the motor end-plate (Fig. 8-12). The axon is expanded slightly and contains numerous mitochondria and vesicles (approximately 45 nm in diameter). At the site of the motor end-plate the surface of the muscle fiber is elevated slightly to form the *muscular element* of the plate, often referred to as the *sole plate* (Fig. 8-12). The elevation results from the local accumulation of granular sarcoplasm beneath the sarcolemma and the presence of numerous nuclei and mitochondria.

The expanded naked axon lies in a groove on the surface of the muscle fiber. Each groove is formed by the infolding of the sarcolemma. The groove may branch many times, each branch containing a division of the axon. It is important to realize that the axons are truly naked; the Schwann cells merely serve as a cap or roof to the groove and never project into it. The floor of the groove consists of sarcolemma, which is thrown into numerous folds, called *junctional folds*; these serve to increase the surface area of the sarcolemma that lie close to the naked axon (Fig. 8-12). The plasma membrane of the axon (the axolemma, or presynaptic membrane) is separated by a space about 20 to 50 μm

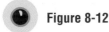

Figure 8-12

Longitudinal section of a neuromuscular junction.

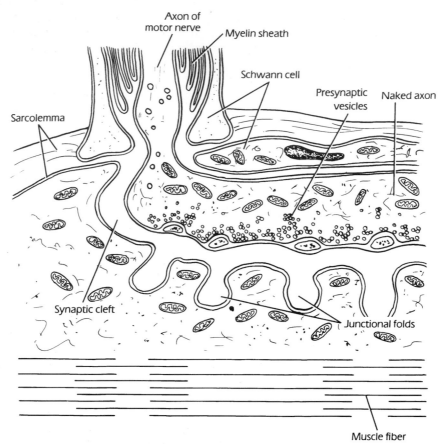

wide from the plasma membrane of the muscle fiber (the sarcolemma, or postsynaptic membrane). This space constitutes the *synaptic cleft*. The synaptic cleft is filled with the basement membranes of the axons and the muscle fiber (Fig. 8-12). The motor end-plate is strengthened by the connective tissue sheath of the nerve fiber, the endoneurium, and becomes continuous with the connective tissue sheath of the muscle fiber, the endomysium.

On reaching a motor end-plate, a nerve impulse causes the release of acetylcholine from some of the axonal vesicles. The acetylcholine discharges into the synaptic cleft by a process of *exocytosis* and diffuses rapidly through the basement membranes to reach the receptors on the postsynaptic membrane. This makes the postsynaptic membrane more permeable to Na$^+$ ions, creating a local potential, called the *end-plate potential*. If the end-plate potential is large enough, an action potential will be initiated to spread along the surface of the sarcolemma. The wave of depolarization is carried into the muscle fiber to the contractile myofibrils through the system of T tubules. This leads to the release of

Ca⁺ ions from the sarcoplasmic reticulum, which in turn causes the muscle to contract.

The amount of acetylcholine released at the motor end-plate will depend on the number of nerve impulses arriving at the nerve terminal. Once acetylcholine crosses the synaptic cleft, it immediately undergoes hydrolysis resulting from the presence of acetylcholinesterase (AChE) in the basement membranes and the postsynaptic membrane or sarcolemma. The acetylcholine remains for about 1 msec in contact with the postsynaptic membrane; then it is rapidly destroyed to prevent re-excitation of the muscle fiber.

Skeletal muscle fiber contraction is thus controlled by the frequency of the nerve impulses that arrive at the motor nerve terminal. A resting muscle fiber shows small occasional depolarizations (end-plate potentials) at the motor end-plate that are insufficient to cause an action potential and make the fiber contract. These weak depolarizations are believed to be due to the sporadic release of acetylcholine (ACh) into the synaptic cleft from a single presynaptic vesicle.

The sequence of events that take place at a motor end-plate on stimulation of a motor nerve can be summarized as follows:

ACh + Receptor (nicotinic) $\rightarrow$ Na⁺ influx $\rightarrow$ End-plate potential

End-plate potential (if large enough) $\rightarrow$ Action potential $\rightarrow$ Increased release of Ca^{2+} $\rightarrow$ Muscle fiber contraction

Immediate hydrolysis of ACh by AChE $\rightarrow$ Repolarization of muscle fiber

Clinical Notes

Effect of Drugs on the Motor End-plate   If drugs having a chemical structure similar to that of acetylcholine were to arrive at the receptor site of a motor end-plate, they might bring about the same changes as acetylcholine and mimic its action. Two examples of such drugs are *nicotine* and *carbamylcholine*. If, on the other hand, drugs having a similar chemical structure to acetylcholine were to arrive at the receptor site of a motor end-plate and were unable to bring about the sequence of changes normally induced by acetylcholine, they would occupy the receptor site and block the access of acetylcholine. Such drugs would be competing with acetylcholine and are called *competitive blocking agents*. An example of such a drug is *d-tubocurarine*, which would cause skeletal muscle to relax and not contract by preventing the action of locally produced acetylcholine (see also p. 261).

Muscle Spindles of Extraocular Muscles

Most of the muscle spindles exist in the proximal or distal third of the muscle. The spindles measure about 900 µm long by about 50 µm in diameter (Figs. 8-13 and 8-14). Each is surrounded by a thin capsule of connective tissue. The intrafusal muscle fibers are of one type and often have central nuclei but no nuclear bag. Small motor end-plates are found on the intrafusal fibers close to the poles. At the equator, nerve fibers and endings have a complex arrangement. In addition to the above simple type of muscle spindle, spiral nerve endings, which wind around extrafusal fibers for about 3 to 8 turns, are also found. They tend to exist in the middle of the muscle. The afferent nerves from the sensory endings ascend to the brain stem in the third, fourth, and sixth cranial nerves and probably have their cell bodies in the mesencephalic nucleus in the brain stem.

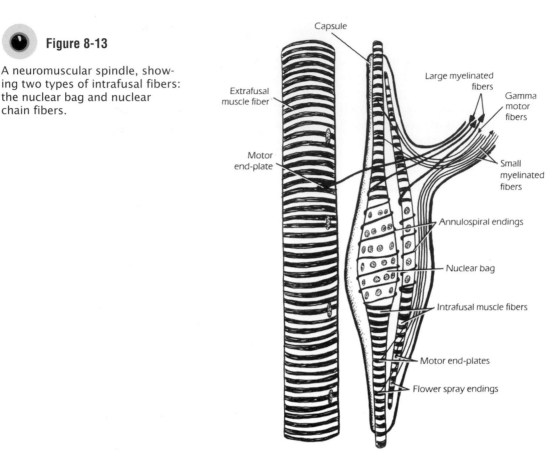

Figure 8-13

A neuromuscular spindle, showing two types of intrafusal fibers: the nuclear bag and nuclear chain fibers.

Under resting conditions, the muscle spindles give rise to continuous afferent nerve impulses ascending to the brain stem. When muscle activity occurs, either actively or passively, the intrafusal fibers stretch, and there is an increased rate of passage of nerve impulses in the afferent neurons. Similarly, if the intrafusal fibers then relax because of cessation of muscle activity, the result is a decreased rate of passage of nerve impulses to the brain stem. The neuromuscular spindle thus plays a very important role in keeping the central nervous system informed about muscle activity—thereby indirectly influencing the control of the extraocular muscles.

Golgi Tendon Organs

The Golgi tendon organs of the extraocular muscles have a similar structure to those found on other skeletal muscles. They vary in size from 70 to 120 μm wide by 300 to 800 μm long (Fig. 8-15). They are found within the tendons having tendinous attachments. Each organ is surrounded by a connective tissue capsule and contains small bundles of tendon collagen fibers. One or more nerves enter the capsule, losing their myelin sheaths, and the naked axons branch many times, to end as enlargements that lie between the bundles of collagen fibers.

Figure 8-14

Photomicrograph of a neuromuscular spindle. ($\times$ 400.)

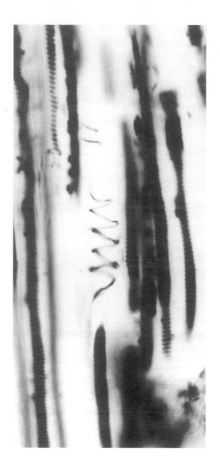

The nerve endings are activated by being squeezed by the adjacent collagen fibers within the spindle when tension develops in the tendon. Unlike the neuromuscular spindle, which is sensitive to changes in muscle length, the neurotendinous organ detects changes in muscle tension.

Muscle Contraction

In skeletal muscle, the nerve impulse reaching the motor end-plate excites the sarcolemma (muscle plasma membrane). The action potential spreads along the sarcolemma and passes into the muscle cell via the tubular indentations, the T tubules (Fig. 8-10). In response, the sarcoplasmic reticulum releases calcium ions, which combine with the proteins *troponin* and *tropomyosin*, which are part of the actin filament. Bridge formation occurs between actin and myosin, and contraction takes place (Fig. 8-10). Once the stimulus has ceased, the calcium ions are withdrawn from the sarcoplasmic matrix back into the sarcoplasmic reticulum, and the muscle begins to relax. Thus, the state of relaxation is thought to be caused by the troponin and tropomyosin, which are now free from the calcium ions and prevent the actin from interacting with myosin filaments. Troponin and tropomyosin are often referred to as the *regulator proteins* of muscle.

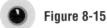 **Figure 8-15**

Neurotendinous spindle.

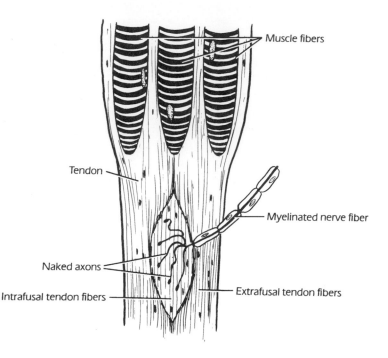

Source of Energy

When a muscle contracts and work is perfomed, large amounts of ATP are broken down by ATPase into ADP, with the liberation of energy. Additional energy is provided by the breakdown of phosphocreatine. The energy so produced in some way causes the actin filaments to move over the myosin filaments so that the sarcomere length decreases. The whole chemical process is initiated by the spread of the action potential over the surface of the muscle cell and the release of calcium ions from the sarcoplasmic reticulum. After the muscle contraction is completed, the oxidation of glycogen provides energy for the resynthesis of phosphocreatine and ATP.

The Four Rectus Muscles

The four rectus muscles arise from a fibrous ring, called the *common tendinous ring* (annulus of Zinn). It is a thickening of the periosteum at the apex of the orbital cavity. The ring is oval in cross-section and encloses the optic foramen and a part of the medial end of the superior orbital fissure (Fig. 8-16). From this common origin the rectus muscles pass forward as a muscle cone to be inserted into the sclera of the eyeball. The superior rectus is the longest, then the medial, then the lateral; the inferior rectus is the shortest. The main anatomic features of the four rectus muscles are summarized in Table 8-1 and may be seen in Figs. 8-26 to 8-31.

Superior Rectus Muscle

The superior rectus muscle arises from the tendinous ring above the optic foramen and its origin is attached to the dural sheath of the optic nerve (Fig.

Figure 8-16

Diagram of the apical region of the right orbit, showing the common tendinous ring, which gives origin to the four rectus muscles. This also shows the origins of the levator palpebrae superioris and the superior oblique muscles. Note the positions of the nerves and blood vessels entering the orbital cavity.

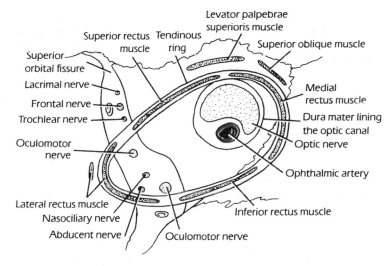

Table 8-1 Summary of the Main Anatomic Features of the Extraocular Muscles

Muscle	Origin	Insertion	Tendon Length (mm)	Nerve Supply
Superior rectus	Tendinous ring	Sclera, 7.7 mm posterior to limbus	5.8	Oculomotor n. (superior div.)
Inferior rectus	Tendinous ring	Sclera, 6.5 mm posterior to limbus	5.5	Oculomotor n. (inferior div.)
Lateral rectus	Tendinous ring	Sclera, 6.9 mm posterior to limbus	8.8	Abducent n.
Medial rectus	Tendinous ring	Sclera, 5.5 mm posterior to limbus	3.7	Oculomotor n. (inferior div.)
Superior oblique	Superomedial to optic canal	Sclera, posterior to equator		Trochlear n.
Inferior oblique	Floor of orbit just posterior to orbital margin and lateral to nasolacrimal canal	Sclera, posterolateral aspect of eyeball		Oculomotor n. (inferior div.)

The function of each muscle is described in detail in the text.

8-16). The muscle passes forward and somewhat laterally and pierces the fascial sheath of the eyeball. It is inserted into the sclera about 7.7 mm posterior to the limbus (corneoscleral junction) by means of a tendon 5.8 mm long. The line of insertion is slightly curved and oblique (Figs. 8-17 and 8-18).

As the muscle pierces the fascial sheath of the eyeball, the fascia is reflected backward around the muscle, providing it with a sheath (Fig. 8-1). The fascial

Figure 8-17

Series of diagrams of the right eyeball, showing the precise insertions of the extraocular muscles. SR = superior rectus; IR = inferior rectus; MR = medial rectus; LR = lateral rectus; SO = superior oblique; IO = inferior oblique.

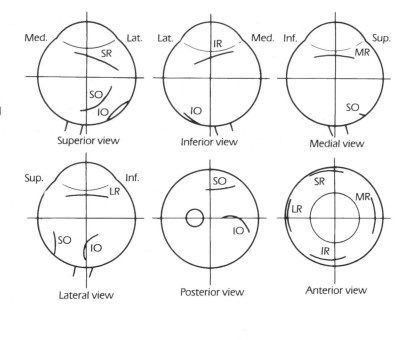

 Figure 8-18

Diagram of right eyeball as seen from front, showing the lengths of the tendons of insertion of the four rectus muscles and the distances between the corneoscleral limbus and tendinous insertions. Note that the distances increase as one passes around the eyeball, as the arrows indicate.

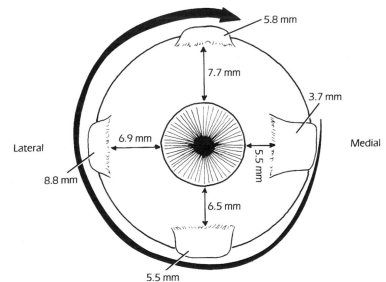

sheath of the superior rectus muscle and that of the levator palpebrae superioris muscle are connected by a band of connective tissue. This connection ensures that the two muscles work synergistically. A further slip of fascia is also connected to the superior fornix of the conjunctiva. This band permits these muscles to raise the superior fornix of the conjunctiva as they contract.

Relations   Superiorly are the levator palpebrae superioris muscle, the frontal nerve, and the roof of the orbit (Fig. 8-28). Inferiorly are the optic nerve, the ophthalmic artery, and the nasociliary nerve embedded in orbit fat (Fig. 8-30). Within the fascial sheath of the eyeball, the tendon is related inferiorly to the tendon of insertion of the superior oblique muscle (Fig. 8-29).

Nerve Supply   The superior rectus is supplied by the superior division of the oculomotor nerve. The nerve enters the inferior surface of the muscle at the junction of its middle and posterior thirds (Fig. 8-27). The nerve usually pierces the muscle and continues to supply the levator palpebrae superioris muscle.

Action   Acting alone (Fig. 8-19), the superior rectus elevates the eye, medially rotates the eye, and rotates the eyeball medially on its anteroposterior axis (intorsion). See discussion of action of extraocular muscles below.

Inferior Rectus Muscle

The inferior rectus muscle arises from the tendinous ring below the optic foramen (Fig. 8-16). It passes forward and somewhat laterally and pierces the fascial sheath of the eyeball. It is inserted into the sclera about 6.5 mm from the limbus by means of a tendon 5.5 mm long. The line of insertion is slightly curved and oblique (Fig. 8-17).

As in the case of the superior rectus, the inferior rectus is covered by a fascial sheath derived from the fascial sheath of the eyeball. The fascial sheaths of the inferior rectus and the inferior oblique are attached to one another and to the suspensory ligament of the eyeball (Fig. 8-1). A band of connective tissue also connects the inferior rectus sheath to the lower eyelid.

Relations   Superiorly lie the oculomotor nerve, the optic nerve embedded in orbital fat, and the eyeball (Fig. 8-27). Inferiorly there lie the floor of the orbit, the infraorbital vessels and nerve in their canal, and the underlying maxillary sinus. At the point where the inferior rectus muscle pierces the fascial sheath of the eyeball, it is related inferiorly to the inferior oblique muscle (Fig. 8-1).

Nerve Supply   The inferior rectus muscle is supplied by the inferior division of the oculomotor nerve, which enters its superior surface at about the junction of the middle and posterior thirds (Fig. 8-27).

Action   Acting alone (Fig. 8-19), the inferior rectus depresses the eye, medially rotates the eye, and rotates the eyeball laterally on its anteroposterior axis (extorsion). See discussion of action of extraocular muscles below.

Lateral Rectus Muscle

The lateral rectus muscle arises from the lateral portion of the tendinous ring as it bridges the superior orbital fissure (Fig. 8-16). A second small head arises from the orbital surface of the greater wing of the sphenoid bone, lateral to the fibrous ring. The muscle passes forward close to the lateral wall of the orbit and pierces the fascial sheath of the eyeball. It is inserted into the sclera about 6.9 mm from the limbus by means of a tendon 8.8 mm long. The line of insertion is nearly vertical (Fig. 8-17).

Figure 8-19

Diagrams showing the actions of the four rectus muscles in producing movements of the eyeball.

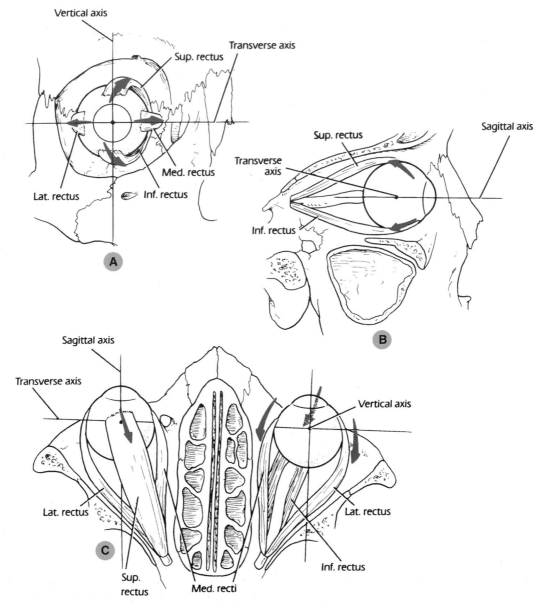

As in the case of the other recti muscles, the lateral rectus is covered by a fascial sheath derived from the fascial sheath of the eyeball. As described elsewhere, the sheath of the lateral rectus sends off an expansion that is attached to the lateral wall of the orbit to form the *lateral check ligament* (Fig. 8-1).

Relations Superiorly lie the lacrimal nerve and lacrimal artery (Fig. 8-27). Inferiorly lies the floor of the orbit. Medially lie the abducent nerve and orbital fat.

Nerve Supply The lateral rectus muscle is supplied by the abducent nerve on its medial surface just behind its middle (Fig. 8-27).

Action The lateral rectus muscle (Fig. 8-19) rotates the eye laterally (abductor). See discussion of action of extraocular muscles below.

Medial Rectus Muscle

The medial rectus muscle is the largest of the extraocular muscles (Fig. 8-27). It arises from the medial portion of the tendinous ring and is attached to the dural sheath of the optic nerve (Fig. 8-16). The muscle passes forward close to the medial wall of the orbit and pierces the fascial sheath of the eyeball. It is inserted into the sclera about 5.5 mm from the limbus by means of a tendon 3.7 mm long (Fig. 8-18). The line of insertion is vertical (Fig. 8-17).

As in the case of the other recti muscles, the medial rectus is covered by a fascial sheath derived from the fascial sheath of the eyeball. The sheath of the medial rectus sends off an expansion that is attached to the medial wall of the orbit to form the *medial check ligament* (Fig. 8-1).

Relations Superiorly lie the superior oblique muscle, the ophthalmic artery and its branches, and the nasociliary nerve (Fig. 8-29). Inferiorly lies the floor of the orbit.

Nerve Supply The medial rectus muscle is supplied by the inferior division of the oculomotor nerve, which enters it on its lateral surface at about the junction of its middle and posterior thirds (Fig. 8-27).

Action The medial rectus (Fig. 8-19) rotates the eye medially (adduction). See discussion of action of extraocular muscles below.

The Two Oblique Muscles

Superior Oblique Muscle

The superior oblique muscle is a long, slender, fusiform muscle that arises from the body of the sphenoid bone above and medial to the optic canal just outside the tendinous ring (Fig. 8-16). The muscle belly runs forward between the roof and medial wall of the orbital cavity and quickly gives rise to a rounded tendon. The tendon then passes through a pulley or *trochlea* of fibrocartilage that is attached to the trochlear fossa of the frontal bone (Fig. 8-27). As the tendon passes through the pulley, it is surrounded by a delicate synovial sheath. After emerging from the trochlea, the tendon bends downward, backward, and laterally. It then pierces the fascial sheath of the eyeball and passes inferior to the superior rectus muscle. The tendon now expands in a fan-shaped manner and inserts into the sclera posterior to the equator of the eyeball (Fig. 8-31). The line of insertion is convex posteriorly and laterally (Fig. 8-17). The tendon of the superior oblique muscle is covered by a fascial sheath derived from the sheath of the eyeball; it extends as far as the trochlea.

Relations   Superiorly lies the roof of the orbit (Fig. 8-27). Inferiorly lie the ophthalmic artery and its branches and the nasociliary nerve. The supratrochlear nerve lies above and lateral to the muscle and lateral to the trochlea.

Nerve Supply   The superior oblique muscle is supplied by the trochlear nerve, which enters its superior surface close to the muscle origin (Fig. 8-28).

Action   The superior oblique muscle (Fig. 8-20) acting alone depresses the eye and turns it laterally (abducts); it also rotates the cornea medially on its anteroposterior axis (intorts). See discussion of action of extraocular muscles below.

Inferior Oblique Muscle

The inferior oblique muscle is the only voluntary muscle within the orbit to take origin from the front of the orbit (Fig. 8-27). It arises from the floor of the orbit just posterior to the orbital margin and just lateral to the nasolacrimal canal; it may also be attached to the fascia covering the lacrimal sac. The muscle passes laterally, posteriorly, and superiorly, following the curve of the lower surface of the eyeball. It runs inferior to the inferior rectus muscle (Fig. 8-27) and reaches the posterolateral aspect of the eyeball, where it inserts into the sclera under cover of the lateral rectus muscle (Fig. 8-31). The line of insertion is convex above and laterally (Fig. 8-17). The inferior oblique muscle is surrounded with a fascial sheath derived from the fascial sheath of the eyeball. The muscle sheath is attached to that of the inferior rectus muscle (Fig. 8-1).

Relations   Superiorly, the muscle is in contact with the orbital fat, the inferior rectus muscle, and the eyeball (Fig. 8-26). Inferiorly, the muscle is in contact with the floor of the orbit, separated by orbital fat.

Nerve Supply   The inferior oblique is supplied by the inferior division of the oculomotor nerve, which enters its superior surface at about its midpoint (Fig. 8-27).

Action   The inferior oblique muscle (Fig. 8-20) acting alone elevates the eye and laterally rotates the eye (abducts); it also rotates the eye laterally on its anteroposterior axis (extorsion). See discussion of action of extraocular muscles below.

The main anatomic features of the two oblique muscles are summarized in Table 8-1 and may be seen in Figs. 8-25 to 8-31.

Further Consideration of the Actions of the Extraocular Muscles

In discussing the action of muscles, it is customary for anatomists to attempt to simplify the process by considering the muscle in isolation, as if it were the only muscle acting on a particular structure (Fig. 8-21). In most situations, this simplified approach works very well. In the movements of the eyeball, however, oversimplification can lead to erroneous conclusions.

It is important to take into consideration the following concepts and laws.

Figure 8-20

Diagrams showing the actions of the superior and inferior oblique muscles in producing movements of the eyeball.

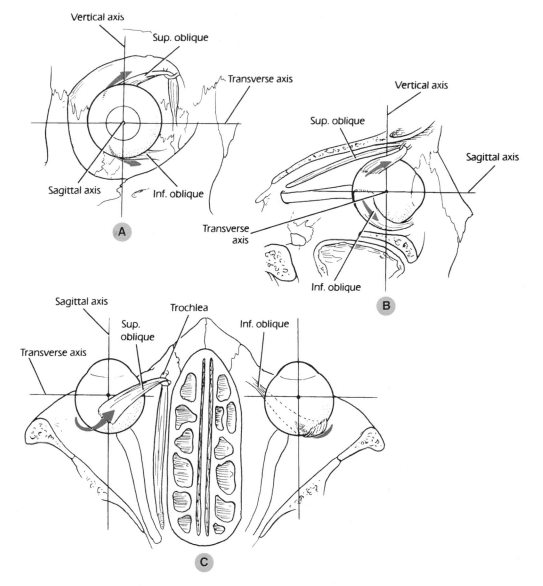

1. Line up the bony origin and the global insertion of each muscle and relate the direction of pull to the various axes on which the eye moves. Note that the superior and inferior rectus muscles pull backward at an angle of 23 degrees to the nasal side of the vertical axis of the eyeball with the eye in the primary position. Note also that the tendon of the superior oblique has a

Figure 8-21

A summary diagram showing the actions of the four rectus and two oblique muscles on each eyeball from the position of rest, if one assumes that each muscle is acting alone. These actions should not be confused with the movements performed by a patient in a test of extraocular muscle action (see Fig. 8-22).

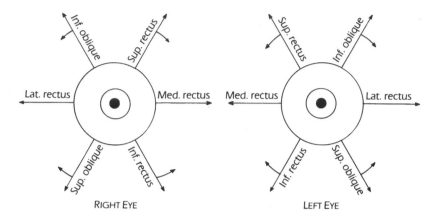

forward pull at an angle of 54 degrees to the nasal side of the vertical axis of the eyeball with the eye in the primary position. The inferior oblique muscle pulls forward at an angle of 51 degrees to the nasal side of the vertical axis of the eyeball with the eye in the primary position.

2. Understand that when a muscle acting on the eyeball contracts, its tone and length change, as do the tone and length of the remaining extraocular muscles. Moreover, once the eyeball moves, the position of the insertions of the other muscles changes relative to their origin, and thus the actions of the remaining muscles change. Thus, for a purposeful movement of the eyeball to be accomplished, the nervous control of all six extraocular muscles must be carefully coordinated within the brain stem. It is here that the muscle spindles and tendon organs are so important in gauging the length and tension of the various muscles.

3. At any one time, the position of the eyeball on its fatty bed, irrespective of the movement, is determined by the tone of all six extraocular muscles. It is thus clear that for the eyeball to move in any given direction, no single muscle acts alone, but groups of muscles must act together as agonists, antagonists, or synergists.

4. When both eyes are focusing on a moving object, it is imperative that there be conjugate movements of both eyeballs so that the image falls on identical positions on both retinae. This necessitates fine coordination of the contraction of all 12 muscles (6 + 6 of each eye) within the central nervous system. The constant feedback of vision will permit fine adjustments to be made to avoid diplopia.

5. *Hering's law*   According to this principle, in voluntary movements of the eye, equal and simultaneous innervation flows from the central nervous system to the muscles of both eyes gazing in a particular direction. For example, during convergence the right and left medial rectus muscles receive equal and simultaneous innervation, and during a gaze to the right, the right lateral rectus and the left medial rectus muscles receive equal and simultaneous innervation.

6. *Sherrington's law of reciprocal innervation*   According to this principle, an increased contraction of the prime mover extraocular muscle is associated with a diminished contractile activity of its antagonist muscle. For example, on gazing to the right there is an increased contraction of the right lateral rectus and left medial rectus muscles, and this is associated with a decreased contractile activity of the right medial rectus and left lateral rectus muscles.

Movements of the Eyeball and the Muscles Used in Producing the Movements ·

Abduction

This is the lateral rotation of the eyeball around an imaginary vertical axis by the contraction of the lateral rectus muscle and the relaxation of the medial rectus muscle.

Adduction

This is the medial rotation of the eyeball around an imaginary vertical axis by the contraction of the medial rectus muscle and the relaxation of the lateral rectus muscle.

Note that in the above two movements the lateral and medial recti are antagonists, and their lengths have to be finely adjusted so that the visual axis can smoothly sweep through a horizontal arc (Fig. 8-19).

Elevation

This is the direct vertical upward movement of the eyeball. It is accomplished by the contraction of the superior rectus muscle assisted by the inferior oblique muscle. Because the superior rectus is obliquely placed in the orbit, the direction of pull is not only upward but posteromedially. Thus, the primary action is elevation on the transverse axis, slight medial rotation on the vertical axis, and very slight intorsion on the anteroposterior axis. The tendency to cause medial rotation and intorsion is countered by the simultaneous contraction of the inferior oblique muscle, which also elevates but tends to rotate laterally and cause extorsion. The sum of all these actions is that the eye rotates vertically upward (Fig. 8-22B).

Depression

This is the direct downward rotation of the eyeball. It is brought about by the contraction of the inferior rectus muscle assisted by the superior oblique muscle.

Figure 8-22

The cardinal positions of the right and left eyes and the actions of the rectus and oblique muscles principally responsible for the movements of the eyes. (A) Right eye, superior rectus muscle; left eye, inferior oblique muscle. (B) Both eyes, superior recti and inferior oblique muscles. (C) Right eye, inferior oblique muscle; left eye, superior rectus muscle. (D) Right eye, lateral rectus muscle; left eye, medial rectus muscle. (E) Primary position, with the eyes fixed on a distant fixation point. (F) Right eye, medial rectus muscle; left eye, lateral rectus muscle. (G) Right eye, inferior rectus muscle; left eye, superior oblique muscle. (H) Both eyes, inferior recti and superior oblique muscles. (I) Right eye, superior oblique muscle; left eye, inferior rectus muscle.

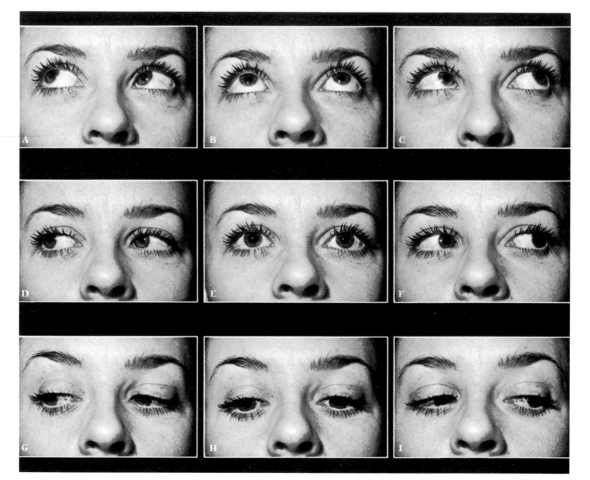

Because the inferior rectus is obliquely placed in the orbit, the direction of pull is not only downward but posteromedially. Thus, the primary action is depression on the transverse axis, slight medial rotation on the vertical axis, and very slight extorsion on the anteroposterior axis. The tendency to cause medial rotation and extorsion is countered by the simultaneous contraction of the superior oblique muscle. The direction of the tendon from the trochlea to its global

Table 8-2 The Many Actions of the Extraocular Muscles

Muscle	Primary Action	Secondary Action	Tertiary Action
Superior rectus	Elevation (transverse axis)	Medial rotation or adduction (vertical axis)	Intorsion or incycloduction (sagittal axis)
Inferior rectus	Depression (transverse axis)	Medial rotation or adduction (vertical axis)	Extorsion or excycloduction (sagittal axis)
Lateral rectus	Lateral rotation or abduction (vertical axis)	—	—
Medial rectus	Medial rotation or adduction (vertical axis)	—	—
Superior oblique	Depression (transverse axis)	Lateral rotation or abduction (vertical axis)	Intorsion or incycloduction (sagittal axis)
Inferior oblique	Elevation (transverse axis)	Lateral rotation or abduction (vertical axis)	Extorsion or excycloduction (sagittal axis)

Note that for completeness, alternative terminologies have been included as well as the various imaginary axes. Note also that the terms sagittal axis and anteroposterior axis are interchangeable.

insertion results in depression of the cornea and also lateral rotation and intorsion. The sum of all these actions is that the eye rotates vertically downward (Fig. 8-22H).

Note that in the movements of elevation and depression, as the agonist muscles shorten, the antagonist muscles have to be lengthened, so that the visual axis can smoothly sweep through a vertical arc.

To assist the reader in understanding the many actions of the extraocular muscles, these actions are summarized in Table 8-2.

Additional Terminology Used in Describing the Movements of Both Eyeballs

Binocular Movements

Binocular movements may be divided into two groups: versions and vergences.

A *version* is the simultaneous movement of both eyes in the same direction, including right and left horizontal and superior and inferior vertical gaze.

Dextroversion occurs as the result of the contraction of the right lateral rectus and the left medial rectus muscles. *Levoversion* is produced by the contraction of the left lateral rectus and the right medial rectus muscles.

Supraversion, or upward gaze, occurs as the result of the contraction of the superior rectus and inferior oblique muscles. *Infraversion*, or downward gaze, is produced by the contraction of the inferior rectus and the superior oblique muscles.

Dextrocycloversion occurs as the result of the contraction of the extorters of the right eye, namely, the inferior rectus and inferior oblique, and the intorters of the left eye, namely, the superior rectus and superior oblique. *Levocycloversion* is produced by the contraction of the extorters of the left eye, namely, the inferior rectus and inferior oblique, and the intorters of the right eye, namely, the superior rectus and the superior oblique.

A *vergence* is the simultaneous movement of both eyes in opposite directions.

Convergence is a medial movement that occurs as the result of contraction of both medial rectus muscles. *Divergence* is a lateral movement that is produced by the contraction of the lateral recti muscles. *Vertical vergences* are produced by the contraction of the elevators of one eye and the depressors of the opposite eye. *Cyclovergence* is simultaneous rotation of the eyeballs so that the superior rims of both corneas move laterally or medially.

Positions of Gaze

The *primary position of gaze* is the position taken up by both eyes fixating on a distant object directly ahead. *Secondary positions of gaze* are any other eye positions, including near-fixation, the cardinal positions, and midline vertical positions.

Position of near-fixation is usually a point about 0.33 m from the eyes. It involves convergence and accommodation. The *cardinal positions* are six in number and compare the vertical and horizontal movements of the eye. The *midline positions* are vertical positions up and down.

Clinical Notes

Disease and Defects in Ocular Movements

For both eyes to move rapidly in a precise, coordinated manner, the connective tissues of the orbit that support the eyeball and the extraocular muscles must function normally. The muscular contractions are controlled by neural activity that originates in the cerebral cortex, the cerebellum, and the brain stem and that is transmitted to the muscles by the third, fourth, and sixth cranial nerves. Disease involving any one of these structures will impair eye movement and result in failure of alignment of both foveas toward targets of visual interest.

Clinical Testing for the Actions of the Superior and Inferior Rectus and the Superior and Inferior Oblique Muscles

Since the actions of the superior and inferior rectus and the superior and inferior oblique muscles are complicated when a patient is asked to look vertically upward or vertically downward, the ophthalmologist tests eye movements in which the single action of each muscle predominates.

The origins of the superior and inferior recti are situated about 23 degrees medial to their insertions; therefore, when the patient is asked to turn the cornea laterally, these muscles are placed in the optimum position to raise the cornea (superior rectus) or lower it (inferior rectus).

Using the same rationale, the examiner tests the superior and the inferior oblique muscles. The pulley of the superior oblique and the origin of the inferior oblique muscles lie medial and anterior to their insertions. The ophthalmologist tests the action of these muscles by asking the patient first to look medially, thus placing these muscles in the optimum position to lower the cornea (superior oblique), or to raise it (inferior oblique). In other words, when you ask a patient to look medially and downward at the tip of his or her nose, you are testing the superior oblique at its best position. Conversely, by asking the patient to look medially and upward, you are testing the inferior oblique at its best position.

Because the lateral and medial recti are simply placed relative to the eyeball, asking the patient to turn his or her cornea directly laterally tests the lateral rectus and turning the cornea directly medially tests the medial rectus.

Infected Surgical Spaces Associated with the Extraocular Muscles

Three spaces may be recognized.

1. The space between the cone of the four rectus muscles and the periorbita lining the orbital walls. This is limited anteriorly by the tarsal plates and the orbital septum.

2. The space within the cone of the four rectus muscles. The connective tissue sheaths of the rectus muscles forming the cone are joined to each other by a membrane of connective tissue forming a wall. This space is limited anteriorly by the eyeball. Collections of fluid in this space lead to exophthalmos and immobility of the eyeball.

3. The space between the sclera and the fascial sheath of the eyeball (Tenon's capsule).

The significance of these spaces is that pus may accumulate within one of them, forming an abscess, and unless an appropriate incision is made, the abscess may not drain adequately.

Strabismus (Squint)

Strabismus is a condition in which the visual axes of both eyes are not straight in the primary position, or the eyes do not follow each other normally in any of the conjugate or disconjugate movements. Two types of strabismus occur, concomitant and incomitant. In concomitant strabismus, the angle of deviation is always the same irrespective of the direction of gaze. In incomitant strabismus, the angle of deviation is unequal in different directions of gaze.

Paralytic Strabismus

This is a form of incomitant strabismus in which the visual axes are not aligned, as the result of weakness or paralysis of one or more of the extraocular muscles. If binocular vision has developed, the patient will have diplopia. Diplopia will not occur if binocular vision has not been developed. Paralytic strabismus is worse when the eyes are moved into the field of action of the paralyzed or weakened muscle. Lesions of the nerves to the extraocular muscles may occur as the result of trauma, neoplasm, aneurysms, ischemia, or demyelination.

Nystagmus

The posture of the eye muscles depends mainly on the normal functioning of two sets of afferent pathways. The first is the visual pathway whereby the eye views the object of interest, and the second is much more complicated and involves the labyrinths, the vestibular nuclei, and the cerebellum. Nystagmus is the involuntary oscillation of the eyes due to irregular motor impulses reaching the extraocular muscles. There are different forms of nystagmus and very many causes.

Jerk Nystagmus

In this condition the eyes move slowly in one direction, followed by a rapid corrective movement (jerk) in the other direction. The rapid corrective movement is used to describe the direction of the nystagmus. Physiologic jerk nystagmus occurs when the vestibular apparatus of the inner ear is stimulated by rotation of the head. Pathologic jerk nystagmus can occur in acute labyrinthitis or with lesions of the cranial nerve nuclei or cerebellum.

Pendular Nystagmus

In this condition the eyes move in both directions with equal amplitude and velocity. Congenital pendular nystagmus is due to reduced visual activity associated with such defects as optic disc involvement with coloboma, congenital cataract, or albinism. The cause of congenital nystagmus is often unknown. Acquired pendular nystagmus may result from demyelinating disease or vascular lesions of the brain stem or cerebellum.

Exophthalmos Associated with Thyrotoxicosis

Thyrotoxicosis may present with the signs and symptoms of bilateral or unilateral exophthalmos and edema of the eyelids. There is now evidence that this condition is a form of autoimmune disease. There is an abnormal production of T-lymphocyte antibody against the thyroid gland and retrobulbar muscle tissue, together with an increase in the mucopolysaccharides and edema of the muscles with an infiltration of lymphocytes. The enlargement of the muscles, which can be seen on CT scans, exerts pressure on the back of the eyeball and produces exophthalmos. As this process continues, there is a partial degeneration of the muscles, with a loss of cross-striation. Later, fibrosis of the extraocular muscles occurs, leading to immobility of the eyeball. Extensive contraction of the inferior rectus muscle is common, causing vertical diplopia and a limitation in elevating the eye.

Retrobulbar Neuritis, the Rectus Muscles, and the Dural Sheath of the Optic Nerve

The origins of the superior and inferior rectus muscles are attached to the dural sheath of the optic nerve. This attachment explains the pain of retrobulbar neuritis experienced when moving the eyeball.

Dysfunction of Ocular Movement Following a Blow-out Fracture of the Orbit

A blow-out fracture of the orbit caused by a frontal blow to the eyeball may result in entrapment of the inferior rectus and inferior oblique muscles and the orbital connective tissues in the fracture line in the orbital floor; such entrapment can seriously limit ocular mobility.

Drugs and Diseases Affecting the Motor End-plates of the Extraocular Muscles

Neuromuscular Blocking Agents

d-Tubocurarine produces flaccid paralysis of skeletal muscle, first affecting the extrinsic muscles of the eyes and then the face, and finally the diaphragm. *Dimethyl tubocurarine, gallamine,* and *benzoquinonium* have similar effects.

These drugs combine with the receptor sites at the postsynaptic membrane, and thus block the neurotransmitter action of acetylcholine. Therefore, they are referred to as *competitive blocking agents,* because they compete for the same receptor site as acetylcholine. They can also be referred to as *nondepolarizing agents* since they do not bring about depolarization. As these drugs are slowly metabolized, the paralysis fades.

Decamethonium and *succinylcholine* also paralyze skeletal muscle, but their action differs from that of competitive blocking agents because they produce their effect by causing depolarization of the motor end-plate. They are commonly referred to as *depolarizing agents.* Acting like acetylcholine, they produce depolarization of the postsynaptic membrane and the muscle contracts once. This is followed by a flaccid paralysis and a blockage of neuromuscular activity. Although the blocking action endures for some time, the drugs are metabolized and the paralysis fades. The actual paralysis is produced by the continued depolarization of the postsynaptic membrane. It must be remembered that continuous depolarization does not produce continuous skeletal muscle contraction. Repolarization has to take place before further depolarization can occur.

Neuromuscular blocking agents are commonly used with general anesthetics to produce the desired degree of muscle relaxation without using larger doses of general anesthetics. Because the respiratory muscles are paralyzed, facilities for artificial respiration are essential.

Anticholinesterases

Physostigmine and *neostigmine* have the capacity to combine with acetylcholinesterase and prevent the esterase from inactivating acetylcholine. In addition, neostigmine has a direct stimulating action on skeletal muscle. The actions of both drugs are reversible and they have been used with success in the treatment of myasthenia gravis.

Bacterial Toxins

Clostridium botulinum, the causative organism in certain cases of food poisoning, produces a toxin that inhibits the release of acetylcholine at the motor end-plate. Death results from paralysis of the respiratory muscles. Small doses of the toxin can be injected into the extraocular muscles to alter contractility. This treatment may be used to correct strabismus and to bring about paralysis of the antagonist muscle in extraocular palsies.

Myasthenia Gravis

Myasthenia gravis is a disease characterized by drooping of the upper eyelids (ptosis), double vision (diplopia), difficulty in swallowing (dysphagia), difficulty in talking (dysarthria), and general muscle weakness and fatigue. Initially, the disease most commonly involves the extraocular muscles of the eye and the pharynx and the symptoms can be relieved with rest. In the progressive form of the disease, the weakness becomes steadily worse and ultimately death occurs.

The condition is an autoimmune disorder in which antibodies are produced against the acetylcholine receptors on the postsynaptic membrane. This results in a reduced amplitude in end-plate potentials. The condition can be temporarily relieved by anticholinesterase drugs such as *neostigmine*, which potentiates the action of acetylcholine.

Table 8-3 gives some examples of drugs and diseases affecting the motor end-plates in the extraocular muscles.

Table 8-3   Examples of Drugs and Diseases Affecting the Motor End-plates in Extraocular Muscles

| Drug or Disease | Increasing ACh Release | Decreasing ACh Release | Acting on Ach Receptors | | AChE Inhibitor |
			Depolarizing Block	Ach Receptor Block	
Drug					
4-Aminopyridines	Yes	—	—	—	—
Guanidine hydrochloride	Yes	—	—	—	—
Succinylcholine	—	—	Yes	—	—
d-Tubocurarine	—	—	—	Yes	—
Dimethyl tubocurarine	—	—	—	Yes	—
Gallamine	—	—	—	Yes	—
Benzoquinonium	—	—	—	Yes	—
Physostigmine	—	—	—	—	Yes
Neostigmine	—	—	—	—	Yes
Disease					
Botulism (botulin toxin)	—	Yes	—	—	—
Myasthenia gravis	—	—	Destruction of receptors		—

ACH = acetylcholine; AChE = acetylcholinesterase.

Figure 8-23

Right eye of a 29-year-old woman. (A) The names of structures seen in examining the eye. (B) An enlarged view of the medial angle between the eyelids. (C) The lower eyelid, pulled downward and slightly everted to reveal the punctum lacrimale.

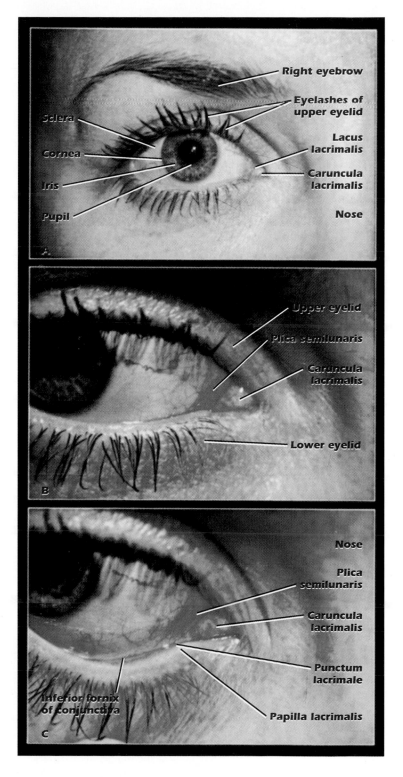

Figure 8-24

Right orbit and the eyelids. (A) Bones of the right orbit, anterior view. (B) Muscles of the eyelids. The lateral part of the upper lid has been removed to reveal the lacrimal gland and its relationship to the tendon of the levator palpebrae superioris muscle and the conjunctiva.

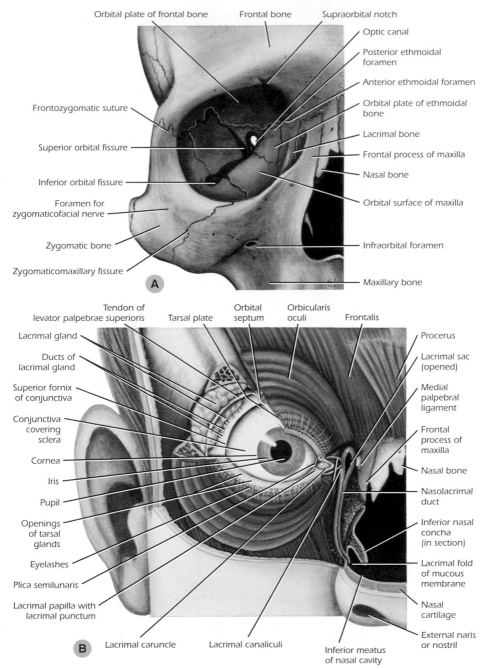

Figure 8-25

Right eye. (A) The superior and inferior tarsal plates, orbital septum, and lacrimal gland. (B) The superior and inferior tarsal plates, conjunctiva, and lacrimal gland, sac, and duct.

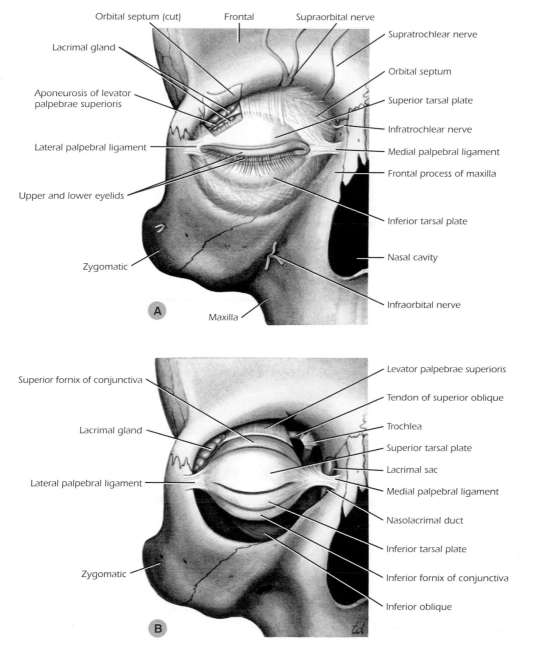

A

Orbital septum (cut) — Frontal — Supraorbital nerve — Supratrochlear nerve — Orbital septum — Superior tarsal plate — Infratrochlear nerve — Medial palpebral ligament — Frontal process of maxilla — Inferior tarsal plate — Nasal cavity — Infraorbital nerve

Lacrimal gland — Aponeurosis of levator palpebrae superioris — Lateral palpebral ligament — Upper and lower eyelids — Zygomatic — Maxilla

B

Superior fornix of conjunctiva — Lacrimal gland — Lateral palpebral ligament — Zygomatic

Levator palpebrae superioris — Tendon of superior oblique — Trochlea — Superior tarsal plate — Lacrimal sac — Medial palpebral ligament — Nasolacrimal duct — Inferior tarsal plate — Inferior fornix of conjunctiva — Inferior oblique

Figure 8-26

Right eye, showing the eyeball exposed from in front. Note the arrangement of the superior and inferior oblique muscles.

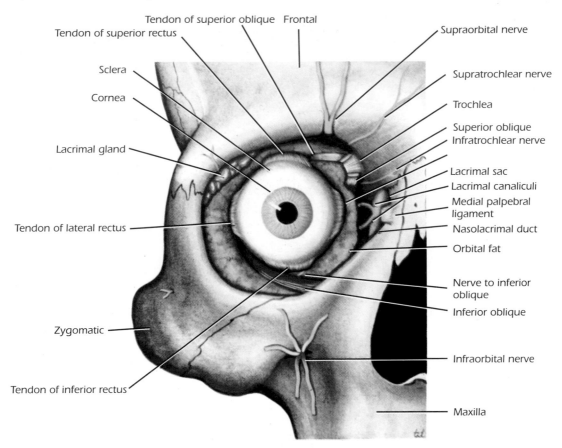

Tendon of superior oblique   Frontal

Tendon of superior rectus

Supraorbital nerve

Sclera

Cornea

Supratrochlear nerve

Trochlea

Superior oblique
Infratrochlear nerve

Lacrimal gland

Lacrimal sac
Lacrimal canaliculi
Medial palpebral ligament
Nasolacrimal duct

Tendon of lateral rectus

Orbital fat

Nerve to inferior oblique
Inferior oblique

Zygomatic

Infraorbital nerve

Tendon of inferior rectus

Maxilla

Figure 8-27

(A) Fascial sheath of the eyeball after eyeball removal. (B) Extrinsic muscles and their related nerves.

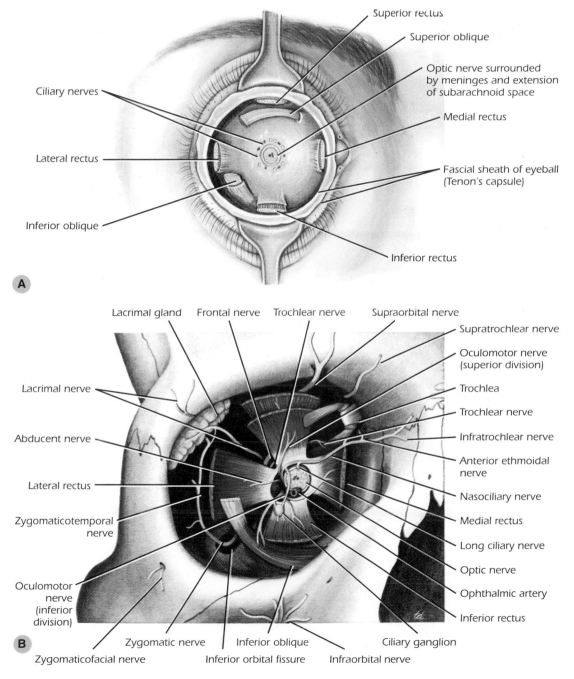

Figure 8-28

Right orbit viewed from above. (A) The periorbita (orbital fascia) after removal of the orbital plate of the frontal bone. (B) Deeper structures after removal of the periorbita.

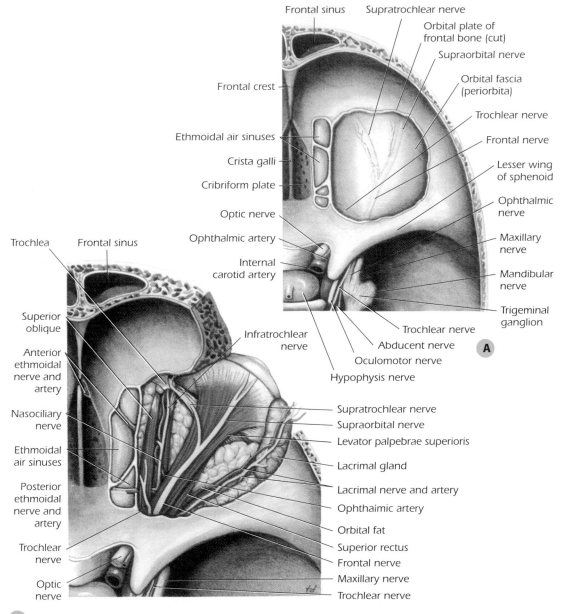

Figure 8-29

Right orbit viewed from above. The frontal nerve and the levator palpebrae superioris muscle have been reflected to show the superior rectus muscle.

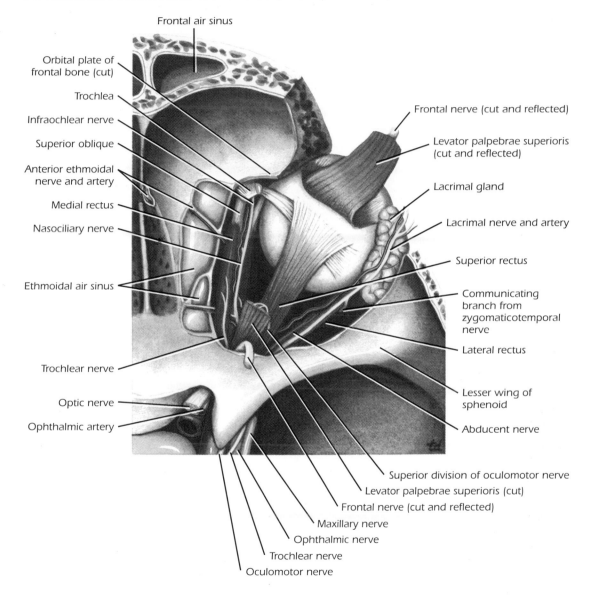

Frontal air sinus

Orbital plate of frontal bone (cut)

Trochlea

Infraochlear nerve

Superior oblique

Anterior ethmoidal nerve and artery

Medial rectus

Nasociliary nerve

Ethmoidal air sinus

Trochlear nerve

Optic nerve

Ophthalmic artery

Frontal nerve (cut and reflected)

Levator palpebrae superioris (cut and reflected)

Lacrimal gland

Lacrimal nerve and artery

Superior rectus

Communicating branch from zygomaticotemporal nerve

Lateral rectus

Lesser wing of sphenoid

Abducent nerve

Superior division of oculomotor nerve

Levator palpebrae superioris (cut)

Frontal nerve (cut and reflected)

Maxillary nerve

Ophthalmic nerve

Trochlear nerve

Oculomotor nerve

Figure 8-30

Right orbit. (A) View from above after reflection of the frontal nerve, levator palpebrae superioris muscle, and superior rectus muscle. (B) View from the lateral side after removal of the lateral wall of the orbit and the lateral rectus muscle.

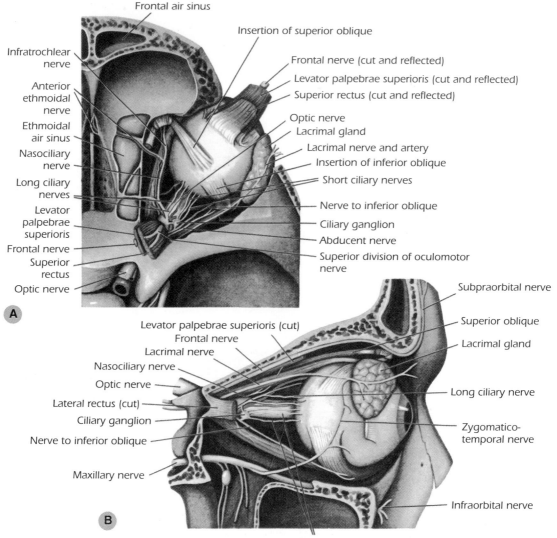

Frontal air sinus

Insertion of superior oblique

Infratrochlear nerve

Frontal nerve (cut and reflected)

Levator palpebrae superioris (cut and reflected)

Superior rectus (cut and reflected)

Anterior ethmoidal nerve

Optic nerve

Lacrimal gland

Ethmoidal air sinus

Lacrimal nerve and artery

Nasociliary nerve

Insertion of inferior oblique

Long ciliary nerves

Short ciliary nerves

Levator palpebrae superioris

Nerve to inferior oblique

Ciliary ganglion

Abducent nerve

Frontal nerve

Superior rectus

Superior division of oculomotor nerve

Optic nerve

A

Levator palpebrae superioris (cut)

Frontal nerve

Subpraorbital nerve

Lacrimal nerve

Superior oblique

Nasociliary nerve

Lacrimal gland

Optic nerve

Lateral rectus (cut)

Long ciliary nerve

Ciliary ganglion

Nerve to inferior oblique

Zygomatico-temporal nerve

Maxillary nerve

Infraorbital nerve

B

Short ciliary nerve

Figure 8-31

Right eyeball. (A) Anterior view, showing the attachment of the extrinsic muscles.
(B) Posterior view, showing the precise insertion of the superior and inferior oblique
muscles.

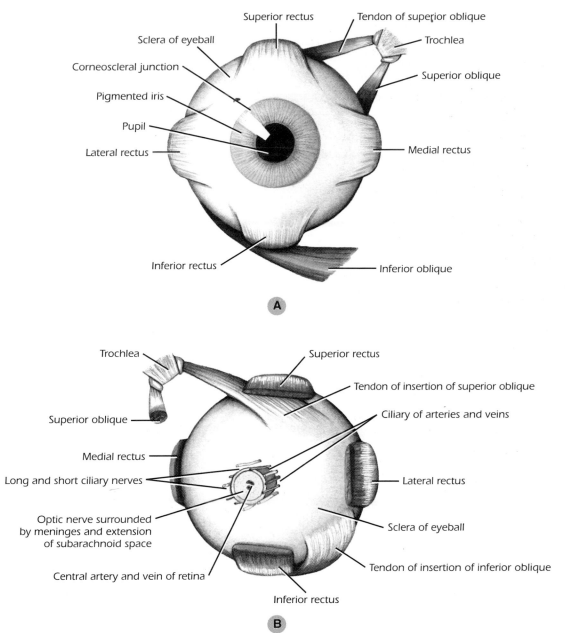

CHAPTER 8
Clinical Problems

Answers on Page 274.

1 When a patient is asked to gaze vertically upward and downward during an ophthalmologic examination, it is noted that the eyelids also move to some extent with the movements of the eyeball. Explain this anatomically.

2 A 38-year-old man visited his physician because he had noticed that his upper eyelid drooped, especially when he was tired or emotionally upset. He had first observed this 8 months earlier. Three months before, he had started to have double vision, which was very slight to begin with and lasted only a few hours. During the past week the double vision had returned, was more severe, and lasted several hours. He commented that his friends have remarked that he does not seem to smile as much as he used to. On questioning he admitted that talking tires him and that his throat feels particularly tired after eating a large meal. On physical examination the patient had slight ptosis (drooping of the upper lid) of the left eye. The eye movements appeared to be normal, but the man's face appeared to be unnaturally immobile. In his attempts to smile the expression was more of a snarl than a happy expression. It was also noted that the patient responded to questions in a rather feeble voice with a nasal quality. When asked to hold his arms outstretched in front of him, the patient became quickly fatigued. What is the diagnosis? What causes this condition?

3 A distinguished author in the field of ophthalmology states that one of the main functions of the inferior oblique muscle is to produce extorsion. Explain the statement.

4 A 50-year-old-woman was seen as an outpatient because she had suddenly developed double vision. She was watching her favorite television program the day before, when double vision suddenly occurred. She had no other symptoms. A complete physical examination revealed that her left eye, when at rest, was turned medially and she was unable to turn it laterally. A moderate amount of glucose was found in her urine, and she had an abnormally elevated blood glucose level. When closely questioned, she admitted that recently she had noticed having to pass water more frequently, especially at night. She also said she often felt thirsty. Without making any efforts to reduce weight, she had lost 30 pounds during the past 3 years. Using your knowledge of neuroanatomy, explain the problem in her left eye. Do you think there is any connection between her glucosuria, high blood glucose, polyuria, polydipsia, and weight loss and her eye condition?

5 A 75-year-old man with a known history of cerebrovascular problems visited his physician because 4 days previously he had begun to have trouble reading the paper. He complained that the print started to tilt and that he was beginning to "see double." He also remarked that he found it difficult to see the steps when he descended the staircase to the physician's office. On physical examination, the patient showed weakness of movement of the left eye both downward and laterally. Using your knowledge of anatomy, explain this patient's signs and symptoms. If we assume that a cranial nerve nucleus is the site of the lesion, is it the right one or the left one that is involved?

6 A 47-year-old woman was admitted to the hospital complaining of severe pain of the left forehead and right eye. The pain had started 3 weeks previously and had progressively increased since then. One week ago she started to have double vision, and this morning her husband had noticed that her left eye was turning out laterally. The physician in charge made a careful neurologic work-up on this patient and found a lateral deviation of the left eye, dilatation of the left pupil with loss of direct and consensual light reflexes, paralysis of accommodation of the left eye, and paralysis of all left-sided ocular movement except laterally. He advised the patient to have a left-sided carotid arteriogram. The film showed an aneurysm of the internal carotid artery on the left side. Explain this patient's signs and symptoms, and relate the signs and symptoms to the aneurysm.

7 After examining a 33-year-old man, the ophthalmologist turned to a fourth-year medical student and said, "This patient has a definite weakness in supraduction and incycloduction of the right eye." What is meant by these terms? Which muscles are used to produce levocycloversion?

8 A 42-year-old man with pyemia secondary to a large carbuncle on the back of his neck suddenly developed a marked fever, chills, and sweating. During the next 48 hours he developed exophthalmos and immobility of his right eye. A CT scan of his orbits showed the presence of a space-occupying lesion behind his right eyeball. Given the history, explain the lesion of the right eye.

9 A 25-year-old student was involved in a head-on collision in his automobile. He was admitted to hospital with severe facial bruising, and an ophthalmology resident was called to examine his eyes. During the examination the resident tested the actions of the extraocular muscles. How would you test the actions of the superior rectus and the superior oblique muscles?

10 A senior ophthalmic surgeon was discussing the surgical treatment of strabismus with his resident. He stated that it was possible to perform a larger recession on the lateral rectus than on the medial rectus muscles without altering the ability of the lateral rectus to rotate the eye. Explain anatomically why this is so.

11 Explain the action of the extraocular muscles used in "rotating the eye upward" or "elevating the eye."

12 Where do the sensory nerve fibers originate in the extraocular muscles? Explain the significance of Hering's law and Sherrington's law of reciprocal innervation relative to the actions of the extraocular muscles.

CHAPTER 8
Answers to Clinical Problems

1 At the point where the tendon of the superior rectus muscle pierces the fascial sheath of the eyeball to pass to its insertion on the sclera, the sheath is reflected backward along the muscle, providing it with a tubular sheath. This muscle sheath is connected by a band of connective tissue to the tendon of the levator palpebrae superioris and to the superior fornix of the conjunctiva. As the result of these connections, the two muscles work together to raise the upper eyelid and raise the superior fornix of the conjunctiva when a person gazes upward.

Similar fascial connections unite the inferior rectus muscle to the inferior tarsal plate and the conjunctiva of the inferior fornix. By this means the lower lid moves downward with the eyeball when a person looks downward.

2 This patient is suffering from myasthenia gravis. The insidious onset of muscle fatigue, with early involvement of the extraocular muscles, the facial muscles, then the pharyngeal and palatal muscles, with exacerbations and remissions, is characteristic of myasthenia gravis, an autoimmune disorder in which there is a reduced responsiveness of the postsynaptic membrane to acetylcholine. The T-lymphocytes produced by the thymus in some way affect the receptor sites. The condition can be temporarily relieved by anticholinesterase drugs such as neostigmine, which potentiate the action of acetylcholine.

3 The movement of torsion can be brought about by the superior and inferior recti and the superior and inferior obliques. This is possible because their direction of pull with the eye in the primary position is not in the line of the vertical axis of the eyeball. This function is greater for the oblique muscles than for the recti, and greatest for the inferior oblique. It will be remembered that the inferior oblique pulls forward at an angle of 51 degrees to the nasal side of the vertical axis of the eyeball, whereas the angle for the superior oblique is 54 degrees.

4 The convergent strabismus of this patient's left eye, the diplopia, and the inability to turn the left eye laterally were due to paralysis of the left lateral rectus muscle, caused by a lesion of the abducent nerve. The glucosuria, high blood glucose, polyuria, polydipsia, and weight loss are the classic signs and symptoms of diabetes mellitus. The lesion of the abducent nerve was an example of diabetic neuropathy, a complication of untreated or inadequately treated diabetes. Once the patient's diabetes was carefully controlled, the left lateral rectus palsy disappeared within 3 months.

5 This patient has a paralysis of the left superior oblique muscle resulting from a lesion of the trochlear nerve. Since the trochlear nerves decussate on emergence from the midbrain, the right trochlear nucleus is the site of the lesion. This patient had a thrombosis of a small artery supplying the right trochlear nucleus. The difficulty in reading, the diplopia, and the difficulty in walking downstairs were due to the paralysis of the left superior oblique muscle.

6 The severe pain over the forehead and the left eye was due to irritation of the ophthalmic division of the trigeminal nerve by the slowly expanding aneurysm of the internal carotid artery lying in the cavernous sinus. The double vision (diplopia) and the lateral deviation of the left eye were due to the unopposed action of the lateral rectus muscle (supplied by the abducent nerve). Pressure on the left oculomotor nerve by the aneurysm caused the dilatation of the left pupil, with loss of direct and consensual light reflexes, paralysis of accommodation, and paralysis of all left-sided ocular movement except laterally. The nerve at this point is situated in the lateral wall of the cavernous sinus. Note that the lateral movement of the eyeball was accomplished by contracting the lateral rectus muscle (abducent nerve); the inferolateral movement, by contracting the superior oblique muscle (trochlear nerve).

7 *Supraduction* is the term used to denote the vertical elevation of the cornea of one eye. *Incycloduction* is the term to denote intorsion, or medial rotation of the upper rim of the cornea of one eye. *Version* is the simultaneous movement of both eyes in the same direction. *Levocycloversion* is produced by contraction of the extorters of the left eye, namely, the inferior rectus and the inferior oblique, and the intorters of the right eye, namely, the superior rectus and the superior oblique.

8 This patient with pyemia developed a retrobulbar abscess of the right eye. The pus had accumulated in the surgical fascial space within the cone of the rectus muscles. Because this space is closed off anteriorly by the eyeball, as the pus accumulated, it pushed the eyeball forward. It also seriously interfered with the mobility of the eyeball. Because the infection was confined within the muscle cone, the inflammation did not involve the conjunctiva or the eyelids.

9 Because the origin of the superior rectus muscle from the apical region of the orbital cavity is situated about 23 degrees medial to its insertion on the eyeball, you first ask the patient to look laterally, so that the muscle is in the optimum position to raise the cornea. Then you ask the patient to look upward from the lateral position.

In the case of the superior oblique muscle, the tendon passes backward and laterally from the trochlea to its insertion on the eyeball on the nasal side of the vertical axis. The patient is first asked to look medially, thus placing the muscle in the optimum position to lower the cornea. Then you ask the patient to look downward to the tip of his nose.

10 According to Dr. Duke Elder (1961), a rectus muscle may be recessed as far as the functional equator without limiting its ability to rotate the eye. Since the lateral and medial recti pass forward obliquely from their origin to their insertion on the eyeball, the lateral rectus tendon first comes into contact with the eyeball 4 mm behind the anatomic equator and then passes forward to its insertion. On the medial side of the eyeball, the medial rectus tendon, however, first comes into contact with the eyeball close to its insertion, about 4 mm in front of the anatomic equator. A circle joining the first points of contact of these two tendons with the eyeball gives you the functional equator.

11 Elevation of the cornea directly upward is accomplished by contraction of the superior rectus muscle assisted by the inferior oblique muscle. Because the superior rectus is obliquely placed in the orbit, the direction of pull is not only upward but posteromedially. Thus the primary action is elevation on a transverse axis, slight medial rotation on a vertical axis, and very slight intorsion on the anteroposterior axis. The tendency to cause medial rotation and intorsion is countered by the simultaneous contraction of the inferior oblique muscle, which also elevates but tends to rotate laterally and cause extorsion. The sum of all these actions is that the cornea moves vertically upward.

12 The sensory nerve fibers originate in the muscle spindles and tendon organs of the extraocular muscles. They play a very important role in keeping the central nervous system informed of the length and tension existing in each muscle. The significance of Hering's law and Sherrington's law of reciprocal innervation is fully discussed on page 255.

The Orbital Blood Vessels

The eye and the orbital contents receive their main arterial supply from the ophthalmic artery. The venous blood of the orbit is drained by the superior and inferior ophthalmic veins. The orbit possesses no lymphatic vessels or lymphoid tissue.*

Arteries of the Orbit

Ophthalmic Artery

The ophthalmic artery is a branch of the internal carotid artery after that vessel emerges from the cavernous sinus medial to the anterior clinoid process (Fig. 9-1). It passes forward through the optic canal below and lateral to the optic nerve. At its origin from the internal carotid artery, the ophthalmic artery lies within the subarachnoid space. As the ophthalmic artery runs forward within the space through the optic canal, it lies within the dural-arachnoid sheath of the optic nerve. On emerging from the optic canal, the artery pierces the meningeal sheath and comes to lie outside it.

In the orbital cavity the artery runs forward for a short distance lateral to the optic nerve (Fig. 9-1) and medial to the lateral rectus muscle, the abducent and oculomotor nerves, and the ciliary ganglion. The artery then turns medially and crosses above the optic nerve, accompanied by the nasociliary nerve. Here it lies inferior to the superior rectus muscle. On reaching the medial wall of the orbit, it runs forward with the nasociliary nerve above the medial rectus muscle and below the superior oblique. At the medial end of the upper eyelid the ophthalmic artery divides into the supratrochlear and dorsal nasal arteries (Fig. 9-1). The course of the ophthalmic artery may be very tortuous, and in 15 percent of people the artery crosses below the optic nerve rather than above it.

Branches

These are as follows:

1. Central artery of the retina
2. Lacrimal artery
3. Muscular branches
4. Ciliary arteries
5. Supraorbital artery
6. Posterior ethmoidal artery
7. Anterior ethmoidal artery
8. Meningeal artery
9. Medial palpebral arteries
10. Supratrochlear arteries
11. Dorsal nasal artery

Central Artery of the Retina   The central artery of the retina is a slender artery that arises from the ophthalmic artery as it lies inferolateral to the optic nerve close to the optic canal (Fig. 9-1). It runs forward beneath the optic nerve, and about 1.25 cm behind the eyeball it turns upward to pierce the dura and arachnoid sheaths

---

*The lacrimal gland is drained by lymphatic vessels that follow those from the eyelids into the parotid lymph nodes.

Figure 9-1

Diagram showing the origin and branches of the ophthalmic artery within the orbital cavity.

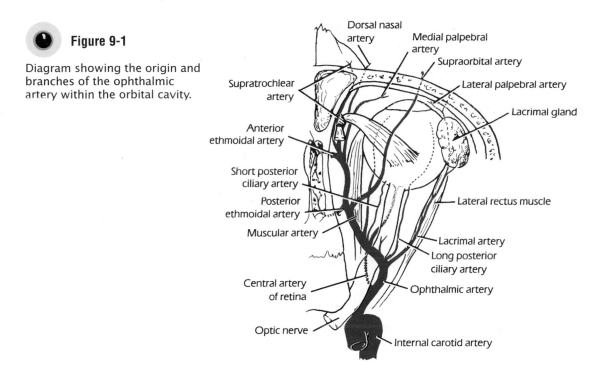

of the optic nerve (Fig. 9-2). It passes obliquely across the subarachnoid space and enters the optic nerve. At the center of the nerve the artery turns forward in company with its vein. It enters the back of the eyeball by piercing the lamina cribrosa. The central artery now divides into two equal superior and inferior branches. After a few millimeters these branches divide into superior, inferior, nasal, and temporal branches. The four arteries now supply a quadrant of the retina and are distributed to its superficial layers as described in the section Blood Supply of the Retina (see p. 188).

Branches of the Central Artery *Small meningeal branches* supply the pial sheath of the optic nerve as the central artery pierces the pia mater (Fig. 9-2). Very small anastomoses occur between the pial vessels at the distal end of the optic nerve and the small vessels in the sclera about the nerve head (circle of Zinn). It should be emphasized that these anastomoses are extremely small, and for practical purposes the central artery of the retina should be considered an end artery (see cilioretinal artery, p. 282).

Central collateral branches have been described arising from the central artery as the central artery enters the optic nerve (Fig. 9-2). A central collateral artery may pass with the central artery toward the lamina cribrosa. A branch of a central collateral artery may pass posteriorly within the optic nerve toward the optic canal and supply the macular nerve fibers.

Lacrimal Artery   The lacrimal artery is a large branch that arises from the ophthalmic artery close to its emergence from the optic canal (Fig. 9-1). Occasionally

Figure 9-2

Diagram showing the blood supply to the optic nerve within the orbital cavity. Note the extensive pial plexus of vessels and the arterial circle of Zinn.

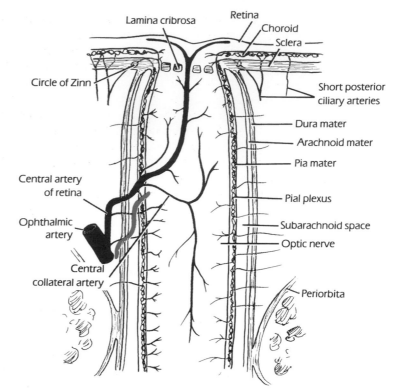

the artery arises from the ophthalmic artery before it enters the orbit. More rarely, the lacrimal artery is a branch of the middle meningeal artery, entering the orbit through the superior orbital fissure.

The lacrimal artery runs forward on the upper border of the lateral rectus muscle accompanied by the lacrimal nerve. It passes through the lacrimal gland, which it supplies, and sends terminal branches to the eyelids and conjunctiva.

Branches of the lacrimal artery include the *lateral palpebral arteries,* which pass medially into the upper and lower eyelids and anastomose with the medial palpebral arteries; the *zygomatic branches,* which pass through the zygomatico-facial and zygomaticotemporal foramina to anastomose with arteries on the face and in the temporal fossa; and a *muscular branch* to the lateral rectus muscle. A *recurrent meningeal branch* runs posteriorly through the lateral part of the superior orbital fissure to anastomose with a branch of the middle meningeal artery.

Muscular Branches   A variable number of muscular branches arise from the ophthalmic artery as it passes forward in the orbital cavity. Most of these branches accompany the branches of the oculomotor nerve. The arteries to the rectus muscles give origin to the anterior ciliary arteries (see below).

Ciliary Arteries   There are three groups of ciliary arteries: the long posterior, the short posterior, and the anterior.

The *long posterior ciliary arteries*, usually two in number, arise from the ophthalmic artery as it crosses the optic nerve (Fig. 9-1). They run forward with the optic nerve and pierce the sclera of the eyeball medial and lateral to the nerve outside the circle formed by the short posterior ciliary arteries (Fig. 9-3). The long posterior ciliary arteries then run forward between the sclera and the choroid to the ciliary body. At the attached margin of the iris they divide into upper and lower branches which encircle the iris and anastomose with corresponding branches of the artery on the other side (Fig. 9-3). In addition, they anastomose with the anterior ciliary arteries to form the *major arterial circle of the iris* (see the discussion of the blood supply of the iris, p. 171). Recurrent branches of the long posterior ciliary arteries and branches from the major arterial circle and the anterior ciliary arteries supply the choroid posteriorly as far as the equator of the eyeball and anastomose with the short posterior ciliary arteries (Fig. 9-3).

 Figure 9-3

Diagram showing the arterial supply and venous drainage of the uveal tract.

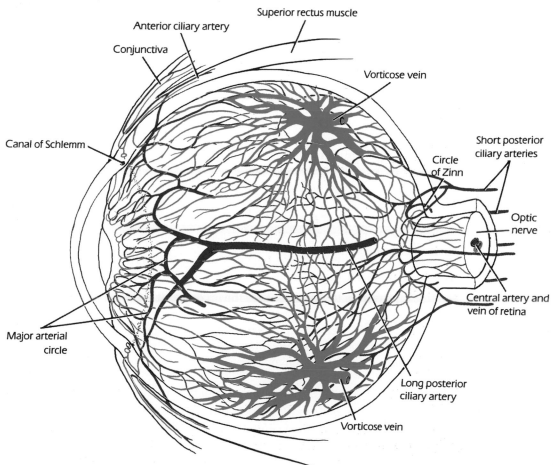

The *short posterior ciliary arteries* are about seven in number. They arise from the ophthalmic artery as it crosses the optic nerve (Fig. 9-1). After dividing into 10 to 20 branches, they run forward around the optic nerve, mingling with the short ciliary nerves. The arteries pierce the sclera around the entrance of the optic nerve and supply the choroid as far forward as the equator of the eyeball (Fig. 9-3). Here they anastomose with the recurrent branches of the long posterior ciliary arteries, branches of the major arterial circle of the iris, and branches of the anterior ciliary arteries.

A number of small branches of the short posterior ciliary arteries form an anastomotic ring (ring of Zinn) around the optic disc (Fig. 9-3). Small branches from the ring anastomose with blood vessels in the pia covering the optic nerve. In approximately 15 to 20 percent of people a *cilioretinal artery* arises from the ciliary circulation. It enters the retina at the lateral border of the optic nerve and supplies an area of the retina between the optic disc and the macula. Its presence is of particular importance in cases of central retinal artery occlusion (see p. 192).

The *anterior ciliary arteries* originate from the muscular branches of the ophthalmic artery to the four rectus muscles (Fig. 9-3). There are two anterior ciliary arteries associated with each rectus muscle, with the exception of the lateral rectus muscle, which is provided only one anterior ciliary artery. These arteries supply the sclera and the conjunctiva, and send branches through the sclera at the insertion of the recti tendons. These latter twigs join the long posterior ciliary arteries to form the *great arterial circle of the iris.*

Supraorbital Artery   The supraorbital artery arises from the ophthalmic artery as it crosses the optic nerve (Fig. 9-1). It passes superiorly round the medial borders of the superior rectus and levator palpebrae superioris muscles. The artery then runs forward with the supraorbital nerve between the levator and the roof of the orbit. It leaves the orbit by passing through the supraorbital notch or foramen and ascends to the scalp deep to the frontalis muscle (Fig. 9-4). Its terminal branches anastomose with branches of the supratrochlear and superficial temporal arteries.

The supraorbital artery supplies the levator palpebrae superioris, the diploë of the frontal bone, the frontal sinus, the upper eyelid, and the skin of the forehead and the scalp.

Posterior Ethmoidal Artery   The posterior ethmoidal artery arises from the ophthalmic artery when the latter reaches the medial wall of the orbit (Fig. 9-1). It passes medially between the upper border of the medial rectus muscle and the superior oblique muscle to enter the posterior ethmoidal canal. The artery supplies the posterior ethmoidal air sinuses, the dura of the anterior cranial fossa, and the upper part of the nasal mucosa.

Anterior Ethmoidal Artery   The anterior ethmoidal artery is larger than the posterior ethmoidal artery. It arises from the ophthalmic artery (Fig. 9-1) and enters the anterior ethmoidal canal accompanied by the anterior ethmoidal nerve. The artery then enters the anterior cranial fossa and passes into the nose through the cribriform plate of the ethmoid. It then descends in a groove on the deep surface

Figure 9-4

Diagram showing the arterial supply to the eyelids.

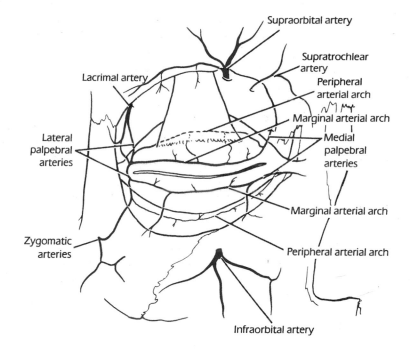

of the nasal bone to enter the face between the nasal bone and the upper nasal cartilage.

During this long course the artery supplies the anterior and middle ethmoidal air cells, the frontal air sinus, the meninges, the mucous membrane of the anterior part of the nasal cavity, and the skin of the nose.

Meningeal Artery   This small artery runs posteriorly through the superior orbital fissure to supply the meninges in the middle cranial fossa.

Medial Palpebral Arteries   The two medial palpebral arteries arise from the anterior part of the ophthalmic artery below the pulley for the superior oblique muscle. They descend behind the lacrimal sac and pierce the orbital septum above and below the medial palpebral ligament (Fig. 9-4). Each artery passes laterally to enter the upper and lower eyelid and divides into two branches, which form the *peripheral and marginal arterial arches* (Fig. 9-4). The arches run laterally between the orbicularis oculi muscle and the tarsal plates. Branches from the arches supply the eyelids and conjunctiva.

Supratrochlear Arteries   The supratrochlear artery, a terminal branch of the ophthalmic artery, leaves the orbit by piercing the orbital septum above the pulley for the superior oblique muscle (Fig. 9-4). It is accompanied by the supratrochlear nerve and supplies the skin of the forehead and scalp.

Dorsal Nasal Artery   The dorsal nasal artery, a terminal branch of the ophthalmic artery (Fig. 9-1), pierces the orbital septum. It passes above the medial palpebral ligament and then descends to the side of the nose. It gives off branches to the lacrimal sac and anastomoses with the facial artery.

Infraorbital Artery

The infraorbital artery arises from the maxillary artery in the pterygopalatine fossa. It enters the orbital cavity through the inferior orbital fissure accompanied by the infraorbital nerve, which is a continuation of the maxillary nerve. Both the artery and the nerve pass forward in the infraorbital groove and canal to emerge on the face through the infraorbital foramen (Fig. 9-4).

Besides supplying the skin and tissues of the face, the maxillary air sinus, and the teeth of the upper jaw (anterior superior alveolar artery), the infraorbital artery gives off *orbital branches* to the inferior rectus and inferior oblique muscles and the lacrimal sac.

Arterial Supply of the Eyeball

Two distinct arterial systems are involved in supplying the eye. The central artery of the retina and its branches are distributed to the inner two-thirds of the retina. The outer-third of the retina, which includes the photoreceptors, is avascular and nourished by tissue fluid derived from the blood vessels in the choroid. The fovea centralis is completely avascular and does not contain a single blood vessel.

As has been emphasized, occlusion of the retinal arteries, which are end arteries, results in the destruction of the inner retinal layers. It has been estimated that irreparable damage occurs in 1 hour. Occlusion of the choroidal arteries leads to damage of the outer part of the retina, even though numerous anastomoses occur between choroidal arteries.

In the anterior segment of the eye, which includes the iris and ciliary body, as well as the insertions of the rectus muscles, the blood supply is profuse owing to the extensive anastomoses that occur between the anterior and long posterior ciliary arteries. For this reason extensive tendon surgery for the correction of strabismus does not result in ischemia.

Nervous Control of the Arterial Supply to the Eyeball

Postganglionic nerves from the superior cervical sympathetic ganglion supply the central artery of the retina up to the lamina cribrosa but not beyond. The choroidal arteries, on the other hand, receive a plentiful supply of postganglionic sympathetic fibers. The parasympathetic innervation of the arteries is derived from the oculomotor nerve via the ciliary ganglion and from the facial nerve via the pterygopalatine ganglion.

Increased sympathetic activity, as occurs at times of stress, is believed to cause arterial vasoconstriction and a reduction in blood flow. The beneficial effect is a reduction in the formation of tissue fluid at the blood-retina barrier and in the formation of aqueous humor. This offsets the general body reaction to increased sympathetic activity at times of stress that causes a rise in blood pressure and an increased production of tissue fluid.

The effect of increased parasympathetic activity on the arteries of the eyeball is not fully understood.

Clinical Notes

The Central Artery of the Retina and Raised Cerebrospinal Fluid Pressure

Unlike the thin-walled central vein of the retina, the thick-walled central artery of the retina is unaffected by a raised cerebrospinal fluid (CSF) pressure. It will be remembered that both these vessels cross the extension of the subarachnoid space around the optic nerve to enter the optic nerve (Fig. 9-2).

Variations in the Anatomy of the Ophthalmic Artery and Its Branches

Rarely, the ophthalmic artery arises not from the internal carotid artery but from the middle meningeal artery. As mentioned, in 15 percent of people, the ophthalmic artery crosses below the optic nerve rather than above it.

Considerable variation exists as to the precise origin of the branches of the ophthalmic artery.

Obstruction of the Internal Carotid or Ophthalmic Arteries and Its Effect on Sight

Multiple anastomoses exist between the branches of the ophthalmic artery and branches of the external carotid artery on the face and scalp (see Table 9-1). These anastomoses provide adequate blood for the central artery of the retina in most people, should the internal carotid or the ophthalmic arteries become blocked. Thus, in most patients these conditions do not result in permanent blindness.

Central Artery Occlusion

The effects of central artery occlusion are discussed on page 192. The artery is susceptible to arteriosclerotic occlusive disease, and most occlusions occur as the artery is emerging from the optic nerve head.

The presence of a cilioretinal artery in approximately 15 to 20 percent of patients is very important in central artery occlusion. The cilioretinal artery arises from the ciliary circulation and enters the retina on the temporal side of the optic disc, between the disc and the macula. In cases of complete central artery occlusion, the presence of a cilioretinal artery will provide for an area of preserved central vision, and thus protect patients from complete blindness.

Table 9-1 Locations of Anastomoses Between Branches of the Ophthalmic Artery and the External Carotid Artery

Ophthalmic Artery	External Carotid Artery	Location
Dorsal nasal branch	Facial artery	Inner canthus
Lacrimal branch	Transverse facial, superficial temporal	Outer canthus
Lacrimal branch	Middle meningeal, deep temporal	Orbital cavity

Foveal Avascular Free Zone

With the advent of laser therapy in recent years, the presence of the foveal avascular free zone has assumed particular importance. In this area, which can be easily seen on fluorescent angiograms, the circulation is vulnerable, because it depends entirely for its nutrition on the underlying choriocapillaries; there are no branches of the central artery at this site.

Central Artery and Vein Relationships Relative to Disease

The fact that the retinal arteries cross the retinal veins and that they are enveloped in a common tight connective tissue covering at these points may explain venous occlusion in arterial disease. For example, in arterial sclerosis the vein can be compressed at the crossing sites.

Blood-Retina Barrier

As noted previously in Chapter 6, page 191, the neural retina, like the brain, is protected from large molecular toxic substances by a barrier. The outer third of the neural retina is protected by the zonulae occludentes that close off the spaces between the pigment epithelial cells of the pigment layer of the retina (Fig. 9-5). The inner two-thirds of the retina that is supplied by the central artery is protected by the zonula occludentes that closes off the spaces between the endothelial cells of the capillaries (Fig. 9-5).

Veins of the Orbit ·

The veins of the orbit are tortuous and freely anastomose with one another; they have no valves. The orbit is drained by the superior and inferior ophthalmic veins, which in turn drain directly into the cavernous sinus. The central retinal vein usually drains directly into the cavernous sinus or into the superior ophthalmic vein.

Superior Ophthalmic Vein

This is the larger of the two ophthalmic veins. The superior ophthalmic vein arises behind the medial part of the upper eyelid by the union of a branch of the supraorbital vein and a branch from the facial vein (Fig. 9-6). The branch from the supraorbital vein enters the orbit through the supraorbital notch, while the branch from the facial vein pierces the orbital septum. The superior ophthalmic vein passes posteriorly in the orbital fat receiving tributaries that correspond to most of the branches of the ophthalmic artery. It communicates with the central vein of the retina and near the apex of the orbit it commonly receives the inferior ophthalmic vein. The superior ophthalmic vein also receives the two *vorticose veins* (*venae vorticosae*) (Fig. 9-6) from the upper part of the eyeball (the vorticose veins correspond to the posterior ciliary veins).

   The superior ophthalmic vein crosses the optic nerve with the ophthalmic artery. It leaves the orbit through the upper part of the superior orbital fissure, above the lateral rectus muscle, to join the cavernous sinus.

Figure 9-5

Diagram showing the nourishment (arrows) of the neural retina. Note that the inner two-thirds is nourished by capillaries fed by the central artery; the outer third is nourished by tissue fluid diffusing from the capillaries in the choroid. Note also that the retina, like the brain, is protected by the blood-retina barrier, formed by the zonulae occludentes of the endothelial cells of the central artery capillaries and those between the cell membranes of the retinal pigment epithelial cells.

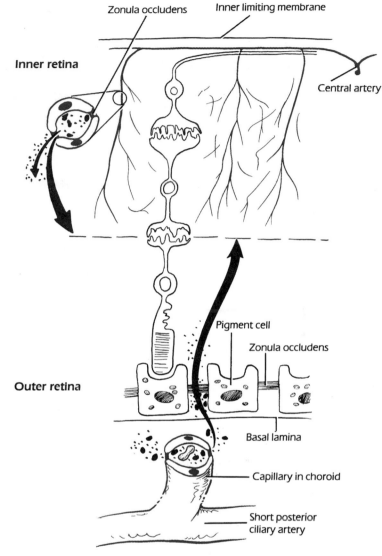

Inferior Ophthalmic Vein

This vein arises from a venous plexus on the anterior part of the floor of the orbital cavity (Fig. 9-6). It communicates with the facial vein over the inferior orbital margin and with the pterygoid venous plexus through the inferior orbital fissure. It passes posteriorly in the orbital fat on the inferior rectus muscle and receives muscular branches and the two inferior *vorticose veins* from the lower part of the eyeball. The inferior ophthalmic vein drains into the cavernous sinus, or it may pass through the lower part of the inferior orbital fissure and empty into the pterygoid venous plexus.

Figure 9-6

A lateral view of the veins draining the right orbit.

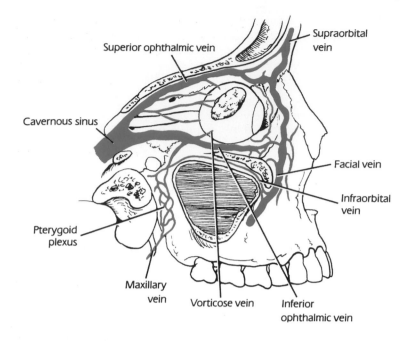

Superior ophthalmic vein

Supraorbital vein

Cavernous sinus

Facial vein

Infraorbital vein

Pterygoid plexus

Maxillary vein

Vorticose vein

Inferior ophthalmic vein

Central Vein of the Retina

The central vein of the retina is formed by the union of tributaries that correspond approximately to the branches of the central artery of the retina (see p. 191). The central vein leaves the eyeball by piercing the lamina cribrosa in company with the artery. The vein now passes backward within the optic nerve. About 10 mm behind the eyeball, the central vein leaves the nerve, crosses the extension of the subarachnoid space around the nerve, and emerges from the dura-arachnoid sheath behind the artery (Fig. 9-2). The vein then drains directly into the cavernous sinus or enters the superior ophthalmic vein. The central vein always communicates with the superior ophthalmic vein.

Infraorbital Vein

The infraorbital vein arises on the face by the union of several tributaries. Accompanied by the infraorbital artery and the infraorbital nerve, it passes posteriorly through the infraorbital foramen, infraorbital canal, and infraorbital groove. It drains through the inferior orbital fissure into the pterygoid venous plexus. It receives tributaries from structures that lie close to the floor of the orbit and communicates with the inferior ophthalmic vein.

Clinical Notes

Papilledema, the Central Vein of the Retina, and Increased Intracranial Pressure

The optic nerve is surrounded by the dura and arachnoid sheaths, and an increase in the intracranial pressure is transmitted through the cerebrospinal fluid along the extension of the subarachnoid space to the lamina cribrosa of the eyeball. Because the central artery and vein of the retina cross the subarachnoid space to enter or leave the optic nerve, they will be subject to a rise in cerebrospinal pressure. The thick-walled artery is unaffected, but the thin-walled vein may be compressed, causing congestion of the retinal veins and edema of the retina; bulging of the optic disc may also occur.

Infection of the Face and Cavernous Sinus Thrombosis

Infection of the facial skin in the area bounded by the eye, the nose, and the upper lip is potentially dangerous. A boil, for example, may cause thrombosis of the facial vein, with spread of infected emboli into the orbit and cavernous sinus. This is possible because of the communications that exist among the facial vein, the superior and inferior ophthalmic veins, and the cavernous sinus. The spread is facilitated by the absence of valves in these veins, so that the blood may carry the emboli upward from the face toward the cavernous sinus. The resulting cavernous sinus thrombosis can be fatal unless adequately treated with antibiotics.

Orbital Cellulitis and Cavernous Sinus Thrombosis

Orbital cellulitis commonly results from bacterial spread from the ethmoidal or maxillary sinuses or spread of infection from the face via the facial and ophthalmic veins (see above). Inflammatory edema of the orbital contents gives rise to impaired ocular movements, pain, and proptosis. Thrombophlebitis of the ophthalmic veins may lead to cavernous sinus thrombosis.

Cavernous Sinus Thrombosis and the Central Vein of the Retina

The central vein of the retina may drain into the cavernous sinus directly or may join the superior ophthalmic vein. In the first situation, the central vein also communicates with the superior ophthalmic vein. This is important in that the central vein has an alternative pathway for the venous blood: The blood may travel into the superior ophthalmic vein and then into the pterygoid venous plexus, and thus bypass the cavernous sinus, should it become thrombosed.

Carotid–Cavernous Sinus Fistulas

Communication between the internal carotid artery and the cavernous sinus results in arteriolization of the cavernous sinus and retrograde flow of arterial blood into the orbit via the ophthalmic veins. This leads to pulsating proptosis, an audible bruit, and dilatation of the conjunctival blood vessels. Paralysis of the cranial nerves with ophthalmoplegia may also occur as the result of increased pressure of the arterial blood on the nerves; the abducent nerve is often involved.

Trauma to the head resulting in laceration of the internal carotid artery as it passes through the cavernous sinus is a common cause of the fistula. The artery may be damaged by a missile or fracture of the sphenoid bone. The exophthalmos and the bruit may be reduced by manual compression of the carotid artery in the neck.

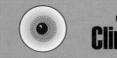

CHAPTER 9
Clinical Problems

Answers on Page 292.

1 A 2-year-old boy was suspected of having hydrocephalus. Explain how the ophthalmoscope can be used to detect a raised intracranial pressure.

2 A 10-year-old girl arrived in the emergency room complaining of pain in her right eye, which was made worse by ocular movement. Her mother had noticed that the child's right eye had been swollen for the past 2 days, and that it was beginning to bulge forward. Her sight appeared to be normal and she did not complain of double vision. On examination, it was seen that the patient had severe edema and congestion of both lids of the right eye with a severe degree of proptosis. Movements of the right eye caused considerable discomfort. The left eye appeared to be normal. Examination of the patient's face showed a small abscess on the right side of the nose with a yellow pustule in its center. What is your diagnosis? Using your anatomic knowledge, explain the etiology of this serious condition.

3 An interesting discussion took place in the cafeteria between a senior ophthalmic surgeon and his resident. The resident maintained that the central artery of the retina supplies the orbital part of the optic nerve and the inner layers of the retina, and that the outer layers of the retina receive their arterial supply from the ciliary arteries. The argument became intense when the resident stated that both sets of blood vessels freely anastomose with each other at the point at which the optic nerve pierces the lamina cribrosa, and at which the inner and outer layers of the retina come together. The surgeon strongly disagreed, and stated that the central artery and the ciliary arteries are distinct arterial systems, and that no functional anastomoses occur between the systems. Who was correct? Why do you think this confusion sometimes exists?

4 A 70-year-old woman was seen in the emergency room complaining of the sudden loss of sight in her right eye. Her daughter told the ophthalmic surgeon that on two previous occasions she had experienced transient loss of vision in the same eye, but sight had returned in a few seconds. A careful examination with the ophthalmoscope revealed that the peripheral retina had a milky white appearance, with the retinal arteries showing fragmentation and constriction of the blood column. The area of the retina between the optic disc and the macula, however, appeared normal. An examination of the eye fields showed that the patient was not completely blind in the right eye but had some central vision. Explain how this patient could have central vision in the presence of complete central retinal artery occlusion? What is the possible explanation for the transient loss of vision on previous occasions?

5 An 85-year-old man complaining of a sudden reduction of vision in his left eye visited an ophthalmologist. Ophthalmoscopic examination showed evidence of severe arteriosclerosis of the central retinal arteries and their branches in both eyes. In the left eye the upper temporal quadrant showed widespread retinal hemorrhages with engorgement of the retinal veins. Examination of the visual fields showed a sectoral field defect. Explain the possible connection between the patient's arteriosclerotic condition and the occurrence of a branch retinal vein occlusion.

6 A 41-year-old man was in a motor vehicle accident and suffered severe trauma to his head. On superficial examination he was found to have a right-sided frontal bone fracture. On recovering consciousness he complained of hearing a "blowing sound" that was found to be synchronous with his pulse. It was also noted that he had right-sided proptosis and difficulty moving his right eye; a florid conjunctivitis was also present on the right. What vascular injury did this patient most likely have?

7 A 62-year-old woman complained that her left eye was red. She had first noticed the condition 3 months previously. On examination she was found to have hypertension and diabetes mellitus. Careful examination of her left eye revealed a subtle conjunctival vascular dilatation and 1 mm of proptosis. On further questioning, she admitted that she heard a "whooshing sound" when she rested her head on a pillow at night. She first heard the sound 2 months previously and it has become progressively worse, so that she has difficulty getting to sleep. Using your knowledge of anatomy, explain this woman's signs and symptoms.

CHAPTER 9
Answers to Clinical Problems

1 In the infant the anterior and posterior fontanelles of the skull can be easily palpated. In cases of raised intracranial pressure, the fontanelles bulge upward. The posterior fontanelle closes by the end of the first year; the anterior fontanelle, at 18 months. For a patient 2 years old the ophthalmoscope can be used to detect raised intracranial pressure, because both optic nerves are surrounded by a tubular extension of the subarachnoid space that reaches forward to the lamina cribrosa of the eyeball. A rise in cerebrospinal fluid pressure will compress the thin walls of the central vein of the retina as it crosses the space, resulting in congestion of the retinal veins, edema of the retina, and bulging of the optic disc (papilledema). These findings will be present in both eyes. The use of MRI may also provide valuable information regarding the state of the ventricles and the general anatomy of the cerebral hemispheres.

2 This girl had a right-sided cavernous sinus thrombosis secondary to an abscess on the side of her nose. A severe pyogenic infection of one of the hair follicles and sebaceous glands had spread into the surrounding tissue, causing a thrombophlebitis of the facial vein. With no valves present, infected emboli had ascended through the anastomosis with the superior ophthalmic vein to lodge in the cavernous sinus. Here further thrombosis occurred, causing extreme congestion of the superior and inferior ophthalmic veins. The congestion and edema of the orbital contents was responsible for the swelling of the eyelids and the proptosis.

3 The surgeon is correct. A small anastomosis does exist between the pial branches of the central artery of the retina and the small ciliary vessels in the sclera around the nerve head. An occasional cilioretinal artery (in 15 to 20 percent of subjects), arising from a short ciliary artery, may enter the retina but does not anastomose with the central artery or its branches.

The branches of the central artery of the retina to the retina are restricted to the inner layers and penetrate only as far as the outer plexiform layer. The outer part of the retina, including the rods and cones, is nourished by tissue fluid that diffuses into the retina from the choroidal capillaries. No choroidal arteries enter the outer layers of the retina.

The central artery of the retina is thus a functional end artery, and the circulation through it is completely separate from that of the ciliary arteries. Confusion sometimes exists, because some accounts exaggerate the importance of the small anastomotic channels at the optic nerve head.

4 This patient was fortunate in having a cilioretinal artery. About 15 to 20 percent of people have a cilioretinal artery. It arises from the ciliary circulation and enters the retina at the lateral border of the optic nerve. It supplies the area of the retina between the optic disc and the macula—and this explains the preservation of an area of central vision in the presence of complete central artery occlusion. The previous episodes of transient loss of vision could have resulted from spasm or thrombosis of the central retinal artery secondary to arteriosclerosis.

5 The branch retinal vein occlusion could be caused by the compression of the vein by the rigid retinal arterial wall secondary to severe arteriosclerosis. Remember that the retinal arteries and the retinal veins are enveloped in a common tight connective tissue covering at the points where the arteries cross the veins. The condition is more likely to occur in patients with preexisting glaucoma.

6 Traumatic carotid–cavernous sinus fistula can follow a severe head injury. In this patient a careful radiologic examination revealed a fracture of the sphenoid bone and showed a spicule of bone projecting into the region of the right cavernous sinus. This high-flow direct fistula between the right internal carotid artery and the right cavernous sinus explained the right-sided pulsating proptosis, the bruit, the ophthalmoplegia, and the dilatation of the conjunctival blood vessels.

Surgical or endovascular closure of the fistula is the treatment of choice and in most patients is successful in eliminating the signs and symptoms.

7 This patient had a left-sided, low-flow carotid–cavernous sinus fistula that apparently occurred spontaneously. The subtle arteriolization of the conjunctival blood vessels in these patients develops slowly over a number of years and can often be mistaken for chronic conjunctivitis. The same signs and symptoms seen in direct high-flow fistula occur much more gradually and are less severe. Unless the diagnosis is suspected, it may be missed. These fistulas may be operated on or they may close spontaneously.

CHAPTER 10

Cranial Nerves—Part I: The Nerves Directly Associated with the Eye and Orbit

CHAPTER OUTLINE

Introduction ·

There are 12 pairs of cranial nerves, which leave the brain and pass through foramina and fissures in the skull. All the nerves are distributed in the head and neck except for the tenth cranial nerve, which also supplies structures in the thorax and abdomen. The cranial nerves are named as follows:

I. Olfactory	VII. Facial
II. Optic	VIII. Vestibulocochlear
III. Oculomotor	IX. Glossopharyngeal
IV. Trochlear	X. Vagus
V. Trigeminal	XI. Accessory
VI. Abducent	XII. Hypoglossal

Organization of the Cranial Nerves

The olfactory, optic, and vestibulocochlear nerves are entirely sensory in function. The oculomotor, trochlear, abducent, accessory, and hypoglossal nerves are entirely motor in function. The trigeminal, facial, glossopharyngeal, and vagus nerves are both sensory and motor nerves. The letter symbols commonly used to indicate the functional components of each cranial nerve are shown in Table 10-1. The cranial nerves have central motor and or sensory nuclei within the brain and peripheral nerve fibers that emerge from the brain and exit from the skull to reach their effector or sensory organs.

The different components of the cranial nerves, their functions, and the openings in the skull through which the nerves leave the cranial cavity are summarized in Table 10-2.

Table 10-1   The Letter Symbols Commonly Used to Indicate the Functional Components of Each Cranial Nerve

Component	Function	Letter Symbols
Afferent nerve fibers	Sensory	
General somatic afferent	General sensations	GSA
Special somatic afferent	Hearing, balance, vision	SSA
General visceral afferent	Viscera	GVA
Special visceral afferent	Smell, taste	SVA
Efferent nerve fibers		
General somatic efferent	Somatic striated muscles	GSE
General visceral efferent	Glands and smooth muscles (parasympathetic innervation)	GVE
Special visceral efferent	Branchial arch striated muscles	SVE

Table 10-2   Cranial Nerves

Number	Name	Components	Function	Opening in Skull
I	Olfactory	Sensory (SVA) plate of ethmoid	Smell	Openings in cribriform
II	Optic	Sensory (SSA)	Vision	Optic canal
III	Oculomotor	Motor (GSE)	Raises upper eyelid, turns eyeball upward, downward, and medially	Superior orbital fissure
		(GVE)	Constricts pupil, accommodates eye	
IV	Trochlear	Motor (GSE)	Assists in turning eyeball downward and laterally	Superior orbital fissure
V	Trigeminal*			
	Ophthalmic division	Sensory (GSA)	Cornea, skin of forehead, scalp, eyelids, and nose; also mucous membrane of paranasal sinuses and nasal cavity	Superior orbital fissure
	Maxillary division	Sensory (GSA)	Skin of face over maxilla; teeth of upper jaw; mucous membrane of nose, the maxillary sinus, and palate	Foramen rotundum
	Mandibular division	Motor (SVE)	Muscles of mastication, mylohyoid, anterior belly of digastric, tensor veli palatini, and tensor tympani	Foramen ovale
		Sensory (GSA)	Skin of cheek, skin over mandible and side of head, teeth of lower jaw and temporomandibular joint; mucous membrane of mouth and anterior part of tongue	
VI	Abducent	Motor (GSE)	Lateral rectus muscle turns eyeball laterally	Superior orbital fissure
VII	Facial	Motor (SVE)	Muscles of face and scalp, stapedius muscle, posterior belly of digastric and stylohyoid muscles	Internal acoustic meatus, facial canal, stylomastoid foramen
		Sensory (SVA)	Taste from anterior two-thirds of tongue, from floor of mouth and palate	
		Secretomotor (GVE) parasympathetic	Submandibular and sublingual salivary glands, the lacrimal gland, and glands of nose and palate	

Table 10-2 (*continued*)

Number	Name	Components	Function	Opening in Skull
VIII	Vestibulo-cochlear			Internal acoustic meatus
	Vestibular	Sensory (SSA)	From utricle and saccule and semicircular canals—position and movement of head	
	Cochlear	Sensory (SSA)	Organ of Corti—hearing	
IX	Glosso-pharyngeal	Motor (SVE)	Stylopharyngeus muscle—assists swallowing	Jugular foramen
		Secretomotor (GVE) parasympathetic	Parotid salivary gland	
		Sensory (GVA) (SVA) (GSA)	General sensation and taste from posterior one-third of tongue and pharynx, carotid sinus (baroreceptor), and carotid body (chemoreceptor)	
X	Vagus	Motor (GVE) (SVE) Sensory (GVA) (SVA) (GSA)	Heart and great thoracic blood vessels; larynx, trachea, bronchi, and lungs; alimentary tract from pharynx to splenic flexure of colon; liver, kidneys, and pancreas	Jugular foramen
XI	Accessory Cranial root	Motor (SVE)	Muscles of soft palate (except tensor veli palatini), pharynx (except stylopharyngeus), and larynx (except cricothyroid) in branches of vagus	Jugular foramen
	Spinal root	Motor (SVE)	Sternocleidomastoid and trapezius muscles	
XII	Hypoglossal	Motor (GSE)	Muscles of tongue (except palatoglossus) controlling its shape and movement	Hypoglossal canal

*The trigeminal nerve also carries proprioceptive impulses from the muscles of mastication and the facial and extraocular muscles.

Motor Nuclei of the Cranial Nerves

Somatic Motor and Branchomotor Nuclei   The somatic motor and branchomotor nerve fibers of a cranial nerve are the axons of nerve cells situated within the brain. These nerve cell groups form motor nuclei and they innervate striated muscle. Each nerve cell with its processes is referred to as a *lower motor neuron*. Therefore, such a nerve cell is equivalent to the motor cells in the anterior gray horns of the spinal cord.

The motor nuclei of the cranial nerves receive impulses from the cerebral cortex through the corticonuclear (corticobulbar) fibers. These fibers originate from the pyramidal cells in the inferior part of the precentral gyrus (area 4) and from the adjacent part of the postcentral gyrus. The corticonuclear fibers descend through the *genu of the internal capsule*. They pass through the midbrain just medial to the corticospinal fibers in the *basis pedunculi* and end by synapsing either directly with the lower motor neurons within the cranial nerve nuclei or indirectly through *connector neurons*.

The majority of the corticonuclear fibers to the motor cranial nerve nuclei cross the median plane before reaching the nuclei. Bilateral connections are present for all the cranial motor nuclei except for part of the facial nucleus that supplies the muscles of the lower part of the face and part of the hypoglossal nucleus that supplies the genioglossus muscle, which is responsible for protruding the tongue.

General Visceral Motor Nuclei   The general visceral motor nuclei form the cranial outflow of the parasympathetic part of the autonomic nervous system (see p. 358, Chap. 12). They are the *Edinger-Westphal nucleus* of the oculomotor nerve, the *superior salivatory nucleus* and *lacrimal nucleus* of the facial nerve, the *inferior salivatory nucleus* of the glossopharyngeal nerve, and the *dorsal motor nucleus* of the vagus nerve. These nuclei receive numerous afferent fibers including descending pathways from the hypothalamus.

Sensory Nuclei of the Cranial Nerves

The sensory nuclei include somatic and visceral afferent nuclei. The sensory or afferent parts of a cranial nerve are the axons of nerve cells outside the brain and are situated in ganglia on the nerve trunks (equivalent to the posterior root ganglia of a spinal nerve) or may be situated in a sensory organ such as the nose, the retina of the eye, or the ear. These cells send central processes into the brain and terminate by synapsing with cells forming the sensory nuclei. Axons from these nuclear cells now cross the midline and ascend to other sensory nuclei, such as the thalamus, where they synapse. The nerve cells from these nuclei send axons that terminate in the cerebral cortex.

Nerves of the Orbital Cavity ·

The nerves of the orbital cavity are motor, sensory, and autonomic in function. In the category of motor nerves are the oculomotor, trochlear, and abducent nerves; in the category of sensory nerves, the ophthalmic and maxillary divisions of the trigeminal nerve. The optic nerve is considered in detail in Chapter 13. The autonomic nerves, which consist of sympathetic and parasympathetic nerves that supply blood vessels, smooth muscle, and glands, are described separately in Chapter 12.

Motor Nerves

The motor nerves to the extraocular muscles are relatively large, the reason for this being the high proportion of nerve fibers to muscle fibers. In other words, a given motor nerve supplies only a few muscle fibers, as compared with other muscles in the body; and this explains how the nervous system has a fine control of eye movements.

Oculomotor Nerve (Cranial Nerve III)

The oculomotor nerve supplies all the extraocular muscles of the orbit except the superior oblique and the lateral rectus; it also supplies the intraocular muscles, the sphincter pupillae, and the ciliary muscle with parasympathetic fibers.

Origin, Course, and Distribution   The oculomotor nerve emerges from the anterior aspect of the midbrain medial to the cerebral peduncle (Fig. 10-1). Lying within the subarachnoid space, it passes between the posterior cerebral and superior cerebellar arteries (Fig. 10-1) and runs forward lateral and parallel to the posterior communicating artery. It pierces the arachnoid and lies between the fixed and free borders of the tentorium cerebelli. On the lateral side of the posterior clinoid process, the nerve perforates the dura mater and comes to lie in the lateral wall of the cavernous sinus above the trochlear nerve (Figs. 10-2 and 10-3). The nerve then runs forward and receives a sensory communicating branch from the ophthalmic division of the trigeminal nerve and a sympathetic branch from the nerve plexus around the internal carotid artery. The nerve is crossed here on its lateral side by the trochlear nerve and farther distally by the ophthalmic division of the trigeminal nerve (Fig. 10-4). The oculomotor nerve now divides into a small superior division and a large inferior division, which enter the orbit through the superior orbital fissure within the tendinous ring (Fig. 10-5).

The superior division of the oculomotor nerve passes upward lateral to the optic nerve and enters the superior rectus muscle at the junction of its proximal and middle thirds. Having supplied the superior rectus muscle, the nerve pierces the muscle and terminates by supplying the levator palpebrae superioris muscle (Fig. 10-6). Sometimes the branch to the levator muscle passes around the medial border of the superior rectus.

The inferior division of the oculomotor nerve divides into three branches, which supply the medial and inferior recti and the inferior oblique muscles (Fig. 10-6). The branch to the medial rectus passes medially below the optic nerve to enter the lateral surface of the muscle at the junction between the proximal and middle thirds. The branch to the inferior rectus runs forward on its upper surface and enters the muscle at the junction of the proximal and middle thirds. The branch to the inferior oblique muscle, the longest branch, passes forward close to the orbital floor and lateral to the inferior rectus muscle. The nerve enters the posterior border of the oblique muscle (Fig. 10-6).

The nerve to the inferior oblique muscle gives rise to a short, thick branch, which passes to the ciliary ganglion (Fig. 10-6). This branch contains parasympathetic fibers of the oculomotor nerve that will synapse in the ciliary ganglion. The postganglionic fibers will pass in the short ciliary nerves to supply the sphincter pupillae and the ciliary muscles.

Nerve Nuclei and Their Central Connections   The oculomotor nerve has two motor nuclei: 1) the main motor nucleus and 2) the accessory parasympathetic nucleus.

Figure 10-1

Diagram of the interior of the skull showing the midbrain (cut) and the origin of the oculomotor and trochlear nerves. Note the long courses taken by these nerves before they enter the lateral wall of the cavernous sinus, and also the relationship between these nerves and the posterior cerebral and superior cerebellar arteries.

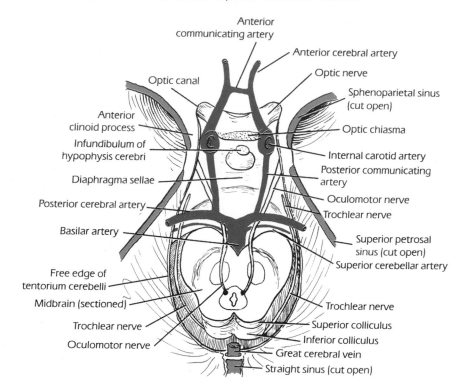

The *main motor nucleus* is situated in the anterior part of the gray matter surrounding the cerebral aqueduct of the midbrain (Fig. 10-7). It lies at the level of the superior colliculus. The nucleus supplies all the extrinsic muscles of the eye except the superior oblique and the lateral rectus. The outgoing nerve fibers pass anteriorly through the red nucleus and emerge on the anterior surface of the midbrain.

Researchers have attempted to divide the large multipolar cells of the main motor nucleus into subgroups having different functions and supplying different muscles. Unfortunately, functional localization within the nucleus has been shown to be complex and uncertain; the reader is referred to the studies of Warwick (1953) and Tarlov and Tarlov (1971).* The following facts, however, appear to

Figure 10-2

Lateral view of the interior of the skull, showing the courses taken by the oculomotor, trochlear, and abducent nerves and the ophthalmic and maxillary divisions of the trigeminal nerve. The dura forming the lateral wall of the cavernous sinus has been removed for clarity.

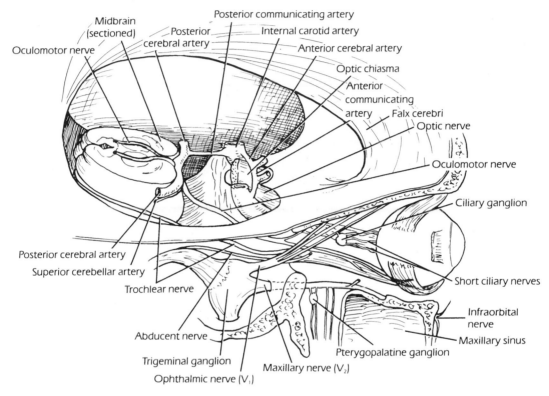

be established: 1) The levator palpebrae superioris muscles of both sides are supplied by a single central group of cells (central caudal nucleus), 2) the superior rectus muscle is supplied by the contralateral oculomotor nucleus, and 3) the remaining muscles innervated by the oculomotor nerve are supplied ipsilaterally.

The main oculomotor nucleus receives corticonuclear fibers from both cerebral hemispheres. It receives tectobulbar fibers from the superior colliculus and through this route is supplied information from the visual cortex. It also receives fibers from the medial longitudinal fasciculus, by which it is connected to the nuclei of the fourth, sixth, and eighth cranial nerves.

The *accessory parasympathetic nucleus* (Edinger-Westphal nucleus) is situated posterior to the main oculomotor nucleus (Fig. 10-7). The axons of the nerve

*R. Warwick, *J. Comp. Neurol.*, 98 (1953), 449. E. Tarlov and S.R. Tarlov, *Brain Res.*, 34 (1971), 37.

Figure 10-3

Coronal section through the body of the sphenoid bone and the cavernous sinuses, showing the position of the cranial nerves and the internal carotid artery.

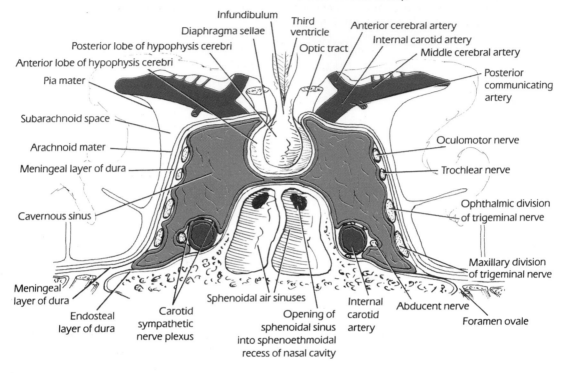

cells, which are preganglionic, accompany the other oculomotor fibers to the orbit. Here they synapse in the *ciliary ganglion*, and postganglionic fibers pass through the short ciliary nerves to the constrictor pupillae of the iris and the ciliary muscles. The accessory parasympathetic nucleus receives corticonuclear fibers for the accommodation reflex and fibers from the pretectal nucleus for the direct and consensual light reflexes (Fig. 10-7).

The oculomotor nerve is therefore entirely motor and is responsible for lifting the upper eyelid; turning the eye upward, downward, and medially; constricting the pupil; and accommodating the eye.

Trochlear Nerve (Cranial Nerve IV)

The trochlear nerve, the most slender of the cranial nerves, supplies the superior oblique muscle in the orbit.

Origin, Course, and Distribution   The trochlear nerve, the most slender of the cranial nerves, and the only one to leave the posterior surface of the brain stem (Fig. 10-8), emerges from the midbrain and *immediately decussates with the nerve of the opposite side.* The nerve passes laterally and forward in the subarachnoid

Figure 10-4

Lateral view of the interior of the skull, showing the oculomotor, trochlear, and abducent nerves entering the orbit through the superior orbital fissure. The three terminal branches of the ophthalmic division of the trigeminal nerve are also seen entering the orbit through the superior orbital fissure.

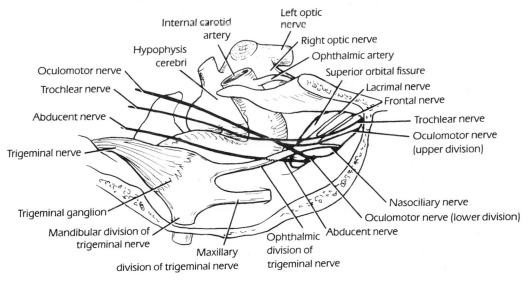

space around the cerebral peduncle (Fig. 10-9) and then pierces the arachnoid and perforates the dura mater just below the free border of the tentorium cerebelli close to the posterior clinoid process. The nerve then passes forward in the lateral wall of the cavernous sinus, lying below the oculomotor nerve and above the ophthalmic division of the trigeminal nerve (Figs. 10-3 and 10-4). At the anterior end of the cavernous sinus the trochlear nerve crosses lateral to the oculomotor nerve and enters the orbit through the superior orbital fissure above the tendinous ring and medial to the frontal nerve (Fig. 10-5). The nerve now passes medially above the origin of the levator palpebrae superioris and enters the upper surface of the superior oblique muscle as a series of small branches (Fig. 10-10).

Nerve Nucleus and Its Central Connections   The trochlear nucleus is situated in the anterior part of the gray matter surrounding the cerebral aqueduct of the midbrain (Fig. 10-11). It lies inferior to the main oculomotor nucleus at the level of the inferior colliculus. The nerve fibers, after leaving the nucleus, pass posteriorly around the central gray matter to reach the posterior surface of the midbrain, where they exit.

The trochlear nucleus receives corticonuclear fibers from both cerebral hemispheres. It receives the tectobulbar fibers, which connect it to the visual cortex through the superior colliculus (Fig. 10-11), and also fibers from the medial longitudinal fasciculus, by which it is connected to the nuclei of the third, sixth, and eighth cranial nerves.

Figure 10-5

Diagram of the apical region of the right orbit, showing the superior orbital fissure and the optic canal. Note the origins of the extraocular muscles and the relative positions of the nerves entering the orbital cavity through the superior orbital fissure.

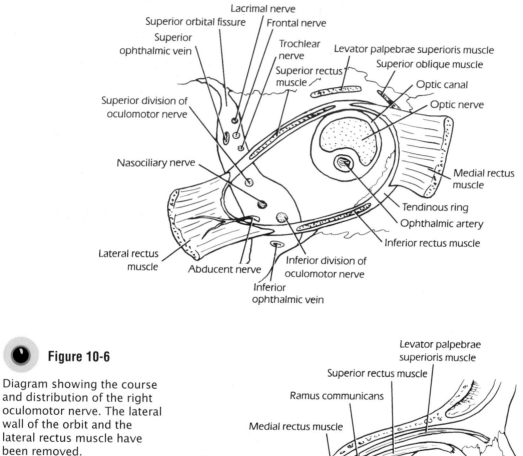

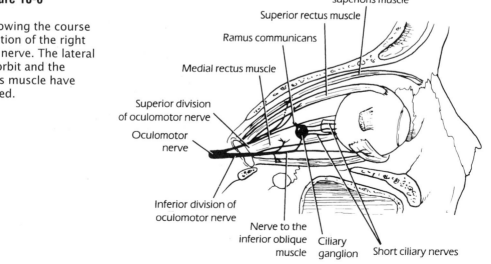 **Figure 10-6**

Diagram showing the course and distribution of the right oculomotor nerve. The lateral wall of the orbit and the lateral rectus muscle have been removed.

Figure 10-7

Diagram showing the oculomotor nuclei and their central nervous connections.

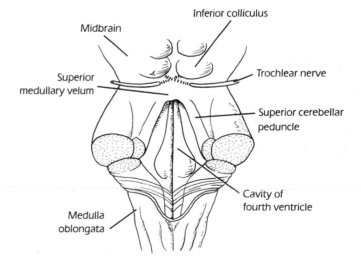 **Figure 10-8**

Diagram showing the trochlear nerve emerging from the
posterior surface of the brain
stem after it has undergone
complete decussation in the
superior medullary velum.
Note that it is the only cranial
nerve to emerge on the dorsal
surface of the brain.

Figure 10-9

Diagram showing the origin and course of the right trochlear nerve from the midbrain at the level of the inferior colliculus to its entrance into the orbit through the superior orbital fissure.

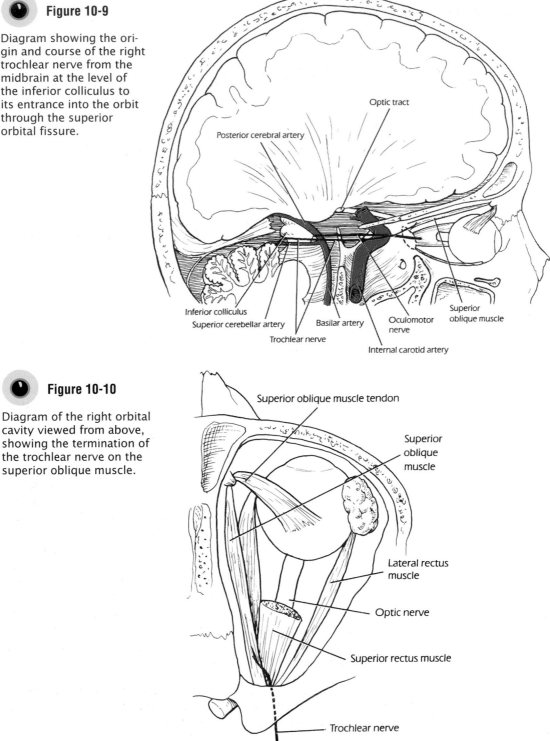

Optic tract

Posterior cerebral artery

Inferior colliculus

Superior cerebellar artery

Basilar artery

Trochlear nerve

Oculomotor nerve

Superior oblique muscle

Internal carotid artery

Figure 10-10

Diagram of the right orbital cavity viewed from above, showing the termination of the trochlear nerve on the superior oblique muscle.

Superior oblique muscle tendon

Superior oblique muscle

Lateral rectus muscle

Optic nerve

Superior rectus muscle

Trochlear nerve

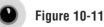

Figure 10-11

Diagram showing the trochlear nucleus and its central nervous connections.

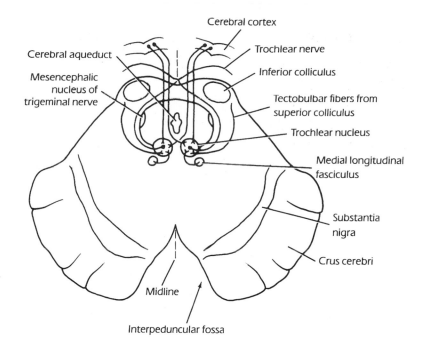

The trochlear nerve is therefore entirely motor. It supplies the superior oblique muscle and thus assists in turning the eye downward and laterally.

Abducent Nerve (Cranial Nerve VI)

The abducent nerve is a small nerve that supplies the lateral rectus muscle of the eyeball.

Origin, Course, and Distribution   The abducent nerve emerges from the anterior surface of the brain stem in a groove between the lower border of the pons and the medulla oblongata. It lies within the subarachnoid space. The nerve runs upward, forward, and laterally and pierces the dura lateral to the dorsum sellae of the sphenoid bone. It now makes an acute bend forward across the sharp upper border of the petrous part of the temporal bone near its apex (Fig. 10-4). The nerve passes forward within the cavernous sinus, covered by endothelium (Fig. 10-4). The nerve lies inferolateral to the internal carotid artery. It enters the orbit through the superior orbital fissure between the two divisions of the oculomotor nerve and within the tendinous ring (Fig. 10-5). The abducent nerve ends by passing forward to enter the medial surface of the lateral rectus muscle (Fig. 10-5).

During the course of the abducent nerve through the cavernous sinus, it receives a sympathetic branch from the internal carotid plexus. Later these fibers leave the abducent nerve to join the ophthalmic nerve.

Nerve Nucleus and Its Central Connections   The motor nucleus is small and situated beneath the floor of the upper part of the fourth ventricle. It lies close to the midline and beneath the *colliculus facialis* (Fig. 10-12).

Figure 10-12

Diagram showing the abducent nerve nucleus and its central nervous connections.

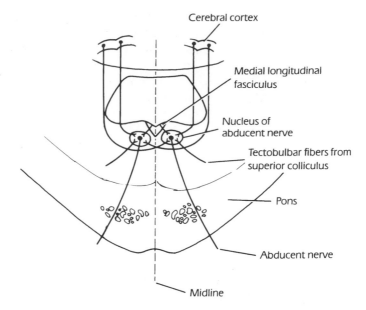

The nucleus receives afferent corticonuclear fibers from both cerebral hemispheres. It receives the tectobulbar tract from the superior colliculus, by which the visual cortex is connected to the nucleus. It also receives fibers from the medial longitudinal fasciculus, by which it is connected to the nuclei of the third, fourth, and eighth cranial nerves (Fig. 10-12).

The abducent nerve is entirely a motor nerve. It supplies the lateral rectus muscle and is therefore responsible for turning the eye laterally.

 Clinical Notes

Oculomotor Nerve

The oculomotor nerve supplies all the extraocular muscles except the superior oblique and the lateral rectus. It also supplies the striated muscle of the levator palpebrae superioris and the smooth muscle concerned with accommodation, namely, the sphincter pupillae and the ciliary muscle.

Lesions In a complete lesion of the oculomotor nerve, the eye cannot be moved upward, downward, or inward. At rest, the eye looks laterally (external strabismus) owing to the activity of the lateral rectus and downward owing to the activity of the superior oblique. The patient has diplopia. There is ptosis of the upper lid due to paralysis of the levator palpebrae superioris. The pupil is widely dilated and nonreactive to light owing to paralysis of the sphincter pupillae and unopposed action of the dilator (supplied by the sympathetic). Accommodation of the eye is paralyzed.

Incomplete lesions of the oculomotor nerve are common and may spare the extraocular muscles or the intraocular muscles. The condition in which the innervation of the extraocular muscles is spared with selective loss of the autonomic innervation of the sphincter pupillae and ciliary muscle is called *internal ophthalmoplegia*. The condition in which the sphincter pupillae and ciliary muscle are spared with paralysis of the extraocular muscles is called *external ophthalmoplegia*. It has been suggested that in the precavernous sinus course of the oculomotor nerve, the parasympathetic autonomic fibers are superficially placed within the nerve and are likely to be first affected by compression, whereas distally they are deeply placed. The nature of the disease also plays a role. For example, in diabetic neuropathy the pupil and ciliary muscle invariably remain unaffected, and in lesions of the oculomotor nerve nucleus the autonomic fibers usually are not affected.

The conditions most commonly affecting the oculomotor nerve are diabetes, aneurysm, tumor, trauma, inflammation, and vascular disease.

Orbital Lesions   Because the two divisions of the oculomotor nerve lie within the muscular cone that passes forward to the eyeball, they are likely to be compressed by a retrobulbar tumor, such as a glioma of the optic nerve, or by a meningioma of the meningeal sheath of that nerve. In addition to proptosis and alteration in sight, signs and symptoms from involvement of the abducent and nasociliary nerves may also become evident.

Cavernous Sinus Lesions   The oculomotor, the trochlear, the abducent, and even the ophthalmic division of the trigeminal nerve are affected by cavernous sinus thrombosis. An aneurysm of the internal carotid artery within the cavernous sinus may press these nerves. Because of the close proximity of the abducent nerve to the artery, that nerve is more likely to be affected first.

As the two divisions of the oculomotor nerve enter the orbit through the superior orbital fissure, they may be involved with the trochlear, abducent, and sympathetic nerves, along with the lacrimal, frontal, and nasociliary nerves. Meningioma, fracture of the skull, and suppuration of the sphenoid air sinus may be the cause.

Interpeduncular Fossa Lesions   In the interpeduncular fossa, the nerve lies close to the posterior cerebral artery, the superior cerebellar artery, and the posterior communicating artery. An aneurysm in any one of these arteries can press on the oculomotor nerve. Chronic meningitis caused by syphilis, tuberculosis, or zoster can involve the nerve in the subarachnoid space. Compression from tumors of the base of the brain also occurs at this site. Traumatic stretching of the nerve as it passes forward to enter the fixed lateral wall of the cavernous sinus may occur with severe head injuries.

Midbrain Lesions   Lesions within the midbrain are often vascular. In *Benedikt's syndrome*, which occurs following occlusion of the blood supply to the midbrain, not only is there a complete lesion of the oculomotor nerve on one side but, because of the involvement of the red nucleus and medial lemniscus on the same side, there are contralateral involuntary movements of the limbs and contralateral hemianesthesia (Fig. 10-13).

In *Weber's syndrome*, caused by occlusion of a branch of the posterior cerebral artery to the midbrain, there is involvement of the oculomotor nerve and the crus cerebri on the same side (Fig. 10-13). There are a complete lesion of the oculomotor nerve on the same side and contralateral paralysis of the lower part of the face, the tongue, and the arm and leg.

Figure 10-13

Diagram showing how pathology of the midbrain can involve the oculomotor nerve. (A) Tumor of the midbrain blocking the cerebral aqueduct and invading the oculomotor nuclei. (B) Weber's syndrome, involving the oculomotor nerve and the crus cerebri following occlusion of the blood supply to the midbrain. (C) Benedikt's syndrome, involving the red nucleus, the oculomotor nerve, and the medial lemniscus following occlusion of the blood supply to the midbrain.

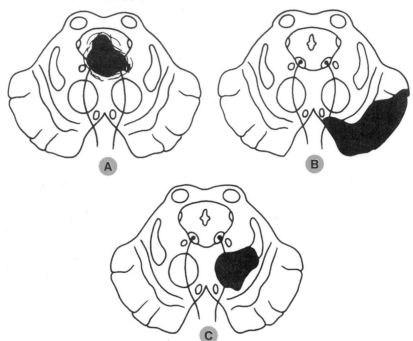

Trochlear Nerve

The trochlear nerve supplies the superior oblique muscle, which rotates the eye downward when it is adducted.

Lesions   In lesions of the trochlear nerve the patient complains of double vision, because the images of the two eyes are tilted relative to each other. Overaction of the antagonistic inferior oblique muscle will cause the paretic eye to be hypertropic in the primary position. The patient characteristically carries the head tilted toward the noninvolved side with the chin depressed. It is an unconscious attempt on the patient's part to compensate for the diplopia, particularly the torsional effects of muscle paresis.

Cavernous Sinus Lesions   The trochlear, the oculomotor, the abducent, and the ophthalmic division of the trigeminal nerve may all be involved in cavernous sinus thrombosis or aneurysm of the internal carotid artery. Tumors encroaching on the superior orbital fissure may also press on these nerves together with the sympathetic nerves.

Subarachnoid Space Lesions Bruising or stretching of the trochlear nerve commonly occurs as a complication of head injuries. The nerve is damaged at the site where it exits on the dorsal surface of the superior medullary velum or as it passes around the midbrain to enter the lateral wall of the cavernous sinus.

Midbrain Lesions Vascular lesions of the dorsal part of the midbrain may involve the trochlear nerve nucleus as well as that of the oculomotor nerve. Because the trochlear nerve fibers decussate in the superior medullary velum, an ipsilateral oculomotor palsy will be associated with a contralateral trochlear nerve palsy.

Abducent Nerve

The abducent nerve supplies the lateral rectus muscle, which rotates the eye laterally.

Lesions In a lesion of the abducent nerve the patient cannot turn the eye laterally. When the patient is looking straight ahead, the lateral rectus is paralyzed and the unopposed medial rectus pulls the eyeball medially, causing esotropia (internal strabismus).

Orbital, Superior Orbital Fissure, and Cavernous Sinus Lesions In the orbit the abducent nerve lies within the cone of extraocular muscles along with the two divisions of the oculomotor nerve, the nasociliary nerve, and the optic nerve. All these nerves can be compressed by a retrobulbar tumor. Similar vulnerability exists in the superior orbital fissure.

In the cavernous sinus, the abducent nerve can be affected by a thrombosis. Because of its close relationship with the internal carotid artery, it can easily be compressed by an aneurysm of that artery.

Subarachnoid Space Lesions The abducent nerve is slender and long, and its course from the lower border of the pons to the cavernous sinus makes it very susceptible to damage in head injuries. It is also likely to be damaged by stretching should the brain stem be displaced by a raised intracranial pressure.

Before the use of antibiotics, middle ear disease commonly spread to involve the petrous part of the temporal bone and the covering meninges. The closeness of the trigeminal and abducent nerves to the tip of the petrous bone often resulted in their involvement (Gradenigo's syndrome). Pain referred to the eye and face and associated with sixth nerve palsy characterized this syndrome.

Pons Lesions Within the pons the facial nerve loops around the nucleus of the abducent nerve. A vascular lesion involving this area can result in an abducent and facial nerve paralysis and contralateral hemiplegia (Millard-Gubler syndrome).

Supramotornuclear Lesions

It will be remembered that the motor nuclei of the third, fourth, and sixth cranial nerves receive the following nerve fibers: 1) corticonuclear fibers from both cerebral hemispheres, 2) tectobulbar fibers from the superior colliculus receiving information from the visual cortex, and 3) medial longitudinal fasciculus fibers connecting the nuclei of the third, fourth, sixth, and eighth cranial nerves to one another and also to the centers for gaze, and possibly to the cerebellum.

These important nerve connections enable both eyeballs, normally, to move together so that they are aligned in parallel.

Lesions of the Cerebral Cortex and Their Pathways   Such lesions permit the eyeball movements to remain aligned and in parallel, and diplopia does not occur. Destructive lesions in the frontal or occipital eye fields result in the eyes turning toward the side of the lesion. Irritative lesions in these eye fields result in the eyes turning toward the opposite side of the lesion.

Vertical Gaze Abnormality (Parinaud's Syndrome)   Tumors in the midbrain or a tumor of the pineal gland may affect the vertical gaze center. With this condition, patients are unable to elevate or depress the eyes on command.

Horizontal Gaze Abnormality   Tumors in the pons may affect the horizontal gaze center in lesions of the medial longitudinal fasciculus. The connections between the third motor nucleus and the sixth motor nucleus are lost. When the patient is asked to look laterally, the eye on the normal side moves correctly, but the opposite eye fails to follow. For example, the eye that should move into the adducted position does not, but the eye that should abduct does, although showing coarse nystagmus. The medial rectus has failed to move the eyeball to the adducted position. If the patient is now asked to converge the eyes, this occurs normally—indicating that the oculomotor nucleus and its peripheral connections are normal, but that the medial longitudinal fasciculus connections are at fault.

Sensory Innervation of the Extraocular Muscles

The extraocular muscles possess typical muscle spindles and tendon organs, which are described in Chapter 8. These endings are important in keeping the central nervous system informed regarding muscle length and muscle tension. The ocular muscles are also sensitive to pain, although specific pain endings have not been described. It is now generally agreed that the afferent nerve fibers travel for part of their course near the muscles within the motor nerves supplying the muscles. Nearer the brain stem, the afferent pathway joins the trigeminal nerve and ends in the mesencephalic nucleus of the trigeminal nerve. It is in the lateral wall of the cavernous sinus that the ophthalmic division of the trigeminal nerve receives communicating branches from the oculomotor, trochlear, and abducent nerves.

Variations in the Innervation of the Extraocular Muscles

These are very rare. The superior oblique has been reported as being supplied by the oculomotor nerve, and, in the absence of the abducent nerve, the lateral rectus also is supplied by the oculomotor nerve. The nerve to the levator palpebrae superioris from the upper division of the oculomotor nerve either pierces the superior rectus to reach the levator or passes around the edge of the superior rectus.

Sensory Nerves ···

Trigeminal Nerve (Cranial Nerve V)

The sensory nerves consist of the ophthalmic and maxillary divisions of the trigeminal nerve.

Ophthalmic Division of the Trigeminal Nerve

The ophthalmic nerve (V_1) is the superior and smallest division of the trigeminal nerve. It is entirely sensory.

Origin, Course, and Distribution   The ophthalmic nerve arises from the antero-medial surface of the trigeminal ganglion and passes forward to enter the lateral wall of the cavernous sinus (Fig. 10-4). Here the nerve lies below the oculomotor and trochlear nerves and above the maxillary nerve (Fig. 10-3). As the nerve passes forward, it is joined by fine branches of the sympathetic internal carotid plexus and by proprioceptive sensory branches from the oculomotor, trochlear, and abducent nerves. The ophthalmic nerve also gives off a meningeal branch to the tentorium cerebelli. Just before the ophthalmic nerve enters the orbit through the superior orbital fissure, it divides into its three main branches—lacrimal, frontal, and nasociliary (Fig. 10-4).

Branches

Lacrimal Nerve   The lacrimal nerve is the smallest of the three branches of the ophthalmic nerve. It enters the orbit through the lateral part of the superior orbital fissure above and lateral to the frontal nerve and the trochlear nerve and close to the superior ophthalmic vein; it lies outside the tendinous ring (Fig. 10-5). The nerve courses forward along the upper border of the lateral rectus muscle with the lacrimal artery (Fig. 10-14). The lacrimal nerve receives a branch from the zygomaticotemporal branch of the zygomatic branch of the maxillary nerve. This branch contains parasympathetic secretomotor fibers from the facial nerve that pass to the lacrimal gland. The lacrimal nerve now enters the lacrimal gland and supplies it with several branches. The nerve gives sensory branches to the conjunctiva and ends by piercing the orbital septum to supply the skin of the upper eyelid. For details concerning the innervation of the lacrimal gland, see page 118.

Frontal Nerve   The frontal nerve is the largest branch of the ophthalmic nerve. It enters the orbit through the superior orbital fissure, where it lies between the lacrimal and trochlear nerves; it lies outside the tendinous ring (Fig. 10-5). The frontal nerve passes forward beneath the roof of the orbit on the upper surface of the levator palpebrae superioris muscle. About halfway between the apex and base of the orbit, the nerve divides into a large supraorbital branch and a small supratrochlear branch (Fig. 10-14).

Branches
- The **supraorbital nerve** leaves the orbit through the supraorbital notch or foramen deep to the orbicularis oculi and the frontalis muscles. It is

Figure 10-14

Diagram of the right orbital cavity viewed from above, showing the course and distribution of the frontal and lacrimal branches of the ophthalmic division of the trigeminal nerve, with a part of the course of the nasociliary branch also shown.

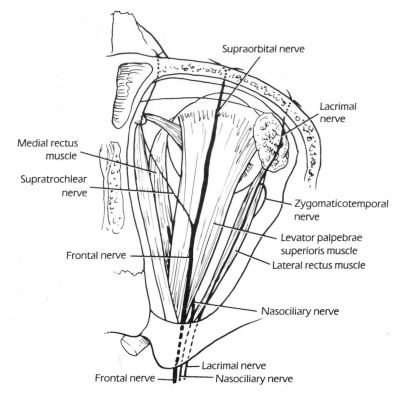

distributed to the skin and conjunctiva of the upper eyelid and to the skin of the forehead and the scalp as far posteriorly as the vertex. As the nerve passes through the supraorbital notch, it supplies a small branch to the mucous membrane of the frontal sinus, which pierces the frontal bone.

- The **supratrochlear nerve** passes forward and medially above the trochlea of the superior oblique muscle (Fig. 10-14). Here it communicates with the infratrochlear branch of the nasociliary nerve. The supratrochlear nerve then leaves the orbit by piercing the orbital septum and turns upward deep to the orbicularis oculi and frontalis muscles. It supplies the skin and conjunctiva of the upper eyelid and the skin of the medial part of the forehead.

Nasociliary Nerve   The nasociliary nerve is intermediate in size between the frontal and lacrimal nerves. It enters the orbit through the medial part of the superior orbital fissure between the two divisions of the oculomotor nerve (Fig. 10-5). It lies within the tendinous ring. The nerve passes forward at first lateral to the optic nerve (Fig. 10-15). It crosses the nerve with the ophthalmic artery to reach the medial wall of the orbit, then passes forward on the upper border of the medial rectus muscle below the superior oblique. The nasociliary nerve ends by passing through the anterior ethmoidal foramen, where it becomes known as the anterior ethmoidal nerve (Fig. 10-15).

The *anterior ethmoidal nerve* supplies the mucous membrane of the anterior ethmoidal air cells and then enters the cranial cavity. It is accompanied by the

Figure 10-15

Diagram of the right orbital cavity viewed from above, showing the course and distribution of the nasociliary branch of the ophthalmic division of the trigeminal nerve.

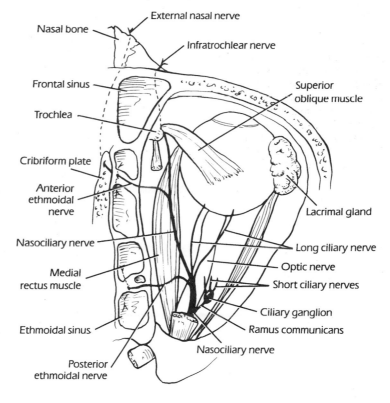

corresponding branch of the ophthalmic artery. The nerve now passes forward and medially on the upper surface of the cribriform plate of the ethmoid bone beneath the dura mater (Fig. 10-15). The nerve leaves the cranial cavity through a slit on the side of the crista galli and enters the nasal cavity. It gives off two *internal nasal nerves,* which are distributed to the mucous membrane of the upper part of the nose. The terminal part of the anterior ethmoidal nerve then descends in a groove on the undersurface of the nasal bone and emerges as the *external nasal nerve* between the lower border of the nasal bone and the lateral nasal cartilage (Fig. 10-15). It supplies the skin on the dorsum of the nose, including the tip and the vestibule.

Branches
The branches of the nasociliary nerve are as follows: 1) ramus communicans to the ciliary ganglion, 2) long ciliary nerves, 3) infratrochlear nerve, and 4) posterior ethmoidal nerve.

- The **ramus communicans to the ciliary ganglion** arises from the nasociliary nerve as soon as it enters the orbital cavity (Figs. 10-15 and 10-16). It passes forward lateral to the optic nerve and after a short course enters the ciliary ganglion. The ramus contains sensory nerve fibers from the eyeball. The sensory fibers reach the ganglion from the eyeball by the short ciliary nerves. They pass without interruption through the ganglion to reach the ramus and so enter the nasociliary nerve.

Figure 10-16

Diagram of the right orbital cavity viewed from above, showing the connections of the ciliary ganglion.

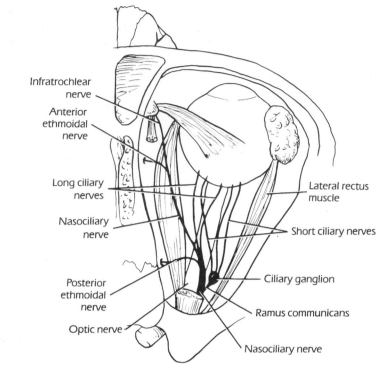

Infratrochlear nerve

Anterior ethmoidal nerve

Long ciliary nerves

Nasociliary nerve

Posterior ethmoidal nerve

Optic nerve

Lateral rectus muscle

Short ciliary nerves

Ciliary ganglion

Ramus communicans

Nasociliary nerve

- The **long ciliary nerves**, usually two in number, arise from the nasociliary nerve as it crosses the optic nerve (Figs. 10-15 and 10-16). They pass forward with the short ciliary nerves from the ciliary ganglion and pierce the sclera of the eyeball close to the attachment of the optic nerve. They then pass forward deep to the sclera in the choroid and are distributed to the ciliary body, iris, and cornea.

    The long ciliary nerves are made up of 1) sympathetic postganglionic fibers to the dilator pupillae muscle and 2) sensory fibers from the cornea.

- The **infratrochlear nerve** arises from the nasociliary nerve close to the anterior ethmoidal foramen (Fig. 10-15). It passes forward along the upper border of the medial rectus muscle and is joined by a branch of the supratrochlear nerve. It passes beneath the trochlear for the superior oblique and pierces the orbital septum and the orbicularis oculi muscle. The infratrochlear nerve supplies the lacrimal sac, the conjunctiva, the skin of the medial parts of the upper and lower eyelids, and the upper part of the lateral aspect of the nose.

- The **posterior ethmoidal nerve** is frequently missing. It arises close to the posterior ethmoidal foramen (Fig. 10-15). It enters the foramen along with the corresponding branch of the ophthalmic artery and supplies the ethmoidal and sphenoidal air sinuses.

Maxillary Division of the Trigeminal Nerve

The maxillary nerve (V_2) is intermediate in position and size between the ophthalmic and mandibular divisions of the trigeminal nerve, it is entirely sensory.

Origin, Course, and Distribution   The maxillary nerve leaves the anterior border of the trigeminal ganglion (Fig. 10-17) and enters the lower part of the lateral wall of the cavernous sinus (Fig. 10-3). The nerve leaves the skull through the foramen rotundum to enter the upper part of the pterygopalatine fossa (Fig. 10-17). Here it is connected by two branches to the pterygopalatine ganglion. The nerve passes laterally and forward and enters the orbit through the inferior orbital fissure.

The maxillary nerve now continues as the *infraorbital nerve*, and, accompanied by the infraorbital artery, it passes forward in the infraorbital groove and canal in the floor of the orbit. It enters the face through the infraorbital foramen (Fig. 10-17). While in the infraorbital groove, it is separated from the contents of the orbit by the orbitalis muscle and from the maxillary sinus by a thin plate of bone. On reaching the face, the nerve divides into several branches beneath the levator labii superioris muscle. By means of its terminal branches, the infraorbital nerve supplies the skin and conjunctiva of the lower eyelid, the skin of the nasal ala, and the skin and mucous membrane of the cheek and upper lip. On the

Figure 10-17

Diagram of the right orbit viewed from the lateral side, with the lateral wall removed, showing the path taken by the postganglionic parasympathetic nerve fibers from the pterygopalatine ganglion, through the maxillary nerve, the zygomatic nerve, the zygomaticofacial nerve, and the lacrimal nerve to the lacrimal gland. The distribution of the maxillary division of the trigeminal nerve is also shown.

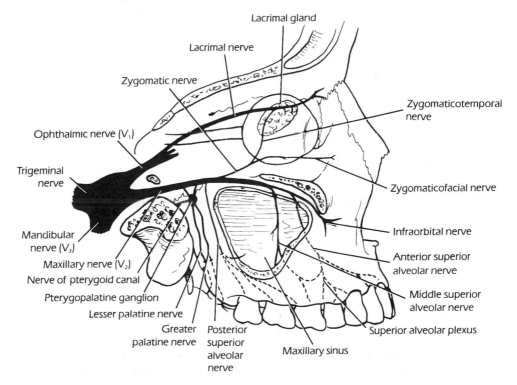

face the nerve receives sensory communicating branches from the facial nerve that are proprioceptive from the muscles of facial expression.

Branches   The branches of the maxillary nerve are as follows: 1) meningeal, 2) ganglionic, 3) zygomatic, and 4) posterior superior alveolar.

Meningeal Branch   The meningeal branch arises from the maxillary nerve close to the foramen rotundum. It supplies the dura mater in the middle cranial fossa.

Ganglionic Branches   The ganglionic branches, two in number, suspend the *pterygopalatine ganglion* from the lower border of the maxillary nerve (Fig. 10-17). They contain sensory fibers from the orbital periosteum and mucous membrane from the nose, palate, and pharynx. They also contain the postganglionic parasympathetic fibers that reach the ganglion from the facial nerve and pass to the lacrimal gland via the zygomatic branch of the maxillary nerve.

Zygomatic Nerve   The zygomatic nerve arises from the maxillary nerve in the pterygopalatine fossa (Fig. 10-17). It enters the orbit through the inferior orbital fissure and runs forward on the lateral wall of the orbit. The nerve then divides into two terminal branches, the zygomaticotemporal and zygomaticofacial nerves.

The *zygomaticotemporal nerve* sends a branch to the lacrimal nerve, which contains postganglionic parasympathetic fibers from the pterygopalatine ganglion to the lacrimal gland (Figs. 10-14 and 10-17). The nerve leaves the orbital cavity by passing through a canal in the zygomatic bone to enter the temporal fossa and supplies the skin on the side of the forehead.

The *zygomaticofacial nerve* leaves the orbital cavity through a canal in the zygomatic bone and supplies the skin on the cheek (Fig. 10-17).

Posterior Superior Alveolar Nerve   The posterior superior alveolar nerve arises from the maxillary nerve in the pterygopalatine fossa (Fig. 10-17). It descends on the posterior surface of the maxilla and pierces that bone to supply the mucous membrane of the maxillary sinus. The nerve then joins the superior dental plexus to supply the upper molar teeth, the gums, and part of the mucous membrane of the cheek.

The branches of the infraorbital nerve (continuation of the maxillary nerve) are as follows: 1) middle superior alveolar, 2) anterior superior alveolar, and 3) facial branches.

Middle Superior Alveolar Nerve   The middle superior alveolar nerve arises from the infraorbital nerve in the infraorbital groove on the floor of the orbital cavity (Fig. 10-17). It runs downward and forward on the lateral wall of the maxillary sinus beneath the mucous membrane that it supplies, and ends by joining the superior dental plexus, supplying the upper premolar teeth and gums.

Anterior Superior Alveolar Nerve   The anterior superior alveolar nerve arises from the infraorbital nerve in the infraorbital canal (Fig. 10-17). It runs downward on the anterior wall of the maxillary sinus beneath the mucous membrane that it supplies. It joins the superior dental plexus and supplies the upper canine and incisor teeth. It also sends off a small branch that enters the nose and supplies a small area of mucous membrane on the anterior part of the lateral wall.

Facial branches   Having emerged on the face through the infraorbital foramen, the infraorbital nerve sends branches to the skin of the lower eyelid, the skin of the cheek, and the skin and mucous membrane of the upper lip. As noted previously, the branches communicate with branches of the facial nerve and contain sensory proprioceptive fibers from the muscles of facial expression.

Trigeminal Nerve Nuclei and Their Central Connections

The trigeminal nerve is the largest cranial nerve. It is the sensory nerve to the greater part of the head and the motor nerve to several muscles, including the muscles of mastication. It has four nuclei: 1) the main sensory nucleus, 2) the spinal nucleus, 3) the mesencephalic nucleus, and 4) the motor nucleus.

Main Sensory Nucleus   This nucleus lies in the posterior part of the pons, lateral to the motor nucleus (Fig. 10-18). It is continuous below with the spinal nucleus.

Spinal Nucleus   This nucleus is continuous superiorly with the main sensory nucleus in the pons and extends inferiorly through the whole length of the medulla oblongata and into the upper part of the spinal cord as far as the second cervical segment (Fig. 10-18).

Mesencephalic Nucleus   This nucleus consists of a column of unipolar nerve cells situated in the lateral part of the gray matter around the cerebral aqueduct. It extends inferiorly into the pons as far as the main sensory nucleus (Fig. 10-18).

Motor Nucleus   This nucleus is situated in the pons medial to the main sensory nucleus (Fig. 10-18).

Sensory Components of the Trigeminal Nerve

The sensations of pain and temperature and touch and pressure travel along axons whose cell bodies are situated in the *trigeminal ganglion* (Fig. 10-18). The central processes of these cells form the large sensory root of the trigeminal nerve. About half the fibers divide into ascending and descending branches when they enter the pons; the remainder ascend or descend without division (Fig. 10-18). The ascending branches terminate in the main sensory nucleus; the descending branches terminate in the spinal nucleus. The sensations of touch and pressure are conveyed by nerve fibers that terminate in the main sensory nucleus. The sensations of pain and temperature pass to the spinal nucleus (Fig. 10-18). It is interesting to note that the sensory fibers from the ophthalmic division of the trigeminal nerve terminate in the inferior part of the spinal nucleus; fibers from the mandibular division end in the superior part of the spinal nucleus.

Proprioceptive sensory impulses from the muscles of mastication and from the facial and extraocular muscles are carried by fibers in the sensory root of the

Figure 10-18

Diagrams of the trigeminal nerve nuclei. (A) The nuclei seen in coronal section of the pons; the corticobulbar fibers to the motor nuclei are also shown. (B) The nuclei in the brain stem; this shows their central nervous connections.

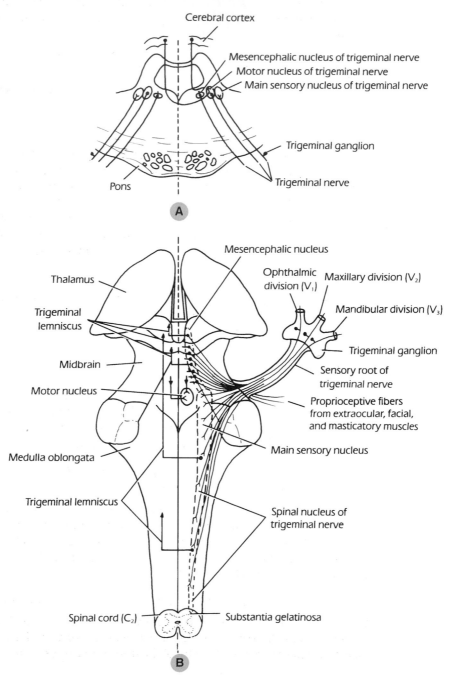

trigeminal nerve that bypass the trigeminal ganglion (Fig. 10-18). These fibers' cells of origin are the unipolar cells of the mesencephalic nucleus (Fig. 10-18).

The axons of the neurons in the main sensory and spinal nuclei, with the central processes of the cells in the mesencephalic nucleus, now cross the median plane and ascend as the *trigeminal lemniscus* to terminate on the nerve cells of the *ventral posteromedial nucleus of the thalamus*. The axons of these cells now travel through the internal capsule to the postcentral gyrus (areas 3, 1, and 2) of the cerebral cortex.

Motor Component of the Trigeminal Nerve

The motor connections of the trigeminal nerve travel in the mandibular division (V_3) and therefore are not of direct interest to the ophthalmologist. Only a brief account is given here.

The motor nucleus receives corticonuclear fibers from both cerebral hemispheres (Fig. 10-18). It also receives fibers from the reticular formation, the red nucleus, the tectum, and the medial longitudinal fasciculus. In addition, the motor nucleus is believed to receive fibers from the mesencephalic nucleus, thereby forming a monosynaptic reflex arc. The cells of the motor nucleus give rise to the axons that form the motor root of the mandibular nerve. The motor nucleus supplies the muscles of mastication, the tensor tympani, the tensor veli palatini, and the mylohyoid and the anterior belly of the digastric muscle.

Clinical Notes

Trigeminal Neuralgia

This is a severe, stabbing pain over the face of unknown cause and involving the pain fibers. The pain is felt most commonly over the skin areas innervated by the mandibular and maxillary divisions of the trigeminal nerve; only rarely is pain felt in the area supplied by the ophthalmic division.

Orbital Compression of the Ophthalmic Nerve

Compression of the terminal branches of the ophthalmic division of the trigeminal nerve may occur with tumors of the orbital cavity or with tumors invading the superior orbital fissure. The common involvement of the optic, oculomotor, trochlear, and abducent nerves helps to localize the lesion.

Involvement of the Ophthalmic and Maxillary Nerves in Diseases of the Cavernous Sinus

Cavernous sinus thrombosis invariably involves the nerves associated with the sinus. These are the oculomotor, trochlear, ophthalmic, and maxillary nerves in its lateral wall and the abducent nerve as it courses through the sinus. Aneurysms of the internal carotid artery and expanding cerebral tumors can also compress these nerves in the sinus.

Hutchinson's Rule in Herpes Zoster of the Ophthalmic Nerve

Hutchinson's rule states that if there is involvement of the eyeball in herpes zoster, there will be skin involvement also along the distribution of the nasociliary nerve, that is, at the tip of the nose. While this dictum is generally true, there are exceptions; it does, however, suggest the path of involvement of this neurotropic virus.

Regional Anesthesia of Branches of the Ophthalmic Nerve

There are no indications for blocking the main stem of the ophthalmic nerve or the lacrimal nerve. The terminal branches of the frontal nerve, namely, the supraorbital and supratrochlear nerves, are commonly blocked.

Supraorbital and Supratrochlear Nerve Block   The *supraorbital nerve* emerges from the orbital cavity in the same vertical plane as the pupil when the patient is looking straight ahead. If the nerve passes through the supraorbital notch, it can be easily palpated on the supraorbital margin. However, if the nerve passes through a foramen, it will be small and difficult to feel. Two to 3 mL of local anesthetic can be infiltrated beneath the skin in the region of the notch or foramen.

The *supratrochlear nerve* winds around the supraorbital margin about one finger's breadth medial to the supraorbital nerve. Two milliliters of anesthetic can be injected into the soft tissue in the vicinity of the nerve.

Retrobulbar and Peribulbar Anesthesia   Blockade of the motor nerve supply to the extraocular muscles and a sensory block of the nerve supply to the eyeball can be achieved by injection of an anesthetic solution behind the globe. Hemorrhage can result if the blood vessels are pierced by the syringe needle, and fibrous septa in the orbital fat can inhibit diffusion of the anesthetic. The latter problem can be largely overcome by the use of hyaluronidase in the anesthetic solution, which hydrolyzes connective tissue mucopolysaccharides. Small amounts of epinephrine can also be added to constrict the blood vessels and retard vascular absorption of the anesthetic.

Retrobulbar Anesthesia   The patient lies supine and is told to look upward, backward, and slightly inward. The lower lateral aspect of the bony orbit is palpated. At its most inferior point, a 3.5-cm, 25-gauge needle is inserted through the lower lid toward the apex of the orbit. The needle should advance between the globe and the lateral bony wall of the orbit. The needle should encounter only minor resistance as it pierces first the orbital septum and then the lateral rectus muscle. On reaching its full depth, the needle end should lie behind the eyeball within the muscle cone between the lateral rectus muscle and the optic nerve. After careful aspiration to test that the needle is not in a blood vessel, 2 to 3 mL of local anesthetic is slowly injected. Larger amounts of the anesthetic may be required for procedures such as enucleation. To assist in the spread of the anesthetic in the retrobulbar tissues, the globe is gently massaged.

The procedure, if successful, should block the oculomotor and abducent nerves, thus paralyzing all the extraocular muscles except the superior oblique (trochlear nerve). It will also block the ciliary ganglion so that the pupil will dilate (constrictor pupillae supplied by the parasympathetic fibers in the ciliary ganglion and the short ciliary nerves). The entire eyeball will be anesthetized owing to blocking of the nasociliary and long ciliary nerves.

Complications   The complications are retrobulbar hemorrhage due to piercing of one of the branches or tributaries of the ophthalmic artery or vein, respectively, during the injection of the anesthetic. This is noticed a short time after the procedure by the occurrence of proptosis, firmness of the globe, and discoloration of the conjunctiva, usually in the lower fornix. This complication is largely avoided by the use of a semisharp needle, careful aspiration prior to the injection of the anesthetic agent, and keeping the tip of the needle away from the globe as it is guided posteriorly.

The effect of the anesthetic on the optic nerve is quite variable, with some patients maintaining reasonably good vision, with paralysis of all the other nerves, and other patients having their vision substantially affected.

Leakage of the anesthetic agent into the subarachnoid space can cause respiratory distress, which is discussed on page 69.

Peribulbar Anesthesia　With this technique, a shorter needle may be used to lessen the chance of piercing the retrobulbar blood vessels, which can occur during the previously described procedure.

The patient looks straight forward and the margins of the bony orbit are carefully palpated as described before. The needle is introduced into the orbit at the lower lateral aspect of the orbital margin, as previously described. The needle is directed backward between the lateral rectus and the inferior rectus muscles. After careful aspiration to test for penetration of blood vessels, as much as 6 mL of the anesthetic agent is introduced. With finger pressure applied on the closed eye, the injected anesthetic agent is gently massaged from the inferolateral region of the orbit toward the superior and nasal regions of the posterior orbit. Additional pressure on the eyeball can be applied with an ophthalmic balloon.

Inadequate anesthesia or muscle paralysis in the superior or medial rectus muscle may require supplementary injections through the nasal portions of the upper and lower eyelids, between the globe and the orbital margin. At these sites the needle may be inserted to a depth of 2.5 cm and only 1 mL of anesthetic agent is required.

Complications　The complications described for retrobulbar anesthesia can also occur with peribulbar anesthesia but less frequently. Introduction of the needle into more than one site of the orbit increases the chance of damage to one of the extraocular muscles, with consequent bleeding.

Topical Anesthesia　Many cataract surgeons are performing phacoemulsification of the cataract with intraocular lens implantation by using a topical anesthetic and a clear corneal incision.

Mild preoperative sedation is used with the anxious patient. Lidocaine in droplet form is added to the conjunctival sac of the patient at 5-minute intervals during the preoperative period and a single drop is administered to the unoperated eye. The lidocaine anesthetizes the sensory innervation of the cornea (long ciliary nerves from the ophthalmic division of the trigeminal nerve) and effectively blocks the corneal blinking reflex. The reflex involves the trigeminal nerve and its connections with the facial nerve that supplies the orbicularis oculi muscle. Since only the cornea is anesthetized, the patient is still able to open and close the eyelids. It is important for the patient to keep both eyes open and fixed on a light source as the operation proceeds.

Although the external topical anesthesia successfully anesthetizes the cornea, it has little or no effect on the ciliary body or iris. Movements of these structures during the operation may cause the patient some discomfort. If the discomfort is excessive, the patient may be sedated. However, a number of surgeons successfully supplement the topical anesthetic by introducing 1% lidocaine directly into the anterior chamber. This anesthetizes the sensory endings of the long and short ciliary nerves in the ciliary body and iris.

Complications   Since ocular motility is preserved with topical anesthesia, movement of the eye during the corneal incision may inadvertently cause a larger incision than necessary. This complication can be prevented by emphasizing to the patient the importance of fixing the eye on the light while the incision is made.

Blow-out Fracture of the Maxilla

The common involvement of the infraorbital continuation of the maxillary nerve in blow-out fractures of the maxilla resulting from severe facial trauma is discussed on page 87.

Malignant Invasion of the Maxillary Nerve

Carcinoma of the mucosa of the maxillary sinus or osteogenic sarcoma of the maxilla can result in extension of the disease through the floor of the orbital cavity or backward into the pterygopalatine fossa. The infraorbital nerve or the maxillary nerve may become involved in the invasive process or have to be sacrificed during surgical ablation of the tumor. In either case, the patient will have sensory loss in the facial skin over the maxilla.

Infraorbital Nerve Block

The infraorbital nerve emerges from the infraorbital foramen as a direct continuation of the maxillary nerve. It sends terminal branches that innervate the lower eyelid, upper lip, and side of the nose. The infraorbital foramen can usually be palpated with gentle pressure just below the infraorbital margin, in line with the pupil. The local anesthetic is injected into the foramen or into the soft tissue over the foramen.

CHAPTER 10
Clinical Problems

Answers on Page 327.

1 A 55-year-old man consulted an ophthalmologist because he had suddenly developed double vision. He was watching his favorite television program the day before, when it suddenly occurred. He had no other symptoms. A complete physical examination revealed that his left eye, when at rest, was turned medially, and that he was unable to turn it laterally. A moderate amount of glucose was found in his urine and he had an abnormally elevated blood glucose level. When closely questioned, he admitted that recently he had noticed having to pass urine more frequently, especially at night. He also said he often felt thirsty. He had lost 25 pounds during the past 18 months. Using your knowledge of anatomy, explain the problem in his left eye. Is there any connection between his glucosuria, high blood glucose, polyuria, polydipsia, and weight loss and his eye condition?

2 A 60-year-old woman with a history of cerebrovascular problems visited her physician because 5 days previously she had begun to have trouble reading the newspaper. She stated that the print started to tilt and she was beginning to see double. She also said that she found it difficult to see the steps when she descended the staircase. On physical examination, the patient had weakness of movement of the left eye both downward and laterally. Using your knowledge of anatomy, explain this patient's signs and symptoms. If we assume that a cranial nerve nucleus is the site of the lesion, is the right one or the left one involved?

3 A 40-year-old man entered the hospital complaining of severe pain over his left forehead and left eye. The pain had started 5 weeks previously and had progressively increased since then. Two weeks ago, he started to see double, and this morning his brother had noticed that his left eye was turning out laterally. The physician in charge made a careful neurologic examination and found a lateral strabismus of the left eye, dilatation of the left pupil with loss of direct and consensual light reflexes, paralysis of accommodation on the left, and paralysis of all left-sided ocular movement except laterally. He advised the patient to have a CT scan of the head. The resulting films showed an aneurysm of the internal carotid artery within the cavernous sinus on the left side. Explain this patient's signs and symptoms. Relate the signs and symptoms to the aneurysm.

4 A 46-year-old woman complaining of pain over the left cheek visited her physician. She had first noticed the pain 3 weeks previously, and it had become progressively worse. The pain was constant in nature. Initially, the pain was relieved by taking aspirin, but later aspirin produced little or no effect; the pain prevented the patient from sleeping at night. In desperation, the patient had consulted her dentist, thinking that she might have a tooth problem, but the dentist could find nothing abnormal. A careful neurologic work-up detected a slight impairment of touch sensation over her left cheek. Both eyes looked and moved normally. An anteroposterior and lateral radiograph of her skull showed a lesion occupying most of the left maxillary air sinus. Superiorly, the roof of the sinus showed invasion by tumor growth. What is the diagnosis? Why did the patient complain of pain over her left cheek and have slight impairment of skin sensation over that area?

5 Intoxicated with alcohol, a 17-year-old boy crashed his sports car into a bridge abutment. Three days later, when he recovered consciousness in the intensive care unit, the neurologist noted that, in addition to extensive skin lacerations of his face, he had an obvious left-sided medial strabismus. All other movements of both eyes were normal. Which cranial nerve to the orbit had been damaged? Where in its intracranial course is this nerve most commonly damaged following head trauma? Why is this nerve the most common orbital nerve to be damaged in head injuries?

6 A 65-year-old man with hypertension was admitted to the hospital with a diagnosis of cerebrovascular hemorrhage. On examination he was found to have paralysis on the right side of the levator palpebrae superioris, superior rectus, medial rectus, inferior rectus, and inferior oblique muscles. Furthermore, his right pupil was dilated and failed to constrict on exposure to light or on accommodation. The left eye was normal in every respect. It was also noted that the lower left part of his face was drooping; the upper part of his face was normal. Examination of his

limbs showed that he had a left-sided hemiplegia. What is the diagnosis? Which area of the brain is involved? How would you explain the signs?

7 Prior to cataract surgery on the right eye, a patient was given a retrobulbar injection of 2% lidocaine solution mixed with 1:100,000 epinephrine. Twenty minutes later the patient was examined and was unable to move his right eye in any direction except for slight movement downward and laterally. His eyeball was completely numb but his eyelids and brow had normal sensation. The patient complained that he was totally blind in his right eye. Which nerves has the local anesthetic affected and which has it spared?

8 Optic nerve tumors confined to the orbital cavity are treated by operating directly on the orbital portion of the optic nerve. Surgeons approach the optic nerve either via the lateral wall or the medial wall of the orbit. The incidence of postoperative pupillary dilatation is much higher after the lateral approach is used. Using your knowledge of anatomy, account for this difference.

CHAPTER 10
Answers to Clinical Problems

1 The medial strabismus of his left eye, the diplopia, and the inability to turn the left eye laterally were due to paralysis of the left lateral rectus muscle caused by a lesion of the left abducent nerve. The glucosuria, high blood glucose, polyuria, polydipsia, and weight loss are the classic signs and symptoms of diabetes mellitus. The lesion of the abducent nerve exemplifies diabetic neuropathy, a complication of untreated or poorly treated diabetes. Once the patient's diabetes was carefully controlled, the left lateral rectus palsy disappeared after 4 months.

2 This patient had a paralysis of the left superior oblique muscle resulting from a lesion of the trochlear nerve. Because the trochlear nerves decussate on emergence from the midbrain, the right trochlear nucleus is the site of the lesion. This patient had a small hemorrhage into the right trochlear nucleus. The difficulty in reading, the diplopia, and the difficulty in walking downstairs were due to paralysis of the left superior oblique muscle.

3 The severe pain over this patient's forehead and left eye was due to irritation of the frontal and nasociliary branches of the ophthalmic division of the trigeminal nerve by the slowly expanding aneurysm of the internal carotid artery lying within the cavernous sinus. The diplopia and the lateral strabismus of the left eye were due to the unopposed action of the lateral rectus muscle (supplied by the abducent nerve). The dilatation of the left pupil, with loss of direct and consensual light reflexes, paralysis of accommodation, and paralysis of all left-sided ocular movement except laterally, was due to pressure on the left oculomotor nerve

by the aneurysm. The nerve at this point is situated in the lateral wall of the cavernous sinus. Note that the lateral movement of the eyeball was accomplished by contracting the lateral rectus muscle (abducent nerve); the inferolateral movement, by contracting the superior oblique muscle (trochlear nerve).

4 At operation the patient was found to have a columnar-celled carcinoma of the mucous membrane lining the left maxillary sinus. The expanding tumor had irritated the sensory nerve supply to the mucous membrane, namely, the anterior and middle superior alveolar nerves, which are branches of the infraorbital nerve. Pain was referred along the distribution of the infraorbital nerve to the skin of the cheek. The tumor had already invaded the infraorbital groove and canal, involving the main trunk of the infraorbital nerve and also invading the orbital fat. The direct involvement of the nerve explained the reduced sensation felt in the skin of the cheek. The patient was treated by complete surgical resection of the left maxilla with removal of the left orbital contents. She is wearing a prosthesis and was very well for 5 years after the operation.

5 The left abducent nerve supplying the left lateral rectus muscle had been damaged in this patient. The most vulnerable of the cranial nerves in head injuries, the abducent nerve is slender and follows a long course in the subarachnoid space in the posterior cranial fossa. It passes forward and laterally and ascends up the posterior surface of the petrous part of the temporal bone near its apex. On reaching the sharp upper border of the bone, it bends forward under the superior petrosal sinus to enter the cavernous sinus.

Any sudden movement of the brain stem can damage this fragile nerve at the point where it turns forward over the sharp upper border of the petrous bone.

6 This patient had the signs of Weber's syndrome, which followed a hemorrhage into the right side of the midbrain, possibly from a branch of the right posterior cerebral artery. The paralyzed right-sided extraocular muscles indicated a lesion of the right oculomotor nerve. The constrictor pupillae muscle on the right side was also paralyzed, further implicating the right oculomotor nerve. The left-sided lower facial paralysis indicated that the paralysis was of the upper motor neuron type, and that the lesion involved the corticobulbar fibers on the right side of the midbrain before they cross the midline. The left-sided hemiplegia can also be explained by the lesion on the right side of the midbrain involving the corticospinal fibers before they cross the midline in the lower part of the medulla oblongata at the decussation of the pyramids.

7 The local anesthetic was infiltrated using the retrobulbar technique described on page 322. Figure 10-5 shows the four rectus muscles and their fascial connections forming a cone behind the bulb. The figure also shows that the muscular cone surrounds a portion of the superior orbital fissure at the apex of the orbit. The frontal, lacrimal, and trochlear nerves enter the orbit through the superior orbital fissure above and outside the muscular cone. Thus, the anesthetic did not reach the frontal, lacrimal, and trochlear nerves, and the skin sensation of the upper lid and forehead as well as the function of the superior oblique muscle remained intact. The nerves within the muscular cone, namely, the oculomotor, the nascociliary, the ciliary ganglion, the ciliary, and the abducent nerves, were blocked. The optic nerve, which also lies within the muscle cone, was temporarily blocked, resulting in visual diminution.

8 The ciliary ganglion commonly lies on the lateral side of the optic nerve (see Fig. 10-16). The ciliary ganglion carries parasympathetic nerve fibers to the sphincter pupillae, which is responsible for pupillary constriction. The ciliary ganglion is more likely to be injured during a lateral approach to the optic nerve than during a medial approach.

Cranial Nerves—Part II: The Nerves Not Directly Associated with the Eye and Orbit

CHAPTER OUTLINE

Introduction

The cranial nerves described in this chapter are the olfactory, facial, vestibulo-cochlear, glossopharyngeal, vagus, accessory, and hypoglossal nerves. The olfactory and vestibulocochlear nerves are entirely sensory in function. The accessory and hypoglossal nerves are entirely motor in function. The facial, glossopharyngeal, and vagus nerves are both motor and sensory. Because these nerves are not directly associated with the eye and orbit, only a brief account of each nerve is given here. The different components of the cranial nerves, their functions, and the openings in the skull through which the nerves leave the cranial cavity are summarized in Table 10-2.

The Sensory Nerves

Olfactory Nerves (Cranial Nerve I)

The olfactory nerves are responsible for conducting the sensations of smell from the upper part of the nasal mucous membrane to the olfactory bulbs in the skull.

Origin and Course

The olfactory nerves arise from the olfactory receptor nerve cells in the olfactory mucous membrane located in the upper part of the nasal cavity above the level of the superior concha (Fig. 11-1). The *olfactory receptor cells* are scattered among supporting cells. Each receptor cell consists of a small bipolar nerve cell with a coarse peripheral process that passes to the surface of the membrane and a fine central process. From the coarse peripheral process a number of short cilia, the *olfactory hairs*, arise and project into the mucus covering the surface of the mucous membrane. These projecting hairs react to odors in the air and stimulate the olfactory cells.

The fine central processes form the *olfactory nerve fibers* (Fig. 11-1). Bundles of these nerve fibers pass through the openings of the cribriform plate of the ethmoid bone to enter the olfactory bulb inside the skull.

Central Connections

Olfactory Bulbs

This ovoid structure lies in the anterior cranial fossa and possesses several types of nerve cells including the large *mitral cell* (Fig. 11-1). The incoming olfactory nerve fibers synapse with the mitral cells. In addition, the olfactory bulb receives axons from the contralateral olfactory bulb through the olfactory tract.

Olfactory Tract

This narrow band of white matter consists of nerve fibers that emerge from the posterior end of the olfactory bulb and run posteriorly beneath the frontal lobe of the brain. It divides into *medial* and *lateral olfactory striae*. The lateral stria carries the axons to the *primary* and *secondary olfactory areas of the cerebral*

Figure 11-1

(A) Distribution of the olfactory nerves on the lateral wall of the nose. (B) Connections between the olfactory cells and the neurons of the olfactory bulb. (C) Connections between the olfactory cell and the rest of the olfactory system.

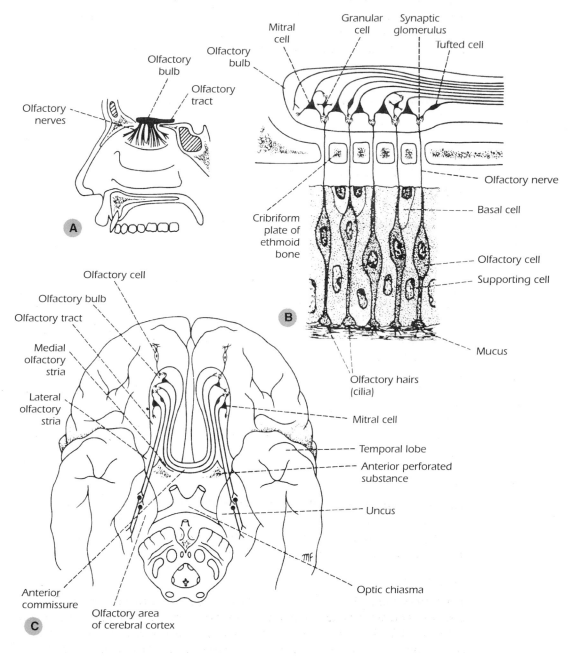

cortex, which are responsible for the appreciation of olfactory sensations (Fig. 11-1). The medial olfactory stria carries the fibers that cross the midline to the olfactory bulb of the opposite side. It is interesting to note that the olfactory afferent pathway reaches the cerebral cortex without synapsing in one of the thalamic nuclei.

Clinical Notes

Testing for the Integrity of the Olfactory Nerves

Once it has been determined that the nasal passages are clear, the examiner applies to each nostril in turn some easily recognizable aromatic substance, such as oil of peppermint or oil of cloves. The patient is asked whether he or she can smell anything. Then the patient is asked to identify the smell.

Bilateral Anosmia

Bilateral anosmia can be caused by disease of the olfactory mucous membrane, such as the common cold or allergic rhinitis.

Unilateral Anosmia

Unilateral anosmia can result from disease affecting the olfactory nerves, bulb, or tract. Fracture of the anterior cranial fossa involving the cribriform plate of the ethmoid could result in a tear in the olfactory nerve. Cerebral tumors of the frontal lobes or meningiomas of the anterior cranial fossa can produce anosmia by pressing on the olfactory bulb or tract.

Vestibulocochlear Nerve (Cranial Nerve VIII)

The vestibulocochlear nerve consists of two distinct parts, the *vestibular nerve* and the *cochlear nerve*, which are concerned with the transmission of afferent information related to the position and movement of the head and hearing, from the internal ear to the central nervous system.

Vestibular Nerve

Origin and Course

The vestibular nerve conducts nerve impulses from the utricle and saccule, which provide information concerning the position of the head. The nerve also conducts impulses from the semicircular canals, which provide information concerning movements of the head.

The nerve fibers of the vestibular nerve are the central processes of nerve cells located in the *vestibular ganglion,* which is situated in the *internal acoustic meatus.* The nerve emerges from the internal acoustic meatus with the cochlear nerve and crosses the posterior cranial fossa with the facial nerve. The vestibular nerve together with the cochlear nerve enters the anterior surface of the brain stem between the pons and the medulla oblongata (Fig. 11-2).

Central Connections

On entering the brain stem, the afferent nerve fibers pass to the vestibular nuclei where they synapse (Fig. 11-3); a small number bypass the nuclei and travel

Figure 11-2

Distribution of the vestibulocochlear nerve.

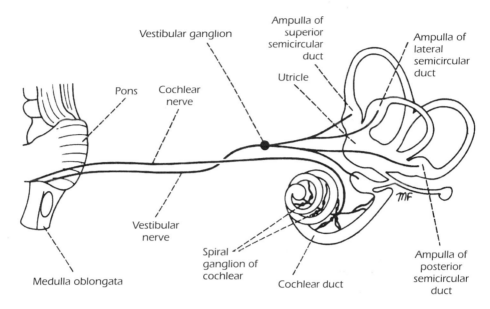

directly to the cerebellum. The efferent nerve fibers from the vestibular nuclei pass to the cerebellum and some descend uncrossed to the spinal cord, forming the *vestibulospinal tract* (Fig. 11-3). In addition, efferent fibers also pass to the nuclei of the oculomotor, trochlear, and abducent nerves through the medial longitudinal fasciculus.

These connections enable the movements of the head and eyes to be coordinated so that visual fixation on an object can be maintained. In addition, information received from the internal ear can assist in maintaining balance by influencing the muscle tone of the limbs and trunk.

Ascending fibers also ascend from the vestibular nuclei to the postcentral gyrus of the cerebral cortex after first synapsing in the thalamus (Fig. 11-3). These connections probably serve to consciously orient the individual in space.

Cochlear Nerve

Origin and Course

The cochlear nerve conducts nerve impulses concerned with sound from the organ of Corti in the cochlea (Fig. 11-2). The fibers of the cochlear nerve are the central processes of nerve cells located in the *spiral ganglion of the cochlea* (Fig. 11-4). The cochlear nerve emerges from the internal acoustic meatus with the vestibular nerve and the facial nerve. It crosses the posterior cranial fossa to enter the anterior surface of the brain stem between the pons and the medulla oblongata alongside the vestibular nerve (Fig. 11-2).

Figure 11-3

Vestibular nerve nuclei and their central connections.

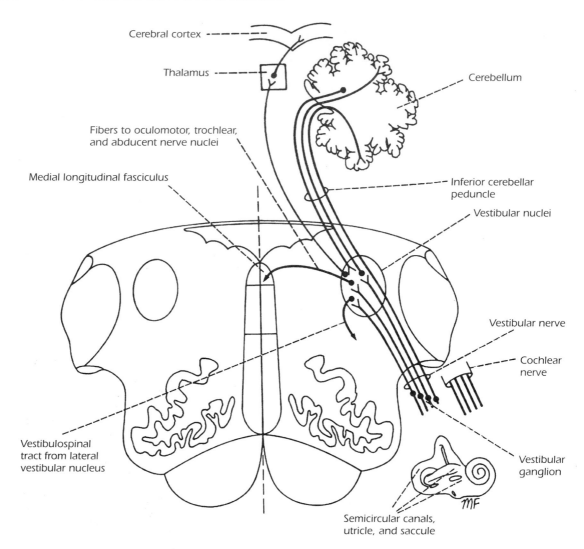

Central Connections

On entering the pons, the nerve fibers divide to enter and synapse with nerve cells in the *anterior* and *posterior cochlear nuclei* (Fig. 11-4). The cochlear nuclei send axons that run medially through the pons to end in the *trapezoid body* and the olivary nucleus. Here they synapse and the new axons ascend through the pons and midbrain as a tract known as the *lateral lemniscus* (Fig. 11-4). As these fibers ascend, some are relayed in nerve cells collectively known as the *nucleus of the lateral lemniscus* (Fig. 11-4). On reaching the midbrain, the fibers of the

Figure 11-4

Cochlear nerve nuclei and their central connections. The descending pathways have been omitted.

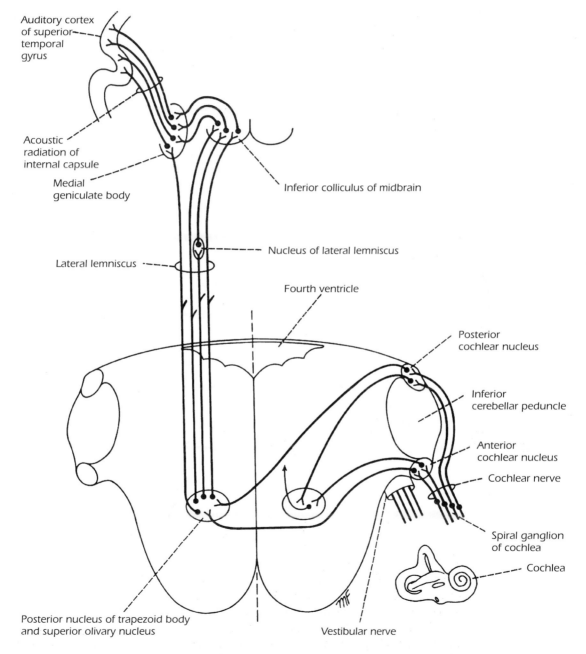

lateral lemniscus either terminate in the *nucleus of the inferior colliculus* or are relayed in the *medial geniculate body* and pass to the *auditory cortex* in the superior temporal gyrus of the cerebral cortex. The recognition and interpretation of sounds on the basis of past experience take place in the secondary auditory area.

Testing for the Integrity of the Vestibular Nerve

Vestibular function can be investigated with the *caloric tests*. These involve the raising and lowering of the temperature in the external auditory meatus, which induces convection currents in the endolymph of the semicircular canals (principally the lateral semicircular canal) and stimulates the vestibular nerve endings.

Disturbances of Vestibular Function

Disturbances of vestibular function include giddiness (*vertigo*) and *nystagmus* (see p. 259).

The causes of vertigo include diseases of the labyrinth of which Meniere's disease is an example. Lesions of the vestibular nerve, the vestibular nuclei, and the cerebellum can also be responsible. Multiple sclerosis, tumors, and vascular lesions of the brain stem also cause vertigo.

Vestibular nystagmus is an uncontrollable rhythmic oscillation of the eyes and the fast phase is away from the side of the lesion. This form of nystagmus is essentially a disturbance in the reflex control of the extraocular muscles, which is one of the functions of the semicircular canals. Normally, the nerve impulses pass reflexly from the canals through the vestibular nerve, the vestibular nuclei, and the medial longitudinal fasciculus, to the oculomotor, trochlear, and abducent nerve nuclei, which control the extraocular muscles; the cerebellum assists in coordinating the muscle movements.

Testing for the Integrity of the Cochlear Nerve

The patient's ability to hear a whispered voice or a vibrating tuning fork should be tested. Each ear should be tested separately.

Disturbances of Cochlear Nerve Function

Disturbances of cochlear function are manifested as *deafness* and *tinnitus*. Loss of hearing may be due to a defect of the auditory conducting mechanism in the middle ear, damage to the receptor cells in the spiral organ of Corti in the cochlea, a lesion of the cochlear nerve, a lesion of the central auditory pathways, or a lesion in the cortex of the temporal lobe of the cerebral hemisphere.

Lesions of the internal ear include *Meniere's disease, acute labyrinthitis*, and *trauma* following head injury. Lesions of the cochlear nerve include *tumor* (*acoustic neuroma*) and *trauma*. Lesions in the central nervous system include *tumors of the midbrain* and *multiple sclerosis*. Only bilateral temporal lobe lesions cause deafness.

The Motor Nerves ·

Accessory Nerve (Cranial Nerve XI)

The accessory nerve brings about movements of the soft palate, pharynx, and larynx and controls the sternocleidomastoid and trapezius muscles in the neck.

Origin

The accessory nerve is formed by the union of a cranial and a spinal root (Fig. 11-5).

Cranial Root (Part) The cranial root is formed from the axons of nerve cells of the *nucleus ambiguus* (Fig. 11-6). The nucleus receives corticonuclear fibers from both cerebral hemispheres.

Course and Distribution The nerve fibers emerge on the anterior surface of the medulla oblongata and run laterally in the posterior cranial fossa and join the spinal root. The two roots unite and leave the skull through the jugular foramen The roots then separate and the cranial root joins the vagus nerve and is distributed in its pharyneal and recurrent laryngeal branches to the muscles of the soft palate, pharynx, and larynx.

Spinal Root (Part)

The spinal root is formed from the axons of nerve cells in the *spinal nucleus,* which is situated in the anterior gray horns of the spinal cord in the upper five

Figure 11-5

Distribution of the accessory nerve.

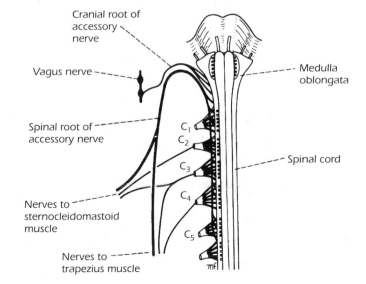

Figure 11-6

Cranial and spinal nuclei of the accessory nerve and their central connections.

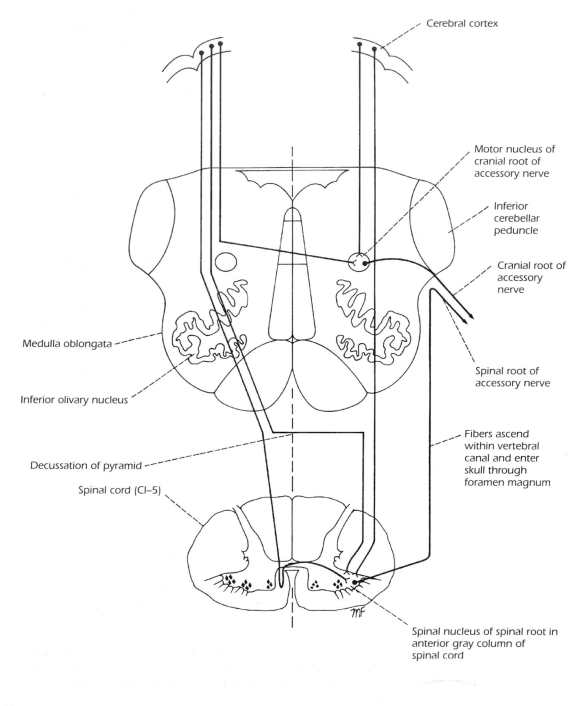

cervical segments (Fig. 11-5). The spinal nucleus receives corticospinal fibers from both cerebral hemispheres (Fig. 11-6).

Course and Distribution   The nerve fibers emerge from the spinal cord to form a trunk that ascends into the skull through the foramen magnum. The spinal root passes laterally and joins the cranial root as they pass through the jugular foramen. The spinal root then separates from the cranial root and runs downward and laterally in the neck to supply the sternocleidomastoid muscle and the trapezius muscle (Fig. 11-5).

The accessory nerve thus brings about movements of the soft palate, pharynx, and larynx and controls the movement of two large muscles in the neck.

Clinical Notes

The Cranial Root of the Accessory Nerve   Since this nerve joins the vagus nerve and is distributed with its branches, it is tested with the vagus nerve and is involved with the same diseases as affect the vagus.

Testing for the Integrity of the Spinal Root of the Accessory Nerve   This involves testing for the activity of the sternocleidomastoid and trapezius muscles. The patient should be asked to rotate the head to one side against resistance, causing the sternocleidomastoid muscle of the opposite side to come into action. Then the patient should be asked to shrug the shoulders, causing the trapezius muscles to come into action.

Lesions of the Spinal Part of the Accessory Nerve   Lesions of the spinal part of the accessory nerve will result in paralysis of the sternocleidomastoid and trapezius muscles. The sternocleidomastoid muscle will atrophy and there will be weakness in turning the head to the opposite side. The trapezius muscle will also atrophy and the shoulder will droop on that side. There will also be weakness and difficulty in raising the arm above the horizontal.

Lesions of the spinal part of the accessory nerve may occur anywhere along its course and may result from tumors or trauma from stab or gunshot wounds in the neck.

Hypoglossal Nerve (Cranial Nerve XII)

The hypoglossal nerve controls the movements and shape of the tongue.

Origin

The hypoglossal nucleus is situated in the medulla oblongata close to the midline immediately beneath the floor of the lower part of the fourth ventricle (Fig. 11-7). It receives corticonuclear fibers from the precentral gyrus of both cerebral hemispheres. However, the cells responsible for supplying the genioglossus muscle only receive corticonuclear fibers from the opposite cerebral hemisphere.

Course and Distribution

The hypoglossal nerve emerges on the anterior surface of the medulla oblongata (Fig. 11-7). It crosses the posterior cranial fossa and leaves the skull through the hypoglossal canal. The nerve then passes downward and forward in the neck and

Figure 11-7

Hypoglossal nucleus and its central connections.

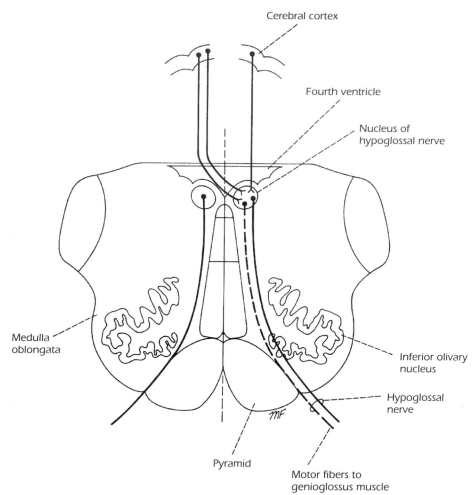

supplies all the intrinsic muscles of the tongue and, in addition, the styloglossus, the hyoglossus, and the genioglossus muscles. The hypoglossal nerve thus controls the movements and shape of the tongue.

Clinical Notes

Testing for the Integrity of the Hypoglossal Nerve   To test the integrity of the nerve, the patient is asked to put out the tongue. If there is a lesion of the nerve, the tongue will be observed to deviate toward the paralyzed side. The tongue will be smaller on the side of the lesion, owing to muscle atrophy. Lesions of the hypoglossal nerve may occur anywhere along its course and may result from tumor, demyelinating diseases, syringomyelia, and vascular accidents within the medulla oblongata. Injury of the nerve in the neck may also follow stab and gunshot wounds.

The Motor and Sensory Nerves ·

Facial Nerve (Cranial Nerve VII)

The facial nerve is both a motor and a sensory nerve. The facial nerve supplies the muscles of the face, scalp, the muscles of the auricle of the ear, the stapedius muscle in the middle ear, and the posterior belly of the digastric and the stylohyoid muscles in the neck. It carries taste fibers from the anterior two-thirds of the tongue, from the floor of the mouth, and from the palate. It also sends secretomotor nerves to the submandibular and sublingual salivary glands, the lacrimal gland, and the glands of the nose and palate.

Facial Nerve Nuclei

The facial nerve has three nuclei: 1) the main motor nucleus, 2) the parasympathetic nuclei, and 3) the sensory nucleus.

Main Motor Nucleus   This lies within the pons (Fig. 11-8). The part of the nucleus that supplies the muscles of the upper part of the face receives corticonuclear

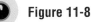 **Figure 11-8**

Facial nerve nuclei and their central connections.

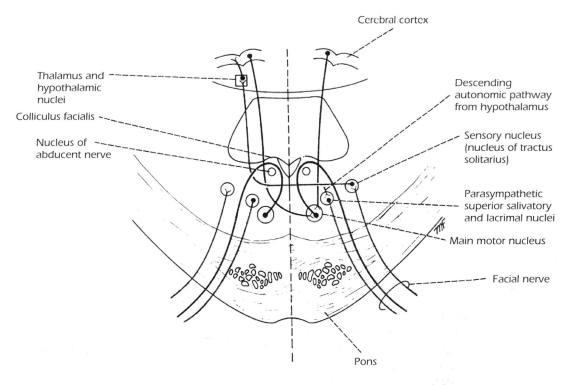

fibers from the precentral gyri of both cerebral hemispheres. The part of the nucleus that supplies the muscles of the lower part of the face receives cortico-nuclear fibers from the opposite cerebral hemisphere.

Parasympathetic Nuclei   These lie posterolateral to the main motor nucleus. They are the *superior salivatory* and *lacrimal nuclei* (Fig. 11-8). The superior salivatory nucleus supplies secretomotor fibers to the submandibular and sublingual salivary glands. The nucleus receives afferent fibers from the hypothalamus. Information concerning taste also is received from the *nucleus of the solitary tract* from the mouth cavity.

The lacrimal nucleus supplies secretomotor fibers to the lacrimal gland. It receives afferent fibers from the hypothalamus for emotional responses and from the sensory nuclei of the trigeminal nerve for reflex lacrimation secondary to irritation of the cornea or conjunctiva.

Sensory Nucleus   This is the upper part of the *nucleus of the tractus solitarius* and lies close to the motor nucleus (Fig. 11-8). Sensations of taste travel from the anterior two-thirds of the tongue and from the floor of the mouth and palate. The sensations travel through the peripheral axons of nerve cells in the *geniculate ganglion* on the seventh cranial nerve. The central processes of these cells synapse on nerve cells in the nucleus. Efferent fibers cross the midline and ascend to the thalamus where they are relayed to the taste area of the cerebral cortex in the lower part of the postcentral gyrus.

Course and Distribution

The facial nerve consists of a motor and a sensory root. The two roots emerge from the anterior surface of the brain stem at the lower border of the pons and pass laterally in the posterior cranial fossa. The facial nerve then accompanies the vestibulocochlear nerve and enters the internal acoustic meatus. At the bottom of the meatus, the nerve enters the facial canal and runs through the inner ear. On reaching the medial wall of the middle ear, the nerve turns sharply backward and descends in the posterior wall of the middle ear to emerge from the skull through the stylomastoid foramen.

Clinical Notes

Testing for the Integrity of the Facial Nerve   To test the facial nerve, the patient is asked to show the teeth by separating the lips with the teeth clenched. Normally, equal areas of the upper and lower teeth are revealed on both sides. If a lesion of the facial nerve is present on one side, the mouth is distorted. A larger area of teeth is revealed on the side of the intact nerve, since the mouth is pulled up on that side. Another useful test is to ask the patient to close both eyes firmly. The examiner then attempts to open the eyes by gently raising the patient's upper lids. On the side of the lesion the orbicularis oculi is paralyzed so that the eyelid on that side is easily raised.

The sensation of taste on each half of the anterior two-thirds of the tongue can be tested by placing on the tongue small amounts of sugar, salt, vinegar, and quinine for sweet, salt, sour, and bitter sensations, respectively.

Facial Nerve Lesions   The facial nerve can be injured anywhere along its course from the brain stem to the face. When the abducent nerve and the facial nerve are not functioning, this would suggest a lesion in the pons of the brain since both nuclei are situated close to one another. When the vestibulocochlear nerve and the facial nerve are not functioning, this would suggest a lesion in the internal acoustic meatus where the nerves lie close together. A firm swelling of the parotid salivary gland caused by a malignant tumor may involve the facial nerve as it passes through the gland. Deep lacerations of the face may involve branches of the facial nerve.

In lesions involving the corticonuclear fibers to the facial motor nucleus, such as might occur with a stroke, only the muscles of the lower part of the face will be paralyzed. This is because the part of the facial motor nucleus that controls the muscles of the upper part of the face receives corticonuclear fibers from both cerebral hemispheres. However, in patients with a lesion of the facial nerve motor nucleus or the facial nerve itself, all the muscles of the affected side of the face will be paralyzed. The lower eyelid will droop and the angle of the mouth will sag. Tears will flow over the lower eyelid, and saliva will dribble from the corner of the mouth. The patient will be unable to close the eye and will be unable to expose the teeth fully on the affected side.

Bell's Palsy   This is a dysfunction of the facial nerve, as it lies within the facial canal; it is usually unilateral. The swelling of the nerve within the bony canal causes pressure on the nerve fibers, which results in temporary loss of function and paralysis. The cause of Bell's palsy is not known; it sometimes follows exposure of the face to a cold draft.

Glossopharyngeal Nerve (Cranial Nerve IX)

The glossopharyngeal nerve is a motor and a sensory nerve. The motor fibers supply the stylopharyngeus muscle, which assists in the process of swallowing. The secretomotor fibers supply the parotid salivary gland. The general sensation and taste arise from the posterior one-third of the tongue and pharynx and from the carotid sinus (baroreceptor) and the carotid body (chemoreceptor).

Glossopharyngeal Nerve Nuclei

The glossopharyngeal nerve has three nuclei: 1) the main motor nucleus, 2) the parasympathetic nucleus, and 3) the sensory nucleus.

Main Motor Nucleus   This nucleus lies in the medulla oblongata and is formed by the superior end of the nucleus ambiguus (Fig. 11-9). It receives corticonuclear fibers from the precentral gyrus of both cerebral hemispheres.

Parasympathetic Nucleus   This nucleus is called the *inferior salivatory nucleus* (Fig. 11-9). It receives afferent fibers from the hypothalamus. Information concerning taste also is received from the mouth cavity. The efferent preganglionic parasympathetic fibers reach the otic ganglion through the *tympanic branch of*

Figure 11-9

Glossopharyngeal nerve nuclei and their central connections.

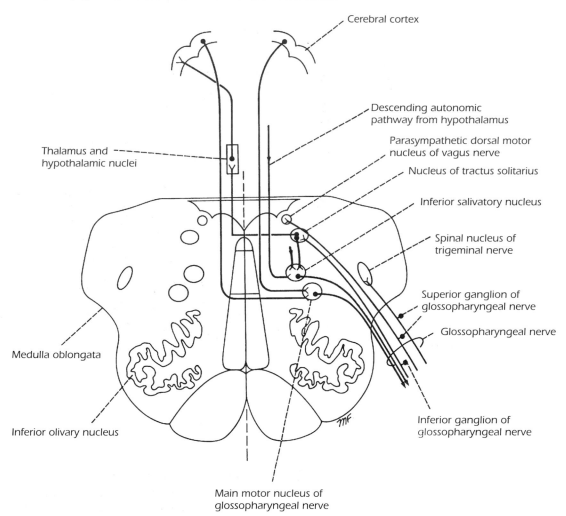

the glossopharyngeal nerve, the tympanic plexus, and the lesser petrosal nerve (Fig. 11-10). The postganglionic fibers pass to the parotid salivary gland.

Sensory Nucleus   This is part of the *nucleus of the tractus solitarius* (Fig. 11-9). Sensations of taste travel through the peripheral axons of nerve cells situated in the *ganglion* on the glossopharyngeal nerve. The central processes of these cells synapse in the nucleus. Efferent fibers cross the midline and ascend to the opposite thalamus where they are relayed to the lower part of the postcentral gyrus of the cerebral cortex.

Figure 11-10

The distribution of the glossopharyngeal nerve.

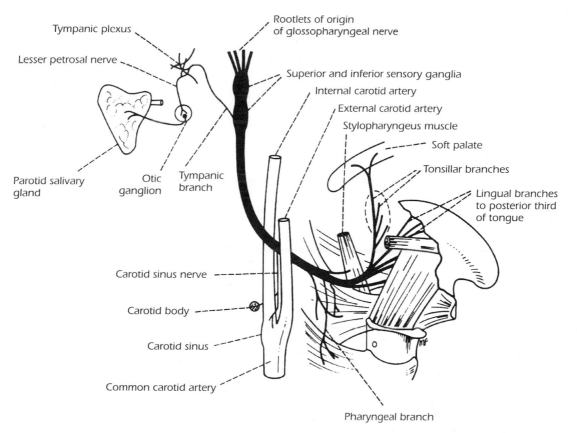

Course and Distribution

The glossopharyngeal nerve leaves the anterior surface of the medulla oblongata. It passes laterally in the posterior cranial fossa and leaves the skull through the jugular foramen. The nerve then descends through the upper part of the neck to reach the posterior border of the stylopharyngeus muscle, which it supplies (Fig. 11-10). The nerve then passes forward into the wall of the pharynx to give sensory branches to the mucous membrane and the posterior third of the tongue. A branch passes to the carotid sinus on the carotid arteries and to the carotid body.

Clinical Notes

Testing for the Integrity of the Glossopharyngeal Nerve   The integrity of this nerve can be evaluated by testing the patient's general sensation and that of taste on the posterior third of the tongue.

Lesions of the Glossopharyngeal Nerve   Isolated lesions of the glossopharyngeal nerve are rare and usually also involve the vagus nerve.

Vagus Nerve (Cranial Nerve X)

The vagus nerve is a motor and a sensory nerve. The nerve fibers supply the heart and great thoracic blood vessels; larynx, trachea, bronchi, and lungs; the alimentary tract from the pharynx to the splenic flexure of the colon; and the liver, kidneys, and pancreas.

Vagus Nerve Nuclei

The vagus nerve has three nuclei: 1) the main motor nucleus, 2) the parasympathetic nucleus, and 3) the sensory nucleus.

Main Motor Nucleus   This nucleus lies in the medulla oblongata and is formed by the nucleus ambiguus (Fig. 11-11). It receives corticonuclear fibers from the precentral gyrus of both cerebral hemispheres. The motor fibers supply the constrictor muscles of the pharynx and the intrinsic muscles of the larynx (Fig. 11-12).

Parasympathetic Nucleus   This nucleus forms the dorsal nucleus of the vagus (Fig. 11-11). It receives afferent fibers from the hypothalamus. The efferent fibers are distributed to the involuntary muscle of the bronchi, heart, esophagus, stomach, small intestine, and large intestine as far as the distal third of the transverse colon (Fig. 11-12).

Sensory Nucleus   This nucleus is part of the *nucleus of the tractus solitarius*. Sensations of taste travel from the sensory ganglion of the vagus to the sensory nucleus (Fig. 11-11). Efferent fibers cross the midline and ascend to the opposite thalamus where they relay and end in the postcentral gyrus of the cerebral cortex.

Course

The vagus nerve leaves the anterior part of the medulla oblongata and passes laterally through the posterior cranial fossa and leaves the skull through the jugular foramen. The vagus nerve possesses a superior and an inferior sensory ganglion. Below the jugular foramen the cranial root of the accessory nerve joins the vagus nerve and is distributed mainly in its pharyngeal and recurrent laryngeal branches.

The vagus nerve descends through the neck (Fig. 11-12) and enters the thorax and contributes branches to the pulmonary and esophageal plexuses. It enters the abdomen through the diaphragm and divides into branches that are distributed to the stomach, small and large intestines, the liver, the pancreas, and the kidneys.

Clinical Notes

Testing for the Integrity of the Vagus Nerve   The vagus nerve innervates many important organs, but the examination of this nerve depends on testing the function of the branches to the pharynx, soft palate, and larynx.

The *pharyngeal* or *gag reflex* can be tested by touching the lateral wall of the pharynx with a spatula. This should immediately cause the patient to gag; that is, the pharyngeal musculature will contract. The innervation of the soft palate can

Figure 11-11

Vagus nerve nuclei and their central connections.

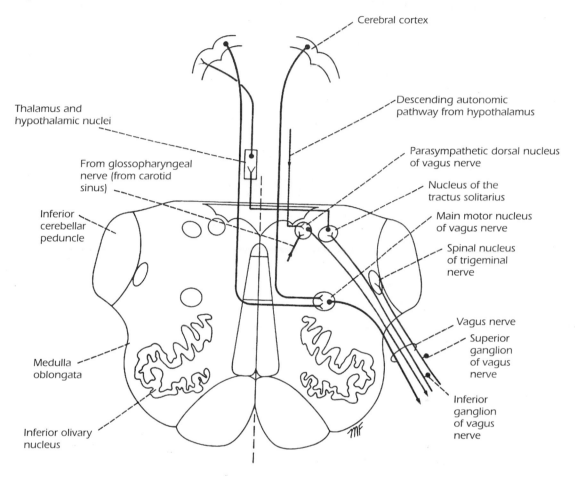

be tested by asking the patient to say "ah." Normally, the soft palate rises and the uvula moves backward in the midline.

Hoarseness or absence of the voice may occur as a symptom of vagal nerve palsy. The movements of the vocal cords may be tested by means of laryngoscopic examination.

Lesions Involving the Vagus Nerve in the Posterior Cranial Fossa   Lesions of the vagus nerve in the posterior cranial fossa commonly involve the glossopharyngeal, accessory, and hypoglossal nerves also. Primary or metastatic tumors, or trauma may be responsible.

Figure 11-12

Distribution of the vagus nerve.

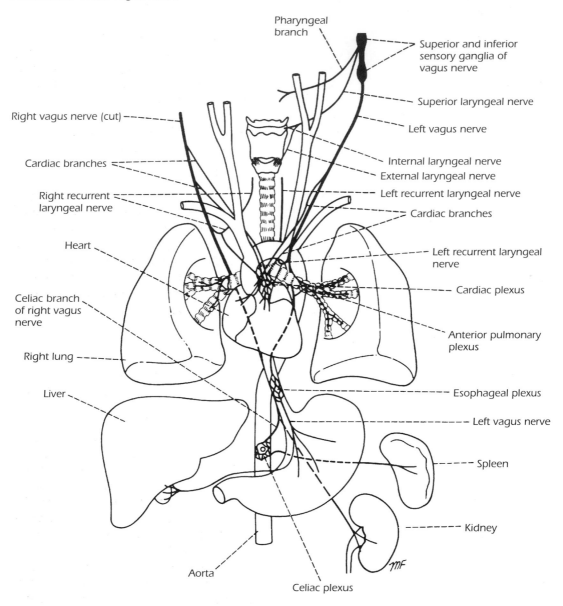

CHAPTER 11
Clinical Problems

Answers on Page 350.

1 An 18-year-old man was seen in the emergency department because of a stab wound at the front of the neck. The entrance wound was located on the right side of the neck just lateral to the tip of the great cornu of the hyoid bone. During the physical examination the patient was asked to protrude his tongue, which deviated to the right. In anatomic terms, explain this finding.

2 A 32-year-old woman had a large abscess located in the middle of the posterior triangle of the neck on the left side. The physician decided to incise the abscess. He found the interior of the abscess to be extensive, and he inserted a drain. Three days later the patient returned to the emergency department for the dressings to be changed. She stated that her neck was no longer painful. However, there was one thing that she could not understand. She could no longer raise her left hand above her head to brush her hair. In anatomic terms, explain this patient's disability.

3 A 48-year-old woman woke up one morning to find the right side of her face paralyzed. When examined by her physician, she was found to have complete paralysis of the entire right side of her face. She was also found to have severe hypertension. The patient talked with a slurred speech. The physician told the patient that she had suffered a mild stroke and that she should be treated in bed. Do you think the diagnosis was correct?

4 A 15-year-old boy was driving his snowmobile at high speed across a snow-covered field when he attempted to negotiate a small opening in the fence. Unfortunately, he lost control and hit a fence post and was thrown to the frozen ground. On arrival at the emergency department, the patient was unconscious. He underwent a complete physical examination including lateral and anteroposterior radiographs of his skull. It was found that he had a fracture involving the anterior cranial fossa. It was also noted that he had a continuous blood-stained watery discharge from his right nostril. Twenty-four hours later, he recovered consciousness and a further physical examination revealed that he could no longer smell. Using your knowledge of anatomy, diagnose what is wrong with this patient.

5 A patient is suspected of having a lesion of the glossopharyngeal and vagus nerves. How would you test the integrity of these cranial nerves?

6 A 65-year-old man complaining of high-pitched noises in his left ear visited his physician. He also said he had recently had attacks of vertigo when he felt he was spinning; this was accompanied by a feeling of nausea. Two days ago he noticed that he was becoming deaf in his left ear. His wife said that she had noticed that the left side of his face was becoming a little distorted and his mouth appeared to be drawn up to the right. Using your knowledge of anatomy, explain these complaints.

CHAPTER 11
Answers to Clinical Problems

1 The protruded tongue pointing to the right side indicated a lesion of the right hypoglossal nerve. The hypoglossal nerve descends in the neck between the internal carotid artery and the internal jugular vein. At the level of the tip of the greater cornu of the hyoid bone, it turns forward and medially toward the tongue. In this patient, the nerve was severed in this location.

2 The spinal root of the accessory nerve crosses the posterior triangle of the neck in a superficial position, being only covered by skin and fascia. The knife opening the abscess in this patient had also cut the nerve, thus paralyzing the left trapezius muscle. To raise the hand above the head, as for brushing your hair, it is necessary for the trapezius muscle, assisted by the serratus anterior muscle, to contract and rotate the scapula.

3 The physician grouped together the facial paralysis, the slurred speech, and the hypertension, and in the absence of other findings made the incorrect diagnosis of cerebral hemorrhage. A lesion of the corticonuclear fibers on one side of the brain will cause paralysis only of the muscles of the lower part of the opposite side of the face. This patient had complete paralysis of the entire right side of the face, which could only be caused by a lesion of the lower motor neuron. The correct diagnosis is Bell's palsy, an inflammation of the connective tissue of the facial nerve.

4 This boy had anosmia secondary to a lesion involving both olfactory tracts. The watery discharge from the nose was due to a leak of the cerebrospinal fluid through the fractured cribriform plate of the ethmoid bone. It was the fracture and the associated hemorrhage that had damaged both olfactory tracts.

5 The glossopharyngeal nerve supplies the posterior third of the tongue with nerve fibers that are concerned with common sensations and taste. This can be easily tested. The vagus nerve, by means of its pharyngeal branch, supplies many muscles of the soft palate and these can be tested by asking the patient to say "ah." Normally the uvula is elevated in the midline. A lesion of the vagus nerve would result in the uvula being elevated to the opposite side. Additional tests may be carried out by observing the movements of the vocal cords through a laryngoscope.

6 The presence of vertigo (vestibular nerve) and tinnitus and deafness (cochlear nerve), combined with facial paralysis on the left side (facial nerve), would strongly suggest the presence of a tumor in the internal acoustic meatus where all three nerves are closely related to one another. These tumors commonly originate from the vestibular portion of the eighth cranial nerve.

The Autonomic Nervous System

CHAPTER OUTLINE

An understanding of the structure and function of the autonomic nervous system is essential for all personnel involved in treating eye diseases. Not only is it important for the ophthalmic surgeon, but it is necessary for all physicians to understand the various light reflexes and accommodation reflexes and the actions of drugs used in clinical practice. For these reasons, a brief outline of the autonomic nervous system follows in this chapter, with special emphasis on the autonomic innervation of the eye.

Organization of the Autonomic Nervous System

The autonomic nervous system exerts control over the functions of many organs and tissues in the body. Along with the endocrine system, it brings about fine internal adjustments necessary for maintenance of the optimal internal environment of the body.

The autonomic nervous system, like the somatic nervous system, has afferent, connector, and efferent neurons. The afferent impulses originate in visceral receptors and travel via afferent pathways to the central nervous system, where they are integrated through connector neurons at different levels and then leave via efferent pathways to visceral effector organs.

The efferent pathways of the autonomic system are made up of efferent preganglionic and postganglionic neurons. The cell bodies of the preganglionic neurons are situated in the lateral gray columns (horns) of the spinal cord and in the motor nuclei of the third, seventh, ninth, and tenth cranial nerves. The axons of these cell bodies synapse on the cell bodies of the postganglionic neurons that are collected together to form *ganglia* outside the central nervous system.

The autonomic nervous system is concerned with the innervation of involuntary structures such as the heart, smooth muscle, and glands. It is distributed throughout the central and peripheral nervous systems. The autonomic system is divided into two parts, called the *sympathetic* and the *parasympathetic*, and both parts have afferent and efferent nerve fibers.

Sympathetic Part of the Autonomic Nervous System

The larger, sympathetic part of the autonomic system is widely distributed throughout the body, innervating the heart and lungs, muscle in the walls of many blood vessels, hair follicles and sweat glands, and many abdomino-pelvic viscera.

The function of the sympathetic system is to prepare the body for an emergency. The heart rate increases, arterioles of the skin and intestine constrict, arterioles of skeletal muscle dilate, and blood pressure rises. There is a redistribution of blood so that it leaves the skin and gastrointestinal tract and passes to the brain, heart, and skeletal muscle. In addition, the sympathetic nerves dilate the pupils, inhibit smooth muscle of the bronchi, intestine, and bladder wall, and close the sphincters. The hair is made to stand on end, and sweating occurs.

The sympathetic part of the autonomic system consists of the efferent outflow from the spinal cord, two ganglionated sympathetic trunks, and important branches, plexuses, and regional ganglia.

Efferent Nerve Fibers (Sympathetic Outflow)

The lateral gray columns (horns) of the spinal cord from the first thoracic segment to the second lumbar segment (sometimes the third lumbar segment) possess the cell bodies of the sympathetic connector neurons (Fig. 12-1). The myelinated axons of these cells leave the cord with the anterior nerve roots and pass into the spinal nerve trunks. They then leave the nerve via the *white rami communicantes* to the *paravertebral ganglia* of the *sympathetic trunk*. Once these (preganglionic) fibers reach the ganglia in the sympathetic trunk, the distribution is as follows:

1. They synapse with an excitor neuron in the ganglion (Figs. 12-1 and 12-2). The gap between the two neurons is bridged by the neurotransmitter

Figure 12-1

Diagram showing the general arrangement of the somatic part of the nervous system (on left) compared with the autonomic part of the nervous system (on right).

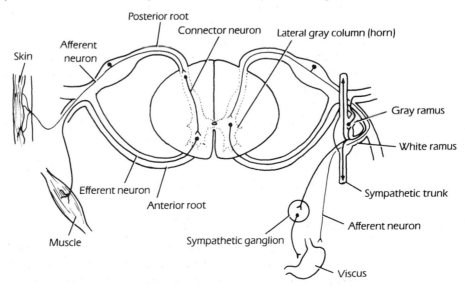

Figure 12-2

Efferent part of the autonomic nervous system. Preganglionic parasympathetic fibers are shown in solid blue, postganglionic parasympathetic fibers in interrupted blue. Preganglionic sympathetic fibers are shown in solid red, postganglionic sympathetic fibers in interrupted red.

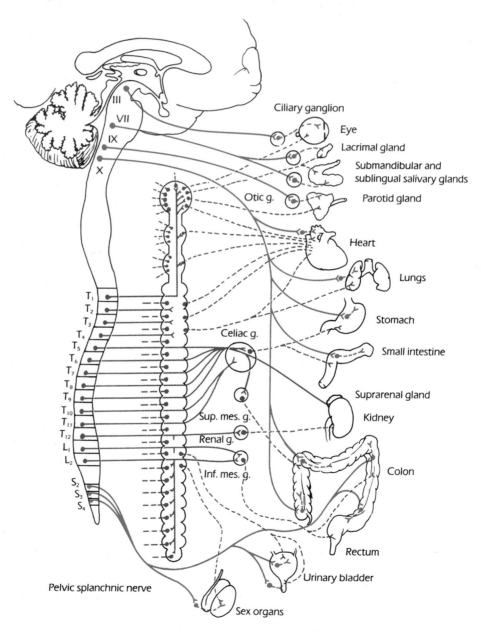

acetylcholine. The postganglionic nonmyelinated axons leave the ganglion and pass to the thoracic spinal nerves as *gray rami communicantes.* They are distributed in branches of the spinal nerves to smooth muscle in the blood vessel walls, sweat glands, and arrector pili muscles of the skin.

2. Axons may travel cephalad in the sympathetic trunk to synapse in ganglia in the cervical region (Fig. 12-2). The postganglionic nerve fibers pass via gray rami communicantes to join cervical spinal nerves. Many of the preganglionic fibers entering the lower part of the sympathetic trunk from the lower thoracic and upper two lumbar segments of the spinal cord travel caudal to synapse in ganglia in the lower lumbar and sacral regions. Here, again, the postganglionic nerve fibers pass via gray rami communicantes to join the lumbar, sacral, and coccygeal spinal nerves (Fig. 12-2).

3. They may pass through the ganglia of the sympathetic trunk without synapsing. These myelinated fibers leave the sympathetic trunk as the *greater splanchnic, lesser splanchnic,* and *lowest or least splanchnic nerves.*

   The greater splanchnic nerve is formed from branches from the fifth to the ninth thoracic ganglia. It descends obliquely on the side of the bodies of the thoracic vertebrae and pierces the crus of the diaphragm to synapse with excitor cells in the ganglia of the *celiac plexus,* the *renal plexus,* and the *suprarenal medulla.*

   The lesser splanchnic nerve is formed from branches of the tenth and eleventh thoracic ganglia. It descends with the greater splanchnic nerve and pierces the diaphragm to join excitor cells in ganglia in the lower part of the *celiac plexus.*

   The lowest splanchnic nerve (when present) arises from the twelfth thoracic ganglion, pierces the diaphragm, and synapses with excitor neurons in the ganglia of the *renal plexus.*

   The splanchnic nerves, therefore, are formed of preganglionic fibers. The postganglionic fibers arise from the excitor cells in the peripheral plexuses and are distributed to the smooth muscle and glands of the viscera. As previously noted, a few preganglionic fibers, travelling in the greater splanchnic nerve, end directly on the cells of the *suprarenal medulla* (Fig. 12-2). These medullary cells, which may be regarded as modified sympathetic excitor neurons, are responsible for epinephrine and norepinephrine secretion.

Afferent Nerve Fibers

The afferent myelinated nerve fibers travel from the viscera through the sympathetic ganglia without synapsing. They pass to the spinal nerve via white rami communicantes and reach their cell bodies in the posterior root ganglion of the corresponding spinal nerve (Fig. 12-1). The central axons then enter the spinal cord and may form the afferent component of a local reflex arc or ascend to higher centers, such as the hypothalamus.

The Sympathetic Trunks

The sympathetic trunks are two ganglionated nerve trunks that extend the whole length of the vertebral column (Fig. 12-2). In the neck, each trunk has three ganglia; in the thorax, 11 or 12; in the lumbar region, four or five; and in the pelvis, four or five. In the neck, the trunks lie anterior to the transverse processes of the cervical vertebrae; in the thorax, they are anterior to the heads of the ribs or lie on the sides of the vertebral bodies; in the abdomen, they are anterolateral to the bodies of the lumbar vertebrae; and in the pelvis, they are anterior to the sacrum and medial to the anterior sacral foramina. Below the two trunks end by joining together to form a single ganglion, the *ganglion impar*.

Cervical Part of the Sympathetic Trunk

This extends upward to the base of the skull and below to the first rib, where it becomes continuous with the thoracic part of the sympathetic trunk. The trunk lies behind the carotid sheath. The cervical part of the trunk possesses three ganglia—the superior, middle, and inferior cervical ganglia (Figs. 12-2 and 12-3). This part of the trunk sends gray rami communicantes to the cervical spinal nerves, but there are no white communicantes.

Superior Cervical Ganglion   This lies immediately below the skull and is joined to the middle ganglion by the connecting trunk.

Branches

1. The *internal carotid nerve*, consisting of postganglionic nerve fibers, accompanies the internal carotid artery into the carotid canal. It divides into branches that form the *internal carotid plexus* around the artery.

2. *Gray rami communicantes*, consisting of postganglionic nerve fibers, pass laterally to the upper four cervical spinal nerves.

3. *Arterial branches* pass to the common and external carotid arteries.

4. *Cranial nerve branches* pass to the ninth, tenth, and twelfth cranial nerves.

5. *Pharyngeal branches*, which join the pharyngeal branches of the ninth and tenth cranial nerves, form the *pharyngeal plexus*.

6. The *superior cardiac branch* descends in the neck to end in the cardiac plexus in the thorax.

Middle Cervical Ganglion   This lies at the level of the cricoid cartilage. It is the smallest of the three cervical ganglia and is connected to the inferior ganglion by two or more nerve bundles.

The anterior bundle crosses anterior to the first part of the subclavian artery and is known as the *ansa subclavia*.

Branches

1. *Gray rami communicantes* pass to the fifth and sixth cervical spinal nerves.

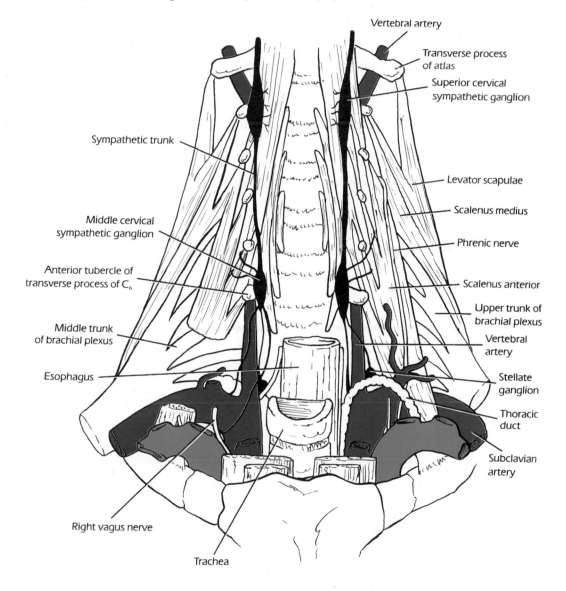

Figure 12-3

The root of the neck, showing the cervical parts of the sympathetic trunks.

2. *Thyroid branches* reach the thyroid gland along the inferior thyroid artery.

3. The *middle cardiac branch* descends in the neck to join the cardiac plexus in the thorax.

4. *Tracheal and esophageal branches.*

Inferior Cervical Ganglion   In most subjects (80 percent), this is fused with the first thoracic ganglion to form the large *stellate ganglion*. It is located between the transverse process of the seventh cervical vertebra and the neck of the first rib. The vertebral artery and the vertebral veins lie anterior to it. Inferior to the ganglion lies the cervical dome of the pleura.

Branches

1. *Gray rami communicantes* pass to the seventh and eighth cervical nerves.

2. *Arterial branches* pass to the subclavian and vertebral arteries.

3. The *inferior cardiac branch* descends to join the cardiac plexus. The portion of the sympathetic trunk that connects the middle cervical ganglion to the inferior or stellate ganglion forms two or more nerve bundles. The preganglionic fibers that supply the head and neck leave the spinal cord through the upper five thoracic nerves (mainly the upper two or three). They ascend the sympathetic trunk to synapse with cells in the cervical ganglia. The postganglionic fibers are distributed as branches of the ganglia as described above.

Medulla of the Suprarenal Gland

Preganglionic sympathetic fibers descend to the gland in the *greater splanchnic nerve*, a branch of the thoracic part of the sympathetic trunk (Fig. 12-2). The nerve fibers terminate on the secretory cells of the medulla, which are comparable to postganglionic neurons. Acetylcholine is the transmitter substance between the nerve endings and the secretory cells, as at any other preganglionic endings. The sympathetic nerves stimulate the secretory cells of the medulla to increase the output of epinephrine and norepinephrine. There is no parasympathetic innervation.

Fig. 12-4 is a summary diagram showing the spinal segmental levels of sympathetic connector neurons associated with different organs in the body.

Parasympathetic Part of the Autonomic Nervous System · · · · · · · · · · · · · · · · · ·

The activities of the parasympathetic part of the autonomic system are directed toward conserving and restoring energy. The heart rate slows, pupils constrict, peristalsis and glandular activity increase, sphincters open, and the bladder wall contracts.

Efferent Nerve Fibers (Craniosacral Outflow)

The parasympathetic part of the autonomic nervous system is located in the nuclei of the oculomotor (Edinger-Westphal nucleus), facial (superior salivary and lacrimatory nuclei), glossopharyngeal (inferior salivatory nucleus), and vagus (dorsal nucleus) cranial nerves and the second, third, and fourth sacral segments of the spinal cord (Fig. 12-2). The axons of the central connector nerve cells are myelinated and emerge from the brain within the cranial nerves. The sacral connector nerve cells give rise to myelinated axons that leave the spinal

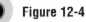 **Figure 12-4**

Diagram showing spinal segmental levels of sympathetic connector neurons associated with different organs in the body.

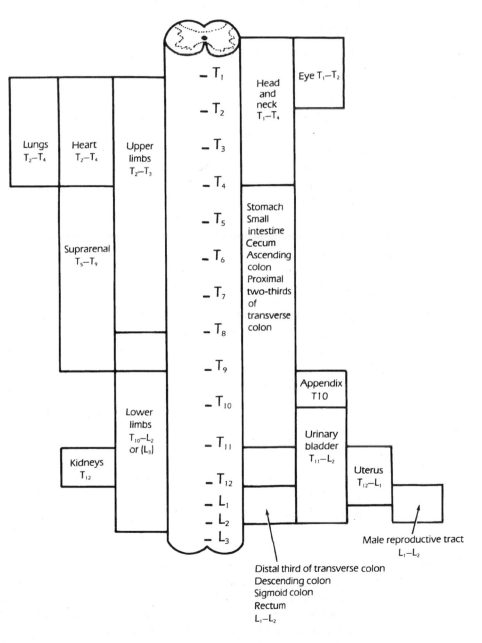

cord in the anterior nerve roots of the corresponding spinal nerves. They then leave the sacral nerves and form the *pelvic splanchnic nerves* (Fig. 12-2).

The efferent fibers of the craniosacral outflow are preganglionic and synapse in peripheral ganglia located close to the viscera they innervate. Here, again, acetylcholine is the neurotransmitter. The cranial parasympathetic ganglia are the *ciliary, pterygopalatine, submandibular,* and *otic.* In certain locations the ganglion cells are placed in nerve plexuses, such as the *cardiac plexus, pulmonary plexus, myenteric plexus* (*Auerbach's plexus*), and *mucosal plexus* (*Meissner's plexus*); the last two plexuses are associated with the gastrointestinal tract. The pelvic splanchnic nerves synapse in ganglia in the hypogastric plexuses. The postganglionic parasympathetic fibers are nonmyelinated and short.

Parasympathetic Ganglia

Ciliary Ganglion   This ganglion, about the size of a pin's head, is situated at the back of the orbital cavity between the optic nerve and the lateral rectus muscle (see Fig. 10-16).

Branches

1. *Parasympathetic preganglionic fibers* arise from the Edinger-Westphal nucleus of the oculomotor nerve. The fibers reach the ganglion via the oculomotor nerve and its branch to the inferior oblique muscle.

2. *Parasympathetic postganglionic fibers* arise from the ganglion nerve cells and pass to the eyeball via the short ciliary nerves. The fibers innervate the ciliary muscle and the sphincter pupillae muscle.

3. *Sensory fibers from the eyeball* reach the ganglion via the short ciliary nerves and pass through it without interruption to join the nasociliary branch of the ophthalmic division of the trigeminal nerve.

4. *Sympathetic postganglionic fibers* arise from the superior cervical sympathetic ganglion and reach the ciliary ganglion via the internal carotid plexus. The fibers pass through the ganglion without interruption to the eyeball via the short ciliary nerves.

Pterygopalatine (Sphenopalatine) Ganglion   This is located in the pterygopalatine fossa and is suspended from the lower border of the maxillary nerve (see Fig. 10-17).

Branches

1. The *parasympathetic preganglionic fibers* arise from the lacrimatory nucleus of the facial nerve. The fibers run in the nervus intermedius of the facial nerve and then travel in the *greater petrosal branch* of the nerve. The greater petrosal nerve now joins with the *deep petrosal nerve* (sympathetic nerve from the internal carotid plexus) to form the *nerve of the pterygoid canal.* The latter nerve of the pterygoid canal now joins the ganglion.

2. The *parasympathetic postganglionic fibers* arise from the ganglion nerve cells

and pass to the maxillary nerve and its zygomatic branch. The zygomatico-temporal branch then gives off a communicating branch to the lacrimal nerve. The lacrimal nerve supplies the parasympathetic fibers to the lacrimal gland.

    Other postganglionic fibers travel with the *palatine* and *nasal branches* of the ganglion to the glands of the pharynx, palate, and nose.

3. The *sympathetic postganglionic orbital branches* are fibers that reach the ganglion via the nerve of the pterygoid canal. They arise from the superior cervical sympathetic ganglion and pass without interruption through the pterygopalatine ganglion, entering the orbit through the inferior orbital fissure to innervate the *orbitalis muscle* (smooth muscle in the back of the orbital cavity whose precise function in humans remains unknown*).

4. The *palatine, nasal,* and *pharyngeal branches* are in reality sensory nerves of the maxillary division of the trigeminal nerve. They leave the maxillary nerve as two bundles that pass uninterrupted through the ganglion and exit as the *greater* and *lesser palatine nerves, lateral posterior superior nasal nerves, medial posterior superior nasal nerves, nasopalatine nerves,* and *pharyngeal nerve.*

Submandibular Ganglion   This lies on the side of the tongue suspended from the lingual nerve. Additional ganglion cells lie in the hilum of the submandibular salivary gland.

Branches

1. The *parasympathetic preganglionic fibers* arise from the superior salivatory nucleus of the facial nerve and pass with the nerve and its chorda tympani branch, which joins the lingual nerve. The fibers leave the lingual nerve to enter the ganglion.

2. The *parasympathetic postganglionic fibers* pass from the ganglion nerve cells to the submandibular and sublingual salivary glands.

3. The *postganglionic sympathetic fibers* pass without interruption through the ganglion to supply the blood vessels of the submandibular and sublingual salivary glands. These fibers originate in the superior cervical sympathetic ganglion.

Otic Ganglion   This lies just below the foramen ovale on the medial side of the mandibular division of the trigeminal nerve. It is attached to the nerve to the medial pterygoid muscle, which is a branch of the mandibular nerve.

Branches

1. The *parasympathetic preganglionic nerve fibers,* which arise from the inferior salivatory nucleus of the glossopharyngeal nerve, pass via the tympanic

---

*In lower animals this muscle is large and takes the place of the lateral wall of the orbit. Together with other pieces of smooth muscle found in the orbit, the orbitalis in these animals is believed to represent the retractor bulbi found in some mammalia (Wolff).

branch of the glossopharyngeal nerve to the tympanic plexus in the middle ear. They leave the plexus via the *lesser petrosal nerve* to reach the ganglion.

2. The *parasympathetic postganglionic nerve fibers*, which arise from the ganglion nerve cells, travel via the auriculotemporal nerve to the parotid salivary gland.

3. The *postganglionic sympathetic fibers* pass without interruption through the ganglion to supply the blood vessels of the parotid salivary gland. These fibers originate in the superior cervical sympathetic ganglion.

Afferent Nerve Fibers

The afferent myelinated fibers leave the viscera and reach their cell bodies in the sensory ganglia of cranial nerves or in posterior root ganglia of the sacral spinal nerves. The central axons then enter the central nervous system and form regional reflex arcs or ascend to higher centers, such as the hypothalamus.

The Large Autonomic Plexuses

Large collections of sympathetic and parasympathetic efferent nerve fibers and their associated ganglia, together with visceral afferent fibers, form autonomic nerve plexuses in the thorax, abdomen, and pelvis. Branches from these plexuses innervate the viscera. In the abdomen the plexuses are associated with the aorta and its branches; thus, the subdivisions of the autonomic plexuses are named according to the branch of the aorta along which they lie. The following are those plexuses, which are not described here: the cardiac, pulmonary, celiac, superior mesenteric, inferior mesenteric, aortic, and superior and inferior hypogastric plexuses.

Structure of Autonomic Ganglia

Autonomic ganglia are situated along the course of efferent nerve fibers of the autonomic nervous system. Sympathetic ganglia form part of the sympathetic trunk or are prevertebral in position. Parasympathetic ganglia, on the other hand, are situated close to or within the walls of the viscera as parasympathetic plexuses.

An autonomic ganglion consists of a collection of multipolar neurons together with capsular or satellite cells and a connective tissue capsule. Nerve bundles are attached to each ganglion and consist of preganglionic nerve fibers that enter the ganglion, postganglionic nerve fibers that have arisen from neurons within the ganglion, and afferent and efferent nerve fibers that pass through the ganglion without synapsing. Preganglionic fibers are small and myelinated; postganglionic fibers are smaller and unmyelinated.

An autonomic ganglion is the site where preganglionic fibers synapse on postganglionic neurons. However, the presence of small interneurons and collateral branches suggests that a ganglion may play a greater role than solely relaying information, and that it probably also serves some integrative function.

Preganglionic Transmitters

The synaptic transmitter that excites the postganglionic neurons in both sympathetic and parasympathetic ganglia is acetylcholine. The action of acetylcholine in autonomic ganglia is terminated by hydrolysis by acetylcholinesterase. The small interneurons of ganglia contain dopamine, which is thought to act as a transmitter. Electron microscopy of synapses in autonomic ganglia shows the characteristic membrane thickening and small, clear vesicles. In addition, there are some larger granular vesicles. The smaller vesicles contain acetylcholine; the content of the granular vesicles is not known.

Ganglion Blocking Agents

There are two types of ganglion blocking agents—depolarizing and nonpolarizing. *Nicotine* acts as a blocking agent in high concentrations, by first stimulating the postganglionic neuron and causing depolarization, and then by maintaining depolarization of the excitable membrane. *Hexamethonium* and *tetraethylammonium* block ganglia by competing with acetylcholine at the receptor sites.

Structure of Postganglionic Nerve Endings

Postganglionic fibers terminate on the effector cells without special discrete endings. The axons run between the gland cells and the smooth and cardiac muscle cells and lose their covering of Schwann cells. At sites where transmission occurs, clusters of vesicles are present within the axoplasm. If the site on the axon is at some distance from the effector cell, transmission time may be slow. The diffusion of transmitter through large extracellular distances causes a given nerve to have action on a large number of effector cells.

Postganglionic Transmitters

Parasympathetic postganglionic nerve endings liberate *acetylcholine* as their transmitter substance. The acetylcholine traverses the synaptic cleft and binds reversibly with the cholinergic receptor on the postsynaptic membrane. Within 2 to 3 msec it is hydrolyzed into acetic acid and choline by the enzyme *acetylcholinesterase*, which is located on the surface of the nerve and receptor membranes. The choline is reabsorbed into the nerve endings and used again for synthesis of acetylcholine.

Most sympathetic postganglionic nerve endings liberate *norepinephrine* as their transmitter substance. In addition, some sympathetic postganglionic nerve endings, particularly those that end on cells of sweat glands, release *acetylcholine*.

Sympathetic endings that use norepinephrine are called *adrenergic endings*. There are two major kinds of receptors in the effector organs, *alpha* and *beta receptors*.

Two subgroups of alpha receptors (alpha-1 and alpha-2 receptors) and two subgroups of beta receptors (beta-1 and beta-2) receptors have been described. Norepinephrine has a greater effect on alpha receptors than on beta receptors.

Phenylephrine is a pure alpha stimulator. The bronchodilating drugs such as *metaproterenol* and *albuterol* mainly act on beta-2 receptors. As a general rule, alpha receptor sites are associated with most of the excitatory functions of the sympathetic system (e.g., smooth muscle contraction, vasoconstriction, diaphoresis), whereas the beta receptor sites are associated with most of the inhibitory functions (e.g., smooth muscle relaxation). Beta-2 receptors are mainly in the lung, and stimulation results in bronchodilation. Beta-1 receptors are in the myocardium, where they are associated with excitation.

The action of norepinephrine on the receptor site of the effector cell is terminated by its reuptake into the nerve terminal, where it is stored in the presynaptic vesicles for reuse. While it is stored in the presynaptic vesicles, it is protected from inactivation by the enzyme *monoamine oxidase.*

Blocking of Cholinergic Receptors

In the parasympathetic and the sympathetic postganglionic nerve endings that liberate acetylcholine as the transmitter substance, the receptors on the effector cells are *muscarinic.* This means that the action can be blocked by *atropine.* Atropine competitively antagonizes the muscarinic action by occupying the cholinergic receptor sites on the effector cells.

Blocking of Adrenergic Receptors

The alpha-adrenergic receptor can be blocked by *phenoxybenzamine* and the beta-adrenergic receptor can be blocked by *propranolol.* The synthesis and storage of norepinephrine at sympathetic endings can be inhibited by *reserpine.*

Higher Control of the Autonomic Nervous System

The sympathetic outflow in the spinal cord (T_1–L_2 or L_3) and the parasympathetic craniosacral outflow (cranial nuclei III, VII, IX, and X; spinal S2, 3, and 4) are controlled by the hypothalamus. The hypothalamus appears to integrate the autonomic and neuroendocrine systems, thus preserving body homeostasis (Fig. 12-5). It receives signals from all parts of the nervous system, afferent input from the viscera, and information concerning blood hormone levels. Within the hypothalamus this input is integrated and transmitted to the lower autonomic centers in the brain stem and spinal cord by descending tracts of the reticular formation. In a similar manner, *releasing factors* or *release-inhibiting factors* are liberated into the circulation to affect hormone levels and endocrine secretions, thus influencing organ activity.

 Figure 12-5

Diagram showing the hypothalamus as the chief center of the brain for controlling the internal milieu of the body.

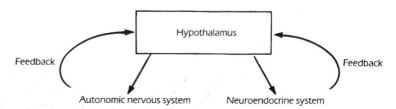

Functions of the Autonomic Nervous System

The autonomic nervous system, along with the endocrine system, maintains body homeostasis. The endocrine control is slower and exerts its influence by means of blood-borne hormones.

The autonomic system should not be regarded as an isolated portion of the nervous system, for it can play a role with somatic activity in expressing emotion, and certain autonomic activities, such as micturition, can be brought under voluntary control.

Table 12-1 shows important anatomic, physiologic, and pharmacologic similarities and differences between the sympathetic and parasympathetic parts of the autonomic nervous system.

Table 12-2 summarizes the effects of the autonomic nervous system on the body organs.

Some Important Autonomic Innervations

Eye

Upper Lid

The upper lid is raised by the levator palpebrae superioris. The major part of this muscle consists of skeletal fibers innervated by the oculomotor nerve. A small part consists of smooth muscle fibers innervated by sympathetic postganglionic fibers from the superior cervical sympathetic ganglion (Fig. 12-6).

Iris

The smooth muscle fibers of the iris consist of circular fibers that form the sphincter pupillae and radial fibers that form the dilator pupillae. The sphincter pupillae is supplied by parasympathetic fibers from the parasympathetic nucleus (Edinger-Westphal nucleus) of the oculomotor nerve (Fig. 12-6). After synapsing in the *ciliary ganglion*, the postganglionic fibers pass forward to the eyeball in the *short ciliary nerves*. (The ciliary muscle of the eye is also supplied by the short ciliary nerves; see p. 164.)

The dilator pupillae is supplied by postganglionic fibers from the superior cervical sympathetic ganglion (Fig. 12-6) that reach the orbit along the internal carotid and ophthalmic arteries. They pass uninterrupted through the ciliary ganglion and reach the eyeball in the *short* and *long ciliary nerves*.

Lacrimal Gland

The parasympathetic secretomotor nerve supply to the lacrimal gland originates in the lacrimatory nucleus of the facial nerve (see Fig. 5-16). Preganglionic fibers reach the *pterygopalatine ganglion* through the *nervus intermedius* and its *great petrosal branch* and through the *nerve of the pterygoid canal*. The postganglionic fibers join the maxillary nerve and pass into its *zygomatic branch* and the *zygomaticotemporal nerve*. They reach the lacrimal gland via the *lacrimal nerve*.

Table 12-1 Important Anatomic, Physiologic, and Pharmacologic Similarities and Differences Between the Sympathetic and Parasympathetic Parts of the Autonomic Nervous System

	Sympathetic	**Parasympathetic**
Action	Prepares body for emergency	Conserves and restores energy
Outflow	T_1–L_2 (3)	CN III, VII, IX, and X; S2, 3, and 4
Preganglionic fibers	Myelinated	Myelinated
Ganglia	Paravertebral (sympathetic trunks); prevertebral (e.g., celiac, superior mesenteric, inferior mesenteric)	Small ganglia close to viscera (e.g., otic, ciliary) or ganglion cells in plexuses (e.g., cardiac, pulmonary)
Neurotransmitter within ganglia	Acetylcholine	Acetylcholine
Ganglion blocking agents	Hexamethonium and tetraethyl-ammonium by competing with acetylcholine	Hexamethonium and tetraethylam-monium by competing with acetylcholine
Postganglionic fibers	Long, nonmyelinated	Short, nonmyelinated
Characteristic activity	Widespread due to many postganglionic fibers and liberation of epinephrine and norepinephrine from suprarenal medulla	Discrete action with few postganglionic fibers
Neurotransmitter at postganglionic endings	Norepinephrine at most endings and acetylcholine at few endings (sweat glands)	Acetylcholine at all endings
Blocking agents on receptors of effector cells	Alpha-adrenergic receptors—phenoxybenzamine; beta-adrenergic receptors—propranolol	Atropine, scopolamine
Agents inhibiting synthesis and storage of neuro-transmitter at post-ganglionic endings	Reserpine	—
Agents inhibiting hydrolysis of neurotransmitter at site of effector cells	—	Acetylcholinesterase blockers (e.g., neostigmine)
Drugs mimicking autonomic activity	Sympathomimetic drugs Phenylephrine: alpha receptors Isoproterenol: beta receptors	Parasympathomimetic drugs Pilocarpine Methacholine
Higher control	Hypothalamus	Hypothalamus

Table 12-2 Effects of the Autonomic Nervous System on the Body Organs

Organ		Sympathetic Action	Parasympathetic Action
Eye	Pupil	Dilates	Constricts
	Ciliary muscle	Relaxes	Contracts
Glands	Lacrimal, parotid, submandibular, sublingual, nasal	Reduces secretion by causing vasoconstriction of blood vessels	Increases secretion
	Sweat	Increases secretion	—
Heart	Cardiac muscle	Increases force of contraction	Decreases force of contraction
	Coronary arteries (mainly controlled by local metabolic factors)	Dilates (beta receptors), constricts (alpha receptors)	—
Lung	Bronchial muscle	Relaxes (dilates bronchi)	Contracts (constricts bronchi), increases secretion
	Bronchial secretion		
	Bronchial arteries	Constricts	Dilates
Gastrointestinal tract	Muscle in walls	Decreases peristalsis	Increases peristalsis
	Muscle in sphincters	Contracts	Relaxes
	Glands	Reduces secretion by vasoconstriction of blood vessels	Increases secretion
Liver	—	Breaks down glycogen into glucose	—
Gallbladder	—	Relaxes	Contracts
Kidney	—	Decreases output due to constriction of arteries	—
Urinary bladder	Bladder wall (detrusor)	Relaxes	Contracts
	Sphincter vesicae	Contracts	Relaxes
Erectile tissue of penis and clitoris	—		Relaxes, causes erection
Ejaculation	—	Contracts smooth muscle of vas deferens, seminal vesicles, and prostate	—
Systemic arteries	—		
Skin	—	Constricts	—
Abdominal	—	Constricts	—
Muscle	—	Constricts (alpha receptors), dilates (beta receptors), dilates (cholinergic)	—
Arrector pili muscles	—	Contracts	—
Suprarenal			
Cortex	—	Stimulates	—
Medulla	—	Liberates epinephrine and norepinephrine	—

Figure 12-6

The autonomic innervation of the upper eyelid and iris.

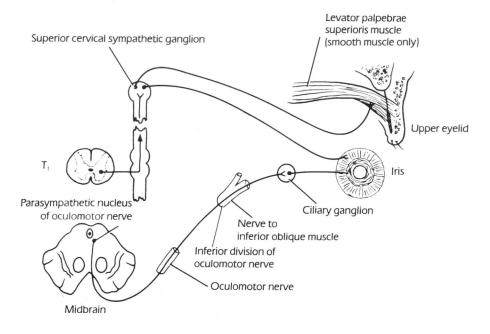

The sympathetic postganglionic fibers arise from the superior cervical sympathetic ganglion and travel in the plexus of nerves around the internal carotid artery. They join the *deep petrosal nerve, nerve of the pterygoid canal, maxillary nerve, zygomatic nerve, zygomaticotemporal nerve,* and, finally, the lacrimal nerve. They function as vasoconstrictor fibers.

Oculo-Cardiac Reflex

This reflex may come into play during eye surgery with the patient under a general anesthetic without retrobulbar anesthesia. Digital massage of the eyeball, which is commonly performed before eye surgery to soften the eye, may cause a marked slowing of the heart. This phenomenon must be monitored by an anesthesiologist, and corrective action must be taken if the cardiac rate becomes too low. Presumably, afferent impulses from the eyeball reach the central nervous system via the nasociliary nerve and the trigeminal nerve and connector neurons link the trigeminal nucleus to the parasympathetic dorsal nucleus of the vagus (see below).

Heart

Sympathetic postganglionic fibers arise from cervical and upper thoracic portions of the sympathetic trunks (Fig. 12-7). Postganglionic fibers reach the heart from the *superior, middle,* and *inferior cardiac branches* of the cervical portion of

Figure 12-7

The autonomic innervation of the heart and lungs.

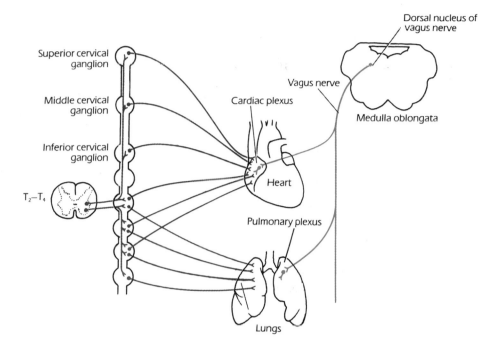

the sympathetic trunk and from a number of *cardiac branches* from the thoracic portion of the sympathetic trunk. The fibers pass via the *cardiac plexuses* to terminate on the *sinoatrial* and *atrioventricular nodes*, cardiac muscle fibers, and coronary arteries. Activation of these nerves results in cardiac acceleration, increased contractile force of the cardiac muscle, and dilatation of the coronary arteries. However, coronary dilatation results mainly in response to local metabolic needs, rather than by direct nerve stimulation.

The parasympathetic preganglionic fibers originate in the *dorsal nucleus of the vagus nerve* and descend into the thorax in the vagus nerves. The fibers terminate by synapsing with postganglionic neurons in the *cardiac plexuses*. Postganglionic fibers terminate on the *sinoatrial* and *atrioventricular nodes* and on the coronary arteries. Activation of these nerves results in a reduction in the rate and force of contraction of the myocardium and constriction of the coronary arteries. Here, again, coronary constriction is produced mainly by reduction in local metabolic needs rather than by neural effects.

Lungs

Sympathetic postganglionic fibers arise from the second to fifth thoracic ganglia of the sympathetic trunk (Fig. 12-7). They pass through the pulmonary plexuses and enter the lung to form networks around the bronchi and blood vessels. The sympathetic fibers produce bronchodilatation and are slightly vasoconstrictor.

Parasympathetic preganglionic fibers arise from the dorsal nucleus of the vagus and descend to the thorax within the vagus nerves. The fibers terminate by synapsing with postganglionic neurons in the pulmonary plexuses that enter the lung, where they form networks around the bronchi and blood vessels. The parasympathetic fibers produce bronchoconstriction and slight vasodilatation and increase glandular secretion.

Some Important Autonomic Reflexes

Visual Reflexes

Direct and Consensual Light Reflexes

Afferent nervous impulses travel from the retina through the optic nerve, optic chiasma, and optic tract (Fig. 12-8). A small number of fibers leave the optic tract and synapse on nerve cells in the *pretectal nucleus,* which lies close to the superior colliculus. The impulses are passed by axons of the pretectal nerve cells to the parasympathetic nuclei (Edinger-Westphal nuclei) of the oculomotor nerve on both sides. Here the fibers synapse and travel through the oculomotor nerve to the *ciliary ganglion* in the orbit. Finally, postganglionic parasympathetic fibers pass through the *short ciliary nerves* to the eyeball and the constrictor pupillae muscle of the iris. Both pupils constrict in the consensual light reflex, because the pretectal nucleus sends fibers to the parasympathetic nuclei on both sides of the midbrain.

Accommodation Reflex

When the eyes are directed from a distant to a near object, contraction of the medial recti brings about convergence of the ocular axes, the lens thickens to increase its refractive power by contraction of the ciliary muscle, and the pupils constrict to limit the light waves to the thickest central part of the lens. The afferent impulses travel through the optic nerve, optic chiasma, optic tract, lateral geniculate body, and optic radiation to the visual cortex (Fig. 12-8). The visual cortex is connected to the eyefield of the frontal cortex. From here, cortical fibers descend via the internal capsule to the oculomotor nuclei in the midbrain. The oculomotor nerve travels to the medial rectus muscles. Some of the descending cortical fibers synapse with the parasympathetic nuclei (Edinger-Westphal nuclei) of the oculomotor nerve on both sides. Here the fibers synapse, and the parasympathetic preganglionic fibers travel through the oculomotor nerve to the *ciliary ganglion* in the orbit. Finally, postganglionic parasympathetic fibers pass through the *short ciliary nerves* to the ciliary muscle and the constrictor pupillae muscle of the iris.

Cardiovascular Reflexes

The *carotid sinus* and the *aortic arch* serve as baroreceptors. As the blood pressure rises, nerve endings situated in the walls of these vessels are stimulated. Afferent fibers from the carotid sinus ascend in the glossopharyngeal nerve and terminate in the *nucleus solitarius.* Afferent fibers from the aortic arch ascend in the vagus nerve. Connector neurons in the medulla oblongata activate the

Figure 12-8

The optic pathway and the visual reflexes. Note the nervous connections of the parasympathetic nucleus of the oculomotor nerve.

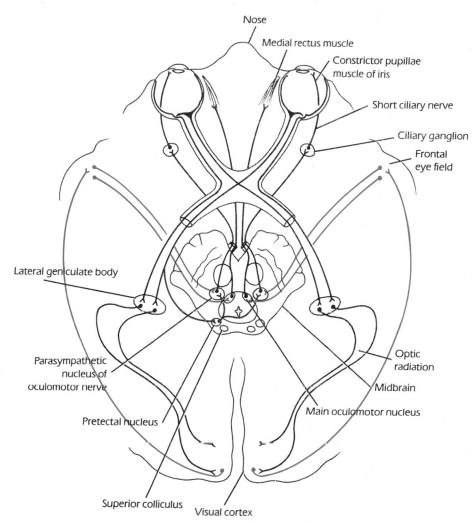

Nose

Medial rectus muscle

Constrictor pupillae muscle of iris

Short ciliary nerve

Ciliary ganglion

Frontal eye field

Lateral geniculate body

Parasympathetic nucleus of oculomotor nerve

Optic radiation

Midbrain

Main oculomotor nucleus

Pretectal nucleus

Superior colliculus

Visual cortex

parasympathetic nucleus (dorsal nucleus) of the vagus, which slows the heart rate. At the same time, reticulospinal fibers descending to the spinal cord inhibit the preganglionic sympathetic outflow to the heart and cutaneous arterioles. The combined effect of stimulation of the parasympathetic action on the heart and inhibition of the sympathetic action on the heart and peripheral blood vessels reduces the rate and force of contraction of the heart and peripheral resistance. As a consequence of this, the blood pressure falls. A person's blood pressure is thus modified by afferent information received from baroreceptors and the modulator of the autonomic nervous system, namely, the hypothalamus; the hypothalamus, in turn, can be influenced by other, higher centers in the central nervous system.

The *Bainbridge right atrial reflex* offers another example of a cardiovascular reflex. When the nerve endings situated in the wall of the right atrium and venae cavae are stimulated by a rise of venous pressure, afferent fibers ascend in the vagus to the medulla oblongata and terminate on the *nucleus of the tractus solitarius*. Connector neurons inhibit the parasympathetic (dorsal) nucleus of the vagus, and reticulospinal fibers stimulate the thoracic sympathetic outflow to the heart, resulting in cardiac acceleration.

Clinical Notes

Injuries to the Autonomic Nervous System

Sympathetic Injuries

The sympathetic trunk in the neck can be injured by stab and bullet wounds. Traction injuries to the first thoracic root of the brachial plexus can damage sympathetic nerves destined for the stellate ganglion. All these conditions may produce a preganglionic type of Horner's syndrome (see p. 373).

Parasympathetic Injuries

The oculomotor nerve is vulnerable when head injuries (herniated uncus) occur and can be damaged by compression by aneurysms in the junction between the posterior cerebral artery and posterior communicating artery. The preganglionic parasympathetic fibers traveling in this nerve are situated in the periphery of the nerve and may be damaged. Surface aneurysmal compression characteristically causes dilatation of the pupil and loss of the visual light reflexes.

The autonomic fibers in the facial nerve may be damaged when fractures of the skull involving the temporal bone occur. The vestibulocochlear nerve is closely related to the facial nerve in the internal acoustic meatus so that clinical findings involving both nerves are common. Involvement of the parasympathetic fibers in the facial nerve may produce impaired lacrimation in addition to paralysis of the facial muscles.

Horner's Syndrome

This syndrome consists of 1) constriction of the pupil (miosis), 2) slight drooping of the eyelid (ptosis), 3) enophthalmus,* 4) vasodilation of skin arterioles, and 5) loss of sweating (anhydrosis), all resulting from an interruption of the sympathetic nerve supply to the head and neck. Pathologic causes include lesions in the brain stem or cervical part of the spinal cord that interrupt the reticulospinal tracts descending from the hypothalamus to the sympathetic outflow in the lateral gray column of the first thoracic segment of the spinal cord. Such lesions include *multiple sclerosis* and *syringomyelia*. Traction on the stellate ganglion due to a *cervical rib*, or involvement of the ganglion in a metastatic lesion, may interrupt the peripheral part of the sympathetic pathway.

*The enophthalmus of Horner's syndrome is often apparent but not real and caused by the ptosis. However, the smooth muscle, the orbitalis, situated at the back of the orbit, is paralyzed and involvement may be responsible.

All patients with Horner's syndrome have miosis and ptosis. However, a distinction should be made between lesions occurring at the first neuron (the descending reticulospinal fibers within the central nervous system), the second neuron (the preganglionic fibers), and the third neuron (postganglionic fibers). For example, the clinical signs suggestive of a first-neuron defect (central Horner's syndrome) could include contralateral hyperesthesia of the body and loss of sweating of the entire half of the body. Signs suggesting second-neuron involvement (preganglionic Horner's syndrome) include loss of sweating limited to the face and neck, and the presence of flushing or blanching of the face and neck. Signs suggesting third-neuron involvement (postganglionic Horner's syndrome) include facial pain or ear, nose, or throat disease.

The presence or absence of other localizing signs and symptoms may assist in differentiating the three types of Horner's syndrome.

Argyll-Robertson Pupil

This condition is characterized by a small pupil, which is of fixed size and does not react to light but contracts with accommodation. It is usually due to a neurosyphilitic lesion interrupting fibers that run from the pretectal nucleus to the parasympathetic nuclei (Edinger-Westphal nuclei) of the oculomotor nerve on both sides. The fact that the pupil constricts with accommodation implies that the connections between the parasympathetic nuclei and the constrictor pupillae muscle of the iris are intact.

Adie's Tonic Pupil Syndrome

In this condition the pupil has a decreased or absent light reflex, a slow or delayed contraction to near vision, and a slow or delayed dilation in the dark. This benign syndrome, which probably results from a disorder of the parasympathetic innervation of the constrictor pupillae muscle, must be distinguished from the Argyll-Robertson pupil (above), which is caused by neurosyphilis. Adie's syndrome can be confirmed by looking for hypersensitivity to cholinergic agents. Drops commonly used for this test are 2.5% methacholine or 0.1% pilocarpine. The Adie's tonic pupil should constrict when these drops are put in the eye. These cholinergic agents do not cause pupillary constriction in mydriasis caused by oculomotor lesions or in drug-related mydriasis.

Frey's Syndrome

Frey's syndrome is an interesting complication that sometimes follows penetrating wounds of the parotid gland. During the process of healing, the postganglionic parasympathetic secretomotor fibers traveling in the auriculotemporal nerve grow out and join the distal end of the great auricular nerve, which supplies the sweat glands of the overlying facial skin. By this means, a stimulus intended to stimulate saliva flow instead produces sweat.

A similar syndrome may follow injury to the facial nerve. During the process of regeneration, parasympathetic fibers normally destined for the submandibular and sublingual salivary glands are diverted to the lacrimal gland. This produces watering of the eyes associated with salivation, so-called *crocodile tears*.

Sympathetic Neural Blockade

Theoretically, sympathetic blockade can be achieved at the following anatomic sites: 1) where the sympathetic preganglionic fibers leave the spinal cord (T_1–L_2 or L_3) in the anterior roots of the spinal nerves (subarachnoid or epidural block); 2) where there is a synapse between the preganglionic fibers and the ganglionic neurons (ganglion block); 3) in a peripheral nerve, where the postganglionic fibers travel to their destination (peripheral nerve block); 4) in a perivascular plexus (perivascular block); and 5) where there is a pharmacologic block at the ganglion or the terminal receptor sites.

Selective sympathetic blockade can be accomplished best by the blockade of sympathetic ganglia. Unfortunately, a sympathetic ganglion blockade is often accompanied by motor and sensory blockade. In the thorax, the ganglia of the sympathetic trunk are closely related to the intercostal nerves, so that differential blockade is difficult, but the cervical ganglia, the celiac ganglia, and the lumbar ganglia lie at some distance from the somatic nerves and are more easily dealt with.

The relay levels between the preganglionic fibers and the ganglionic neurons described in this test are those most often quoted in the literature. However, variations do occur, and this may explain the poor results that sometimes follow a technically successful block.

Botulinum Toxin

A very small amount of this toxin binds irreversibly to the nerve plasma membranes and prevents the release of acetylcholine at cholinergic synapses and neuromuscular junctions, producing an atropine-like syndrome with skeletal muscle weakness.

Black Widow Spider Venom

The venom causes a brief release of acetylcholine at the nerve endings followed by a permanent blockade.

Anticholinesterase Agents

Acetylcholinesterase, which is responsible for hydrolyzing and limiting the action of acetylcholine at nerve endings, can be blocked by certain drugs. Physostigmine, neostigmine, pyridostigmine, and carbamate and organophosphate insecticides are effective acetylcholinesterase inhibitors. Their use results in excessive stimulation of the cholinergic receptors, producing the "SLUD syndrome"—salivation, lacrimation, urination, and defecation.

CHAPTER 12
Clinical Problems

Answers on Page 377.

1 A 43-year-old man was standing on a ladder and sawing off the limb of a tree when he lost his footing and slipped. As he began to fall, he grabbed at a branch with his left hand and held on until he was rescued some minutes later. Careful examination of his left upper limb showed paralysis of his flexor carpi ulnaris and flexor digitorum profundus and weakness of the palmar and dorsal interossei and the thenar and hypothenar muscles. There was also some loss of sensation on the medial side of the forearm and hand. It was noted that the pupil of his left eye was constricted and that he had ptosis of the left upper lid. A slight degree of left-sided enophthalmus was also present. The skin of his left cheek felt warmer and drier than the right cheek. How can you account for these widespread physical signs?

2 A 19-year-old woman with a history of experiencing severe attacks of painful discoloration of the fourth and fifth fingers of both hands, especially during cold weather, visited her physician. A diagnosis of Raynaud's disease was made. In view of the severity of her symptoms and the possibility of gangrene of the fingertips, it was decided to recommend a cervicodorsal preganglionic sympathectomy. What is the innervation of the arteries of the upper limb?

3 Explain the following anatomic facts: (a) the presence of sympathetic nerve fibers in a parasympathetic ganglion; (b) the large intestine's innervation by the vagus nerves down as far as the splenic flexure, although the vagal nerve trunks apparently come to an end very soon after piercing the diaphragm with the esophagus; and (c) how the sacral parasympathetic outflow reaches the splenic flexure of the colon.

4 A 4-year-old boy with a history of chronic constipation and abdominal distention was taken to a pediatrician. The child's mother said that the constipation was getting progressively worse. It was not responding to laxatives, and she was finding it necessary to give her son an enema once a week to relieve his abdominal distention. On physical examination, the child's abdomen was obviously distended and a dough-like mass could be palpated along the course of the descending colon in the left iliac fossa. Examination of the rectum showed it to be empty and not dilated. After an enema and repeated colonic irrigation with saline solution, the patient was given a barium enema followed by a radiographic examination. The radiograph showed a grossly distended descending colon and an abrupt change in lumen diameter where the descending colon joined the sigmoid colon. It was interesting to note that the child failed to empty the colon of the barium enema. Using your knowledge of the autonomic nerve supply to the colon, you would find what diagnosis? How would you treat this patient?

5 Examination of a patient with neurosyphilis indicated that the pupil of her left eye was small and fixed and did not react to light, but contracted when she was asked to look at a near object. What is the innervation of the iris? Using your knowledge of neuroanatomy, state where you believe the neurologic lesion to be situated to account for these defects.

6 What transmitter substances are liberated at the following nerve endings? (a) Preganglionic sympathetic, (b) preganglionic parasympathetic, (c) postganglionic parasympathetic, (d) postganglionic sympathetic fibers to the heart muscle, and

(e) postganglionic sympathetic fibers to the sweat glands of the hand.

7 During a neurologic examination of a patient aged 18 years, the resident noted that her right pupil failed to react to the direct and consensual light reflexes. Moreover, the same pupil contracted very slowly when the patient was asked to focus on a near object. The pupillary reflexes were normal in her left eye. Explain this finding. What test could you perform to confirm the diagnosis? Explain the possible underlying anatomic defect in this condition. Can the condition become bilateral? How does this condition differ from an Argyll-Robertson pupil?

8 A 5-year-old girl with right-sided medial strabismus was undergoing surgery under general anesthesia. During dissection of the medial rectus muscle, the resident placed gentle traction on the muscle. The child's heart rate immediately plummeted to 20 beats per minute but recovered within a minute when the resident stopped manipulating the muscle. What reflex was triggered by this procedure?

CHAPTER 12
Answers to Clinical Problems

1 This man had sustained a severe traction injury of the eighth cervical and first thoracic roots of the brachial plexus on the left side. The various paralyzed muscles and the sensory loss were characteristic of Klumpke's paralysis. In addition, the white ramus communicans passing from the first thoracic nerve to the stellate ganglion was torn, cutting off the preganglionic sympathetic fibers to the head and neck and producing a left-sided Horner's syndrome.

2 The arteries of the upper limb are innervated by sympathetic nerves. The preganglionic fibers originate from the nerve cells in the lateral gray columns of the second to the eighth thoracic segments of the spinal cord. They reach the sympathetic trunk via the white rami communicantes and ascend in the trunk to synapse in the middle cervical, inferior cervical, and first thoracic or stellate ganglia. The postganglionic fibers join the spinal nerves that form the brachial plexus traveling in the gray rami communicantes. The sympathetic fibers are distributed to the digital arteries within the branches of the brachial plexus.

3 (a) It is not uncommon to find sympathetic preganglionic and postganglionic fibers passing through a parasympathetic ganglion without interruption. The nerve fibers are merely using the ganglion as a conduit en route to their destination. Visceral sensory nerve fibers travel in a similar manner.

(b) The vagal nerve trunks, on reaching the abdominal cavity, split up after a short course on the esophagus into their terminal branches. The posterior vagal trunk (right vagus) gives off an important branch that passes to the celiac and superior mesenteric plexuses. The terminal fibers are distributed with the branches of the celiac and superior mesenteric arteries to the small and large intestine as far as the splenic flexure.

(c) The sacral parasympathetic outflow (S_2, S_3, and S_4) leaves the anterior rami of the sacral nerves as the pelvic splanchnic nerve. These preganglionic fibers pass through the hypogastric and aortic plexuses to reach the inferior mesenteric plexus. The fibers are then distributed to the splenic flexure and descending colon along with the branches of the inferior mesenteric artery.

4 This child has Hirschsprung's disease, a congenital condition in which there is a failure of development of the myenteric plexus (Auerbach's plexus) in the distal part of the colon. The proximal part of the colon is normal but becomes greatly distended because of accumulated feces. In this patient, the lower pelvic colon, later at operation, was shown to have no parasympathetic ganglion cells. Thus, this segment of the bowel had no peristalsis and effectively blocked the passage of feces. Once the diagnosis had been confirmed by taking a biopsy of the distal segment of the bowel, the treatment was to remove the aganglionic segment of the bowel by surgical resection.

5 This patient had an Argyll-Robertson pupil, which is a small, fixed pupil that does not react to light but contracts with accommodation. The condition usually is due to a syphilitic lesion. The innervation of the iris is described on page 172. The neurologic lesion in this patient interrupted the fibers running from the pretectal nucleus to the parasympathetic nuclei of the oculomotor nerve on both sides.

6 (a) Acetylcholine, (b) acetylcholine, (c) acetylcholine, (d) norepinephrine, and (e) acetylcholine.

7 This young woman had a condition known as Adie's tonic pupil syndrome. The syndrome can be confirmed by looking for hypersensitivity to cholinergic agents such as 2.5% methacoline or 0.1% pilocarpine. The Adie's pupil should constrict when the drops are put in the eye. These cholinergic agents do not cause pupillary constriction in mydriasis caused by oculomotor lesions or in drug-related mydriasis. Adie's syndrome is a benign disorder that is probably caused by a lesion of the parasympathetic innervation of the constrictor pupillae muscle. The condition can become bilateral, although initially it is uniocular. The Argyll-Robertson pupil is caused by neurosyphilis, the lesion interrupting the nerve fibers that run from the pretectal nucleus to the parasympathetic nuclei of the oculomotor nerve on both sides (see p. 373). It is characterized by the pupil being small and fixed; the pupil does not react to light but contracts with accommodation.

8 The oculo-cardiac reflex can produce severe bradycardia. Even gentle manipulation of the eyeball, the extraocular muscles, or the orbital fascia can trigger afferent sensory impulses that travel to the central nervous system via the ophthalmic division of the trigeminal nerve. These impulses reach the parasympathetic dorsal nucleus of the vagus nerve and the bradycardia is initiated (see Fig. 12-7). The reflex action is generally of short duration and often responds to atropine.

CHAPTER 13

The Visual Pathway

CHAPTER OUTLINE

Definition of the Visual Pathway

The retina, the optic nerve, the optic chiasma, the optic tracts, the lateral geniculate bodies, the optic radiations, and the visual cortical areas make up the visual
pathway. This entire pathway may be regarded as part of the central nervous system, and during development it has extended forward into the orbital cavities of
the skull. The retina is an outgrowth from the forebrain, and the optic nerve is
white matter. Microscopically, the optic nerve possesses oligodendrocytes, astrocytes, and microglia, whereas true peripheral nerves contain Schwann cells,
fibroblasts, and macrophages. Because the optic nerve is identical to white matter, it has no powers of regeneration. Like other parts of the central nervous system, the optic nerve is covered with pia, arachnoid, and dura mater.

It is interesting to note that the forward extension of this specialized afferent
pathway crosses at right angles the main descending motor systems and the
main ascending sensory systems of the cerebral hemispheres (Fig. 13-1).

The structure of the retina has already been described in detail in Chapter 6
(p. 175).

Anatomy of the Visual Pathway

Optic Nerve

For purposes of description, the optic nerve may be divided into four parts:
1) intraocular (1 mm), 2) intraorbital (25 mm), 3) intracanalicular (5 mm), and
4) intracranial (10 mm).

Intraocular Portion

The intraocular portion includes the *optic disc* and that portion of the optic nerve
that lies within the sclera. The optic disc lies about 3 mm nasally to the macula
lutea and slightly above the posterior pole of the eyeball. It measures about 1.5
mm in diameter and has a pale pink color; it is much paler than the surrounding
retina. The edge of the disc is flat or very slightly raised; the central part has a
slight depression. It is in the depression that the central retinal vessels enter and

Figure 13-1

Diagram showing the visual pathway crossing at right angles to the main motor and sensory systems of the cerebral hemispheres.

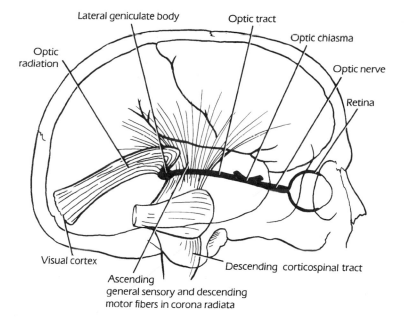

leave the eye. The optic disc is sometimes referred to as the *optic nerve head*. The term "optic papilla" is a misnomer, because the disc is not elevated above the surrounding retina.

The optic disc is composed of all the retinal ganglion cell axons. The axons from the cone's system, which dominate the posterior part of the retina, pass directly to the lateral aspect of the optic disc. Other axons originating in the lateral retina do not mix with the cone system axons, but curve above and below them, forming *superior and inferior arcuate bands*. Axons originating from peripheral and central areas of the retina are mixed together, but on reaching the optic nerve the peripheral retinal axons take up a peripheral position in the optic nerve, and those of central retinal origin come to lie in the center of the nerve. The complete absence of rods and cones at the disc makes this area of the retina insensitive to light, and thus it is referred to as the *blind spot*.

As the retinal ganglion cell axons bend sharply posteriorly at the disc, they are seen to be unmyelinated and supported by astrocytes; at the periphery of the disc these axons are covered by the internal limiting membrane of the retina. At this site the pigment cells of the retina and the choroid are absent.

The bundles of axons or optic nerve fibers finally exit from the eyeball (Fig. 13-2), by passing backward through the orifices of the lamina cribrosa, the central retinal vessels passing through individual holes. The lamina cribrosa represents the sclera at this site and consists of fibrous tissue and elastic tissue.

Orbital Portion

As the optic nerve fibers traverse the lamina cribrosa, they acquire myelin sheaths, which are formed by oligodendrocytes. The presence of the myelin and the oligodendrocytes causes the optic nerve to increase in diameter to 3 to 4 mm.

Figure 13-2

Photomicrograph of a section through the optic disc and the commencement of the optic nerve. The arrow indicates the site of the lamina cribrosa. (H&E; × 40.)

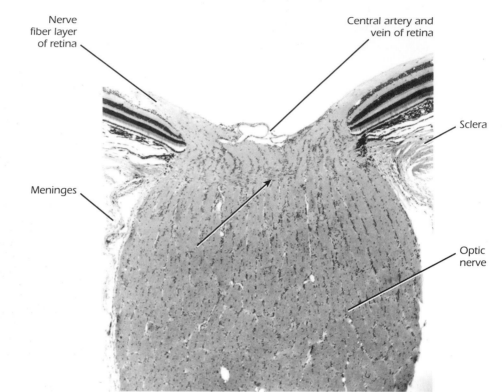

The orbital portion of the optic nerve is about 25 mm long, which is about 6 mm longer than the distance between the eyeball and the optic canal. This allows the nerve to have a slightly sinuous course and permits freedom of movement to the eyeball. The optic nerve is surrounded by a dense sheath of dura mater, a middle delicate sheath of arachnoid, and an innermost vascular sheath of pia (Fig. 13-3). These sheaths, together with an extension of the subarachnoid space, extend anteriorly to the eyeball. Here the sheaths blend with the sclera. Posteriorly, the sheaths are continuous through the optic canal with the meningeal coverings of the brain.

To begin with, the optic nerve is surrounded and supported by orbital fat in which are embedded the ciliary vessels and nerves. The ciliary ganglion lies between the lateral border of the nerve and the lateral rectus muscle (see Fig. 10-16). Posteriorly, the nasociliary nerve and the ophthalmic artery run forward and then pass medially to cross above the optic nerve. At about the same position, the nerve to the medial rectus muscle from the inferior division of the oculomotor nerve crosses below the optic nerve.

● **Figure 13-3**

Photomicrograph of cross-section of the optic nerve, showing bundles of optic nerve fibers separated by connective tissue septa. Note the position of the central artery and vein of the retina and the surrounding meningeal sheath, and also the extension of the subarachnoid space filled with cerebrospinal fluid. (H&E; x 40.)

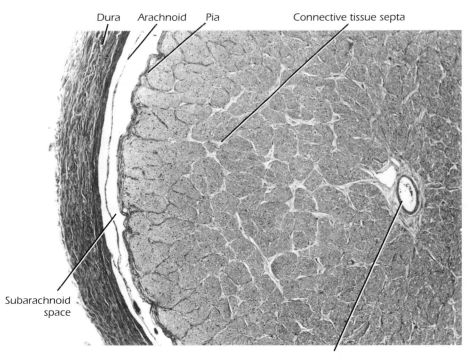

About 12 mm behind the eyeball, the inferomedial surface of the dural sheath is pierced by the central artery and vein of the retina (Fig. 13-4). The artery crosses the subarachnoid space obliquely before entering the optic nerve. The vein has a more prolonged course in the subarachnoid space lying posterior to the artery. The central vessels now assume an axial position and pass forward to emerge on the optic disc. At the apex of the orbital cavity, the optic nerve lies within the muscular cone formed by the four recti and is surrounded by their tendinous origin.

The optic nerve axons or fibers are grouped together into bundles separated by fine septa derived from the inner surface of the pial sheath (Fig. 13-3). It has been estimated that about 1000 bundles are visible on cross-section of the optic nerve. The septa also provide a supporting sheath for the central vessels of the retina as far forward as the optic disc.

Intracanalicular Portion

The optic canal lies within the lesser wing of the sphenoid bone and is about 5 mm long. The optic nerve passes through the optic canal surrounded by its three

Figure 13-4

Diagram showing the arterial
supply and venous drainage
of the optic disc and optic
nerve.

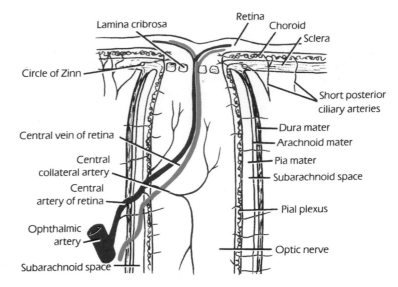

meningeal sheaths. The dural sheath fuses with the periorbita lining the canal,
thus fixing the nerve (see Fig. 3-5). The subarachnoid space filled with cerebrospinal fluid around the optic nerve communicates and is continuous with the
intracranial subarachnoid space.

Also passing through the optic canal are the ophthalmic artery on the inferolateral border of the optic nerve and the postganglionic sympathetic nerves
accompanying the artery.

As the nerve traverses the canal it is separated on its medial side from the
sphenoidal and posterior ethmoidal air sinuses by a thin layer of bone.

Intracranial Portion

The optic nerve leaves the canal and passes backward, upward, and medially within the subarachnoid space to reach the optic chiasma in the floor of the third ventricle (Figs. 13-5 and 13-6). It is related above to the olfactory tract, the gyrus rectus,
and the anterior cerebral artery; it is related laterally to the internal carotid artery.

Structure

The optic nerve is composed of about 1,200,000 myelinated axons, about 90 percent of these being of small diameter (1 μm) the remainder measuring from 2 to
10 μm in diameter. The smaller axons originate from the midget ganglion cells
that are associated with the cones; the larger axons are related to the ganglion
cells associated with the rods at the peripheral retinal areas.

Blood Supply

Intraocular Portion   This is supplied by branches of the anastomotic circle of Zinn
in the sclera around the optic nerve (Fig. 13-4). This incomplete circle receives its
blood supply from the short posterior ciliary arteries. The central artery of the
retina does not supply the intraocular portion of the optic nerve.

Figure 13-5

Diagram showing the visual pathways as seen from the under aspect of the brain. The temporal and occipital lobes of the cerebral hemisphere have been dissected to show the optic radiation.

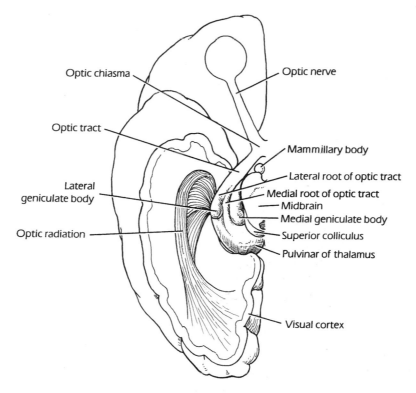

Orbital Portion　This receives its blood supply from the pial plexus of vessels; branches of the plexus pass into the nerve along the pial septa. The pial plexus receives its arterial supply from neighboring branches of the ophthalmic artery (Fig. 13-4).

　　The extraneural part of the central artery of the retina also contributes a few branches (central collateral arteries; see p. 279). The intraneural part of the central artery gives off only a few small branches.

Intracanalicular Portion　This is supplied by branches from the pial plexus. Here the plexus receives recurrent branches from the ophthalmic artery.

Intracranial Portion　This also receives its blood supply from the pial plexus. This part of the plexus is supplied by branches from the superior hypophyseal artery from the internal carotid, and from the ophthalmic artery (Fig. 13-7).

Figure 13-6

Diagram of a sagittal section of the optic chiasma, showing its important relationships.

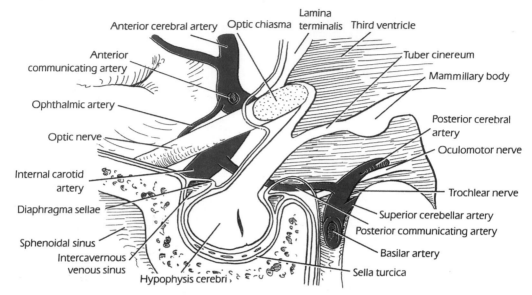

Anterior cerebral artery   Optic chiasma   Lamina terminalis   Third ventricle

Anterior communicating artery

Ophthalmic artery

Optic nerve

Internal carotid artery

Diaphragma sellae

Sphenoidal sinus

Intercavernous venous sinus

Hypophysis cerebri

Tuber cinereum

Mammillary body

Posterior cerebral artery

Oculomotor nerve

Trochlear nerve

Superior cerebellar artery

Posterior communicating artery

Basilar artery

Sella turcica

Optic Chiasma

The optic chiasma is situated at the junction of the anterior wall and floor of the third ventricle (Fig. 13-6). It is essentially a flattened bundle of nerve fibers measuring about 12 mm wide and 8 mm from before backward. It is covered with pia mater and projects downward into the subarachnoid space. Its anterolateral angles are continuous with the optic nerves and the posterolateral angles with the optic tracts (Fig. 13-5).

The optic chiasma has important relationships and these are as follows: *Anteriorly* lie the anterior cerebral arteries and the anterior communicating artery (Fig. 13-6). *Posteriorly* lies the tuber cinereum, with the infundibulum below and the cavity of the third ventricle above. *Laterally* lies the internal carotid artery after it leaves the cavernous sinus and ascends between the optic nerve and the optic tract; there is also the anterior perforated substance. *Superiorly* lie the lamina terminalis (anterior wall of the third ventricle) and the cavity of the third ventricle (Fig. 13-6). *Inferiorly* lie the diaphragma sellae and the hypophysis cerebri (Fig. 13-6). The inferior relationships vary somewhat and depend on the relative lengths of the intracranial part of the optic nerve. In a small number of individuals, when the nerves are short, the anterior border of the chiasma rests directly in the optic groove of the sphenoid bone. In most people, who have longer optic nerves, the chiasma lies partly or wholly above the diaphragma sellae.

In the chiasma the nerve fibers from the nasal half of each retina (including the nasal half of the macula) cross the midline and enter the optic tract of the opposite side; the nerve fibers from the inferior nasal retina cross at the anterior

Figure 13-7

The arterial supply to the visual pathway as seen from below.

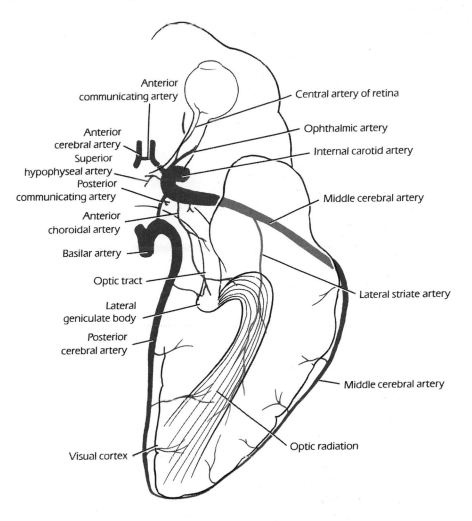

part of the chiasma, whereas the nerve fibers from the superior nasal retina cross at the posterior part of the chiasma. The nerve fibers from the temporal half of the retina pass backward into the optic tract of the same side. The partial crossing of the optic nerve fibers in the optic chiasma is essential for binocular vision.

Blood Supply

The nervous tissue is supplied by small branches from the plexus of vessels in the covering pia mater. This pial plexus is supplied by branches from the internal carotid, the superior hypophyseal branch of the internal carotid, the posterior communicating artery, the anterior cerebral artery, and the anterior communicating artery (Fig. 13-7).

Figure 13-8

The right visual pathway, lateral view. Note the position of the optic nerve, optic chiasma, optic tract, and lateral geniculate body. Note also the optic tract sweeping around the lateral surface of the crus cerebri of the midbrain.

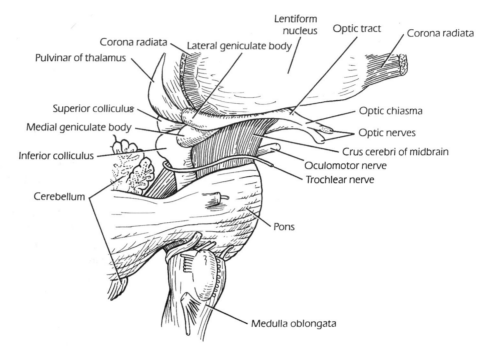

Optic Tracts

The optic tracts emerge from the posterolateral angles of the optic chiasma as cylindrical bands (Fig. 13-5). Each passes posterolaterally between the tuber cinereum medially and the anterior perforated substance laterally. Here, the tract becomes flattened and winds around the lateral margin of the upper part of the cerebral peduncle (Fig. 13-8). It is here adherent to the midbrain and overlapped by the uncus and the parahippocampal gyrus.

Most of the nerve fibers in the optic tract terminate in the lateral geniculate body and are concerned with conscious visual sensation; these fibers constitute the lateral root of the optic tract. The smaller medial root contains fibers of unknown function.

Just before the nerve fibers of the optic tract enter the lateral geniculate, about 10 percent pass medially in the *superior brachium* below the pulvinar of the thalamus to enter the superior colliculus and the pretectal nucleus (Fig. 13-5). These fibers are not concerned with visual sensations, but are involved, respectively, in visual body reflexes and light reflexes (see p. 370).

Blood Supply

Each optic tract is supplied by pial arteries, which receive branches from the anterior choroidal artery and the posterior communicating artery; the middle cerebral artery also sends branches (Fig. 13-7).

Lateral Geniculate Bodies

The lateral geniculate body is a small ovoid swelling on the undersurface of the pulvinar of the thalamus (Figs. 13-5 and 13-8). It is connected to the superior colliculus by the *superior brachium*, which is formed by the nerve fibers that do not terminate in the lateral geniculate body, but pass to the superior colliculus and the pretectal nucleus (referred to above). The lateral geniculate body receives the caudal termination of the lateral root of the optic tract.

The *dorsal or main lateral geniculate nucleus* has a laminated structure and consists of six curved layers of cells oriented in a dome-shaped mound, similar to a stack of hats set one on another. The layers are best seen on coronal section (Fig. 13-9). The layers of cells are separated by white bands of optic nerve fibers and are numbered 1 to 6 beginning at the hilus and continuing dorsally to the crest of the geniculate body. The nerve fibers are the axons of the ganglion cell layer of the retina and come from the temporal half of the ipsilateral eye and from the nasal half of the contralateral eye, the latter fibers crossing the midline in the optic chiasma. The nerve fibers that cross the midline terminate in layers 1, 4, and 6, while the optic nerve fibers that do not cross terminate in layers 2, 3, and 5. Each lateral geniculate body, therefore, receives visual information from both retinas.

It is interesting to note that each lateral geniculate body contains about 1 million nerve cells, about the same number as the nerve fibers in the optic nerve and the optic tract. Although it is tempting to postulate that each optic nerve fiber terminates on a single geniculate nerve cell, this has not yet been substantiated. Moreover, it has long been known that each retinal ganglion cell axon may divide into as many as six branches, which synapse with six separate geniculate neurons in one lamina.

Blood Supply

The lateral geniculate body receives the anterior choroidal branch of the middle cerebral artery (Fig. 13-7), the thalamogeniculate branches of the posterior cerebral artery, and the lateral choroidal arteries.

Optic Radiations

The optic radiations, or *geniculocalcarine tracts*, are formed of nerve fibers that originate from the nerve cells in the laminae of the lateral geniculate bodies. Those fibers arising from the lateral portions of the lateral geniculate body, receiving impulses from the inferior retinal quadrants (superior visual field), fan out laterally and inferiorly around the anterior tip of the inferior (temporal) horn of the lateral ventricle, before swinging posteriorly (Fig. 13-5). The fibers associated with the peripheral part of the retina swing farthest forward, and those related to the macula loop very little.

Figure 13-9

Diagram showing the retinal projections to the different laminae of the lateral geniculate body. Note that the macular fibers end in the center and posterior part of the nucleus.

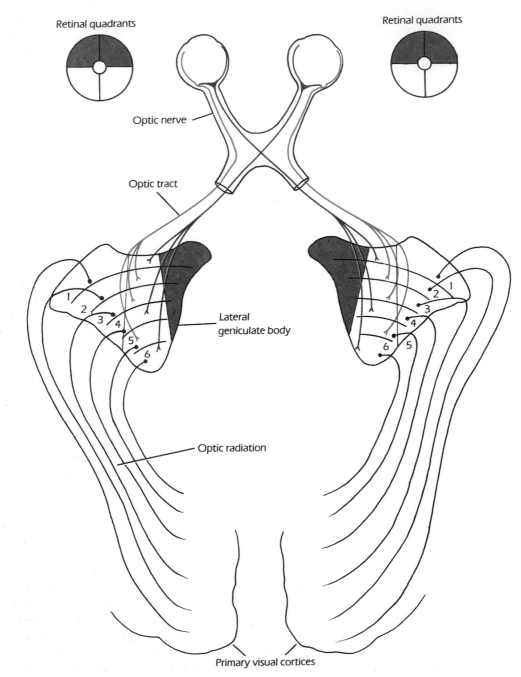

These forward-looping fibers form the *loop of Meyer*. The fibers continue posteriorly in the retrolentiform part of the internal capsule, lying lateral to the inferior (temporal) and posterior (occipital) horns of the lateral ventricle. They terminate by turning medially to enter the occipital cortex. Here, the fibers end on the inferior lip of the calcarine fissure.

Fibers originating from the medial portions of the lateral geniculate body, receiving impulses from the superior retinal quadrants (inferior visual field), turn almost directly posteriorly and accompany the other fibers in the retrolentiform part of the internal capsule. On entering the occipital cortex, the fibers terminate in the superior lip of the calcarine fissure.

Blood Supply

The anterior portion of the optic radiations is supplied by the anterior choroidal branch of the internal carotid artery; the posterior portion is supplied by the middle cerebral artery and the posterior cerebral artery (Fig. 13-7).

Visual Cortical Areas

The visual cortex (Fig. 13-10) may be divided into the primary visual area (Brodmann's area 17) and the secondary visual area (Brodmann's areas 18 and 19).

Primary Visual Area (Area 17)

The primary visual area occupies the walls of the deep calcarine sulcus on the medial surface of the hemisphere and extends onto the cortex above and below the sulcus (Fig. 13-10). It extends posteriorly as far as the occipital pole, and a small portion of the variable size extends onto the posterolateral aspect of the pole. Anteriorly, the area extends forward above the calcarine sulcus as far as the parieto-occipital sulcus; below the calcarine sulcus, it extends forward a little farther.

On sectioning a fresh brain, the primary visual cortex can be recognized by its thinness and the characteristic presence of a white line or stria (of Gennari) in the gray matter (hence the term *striate cortex*) (Fig. 13-11). The white line is formed in the fourth layer of the cortex by the presence of myelinated fibers from the optic radiation and association fibers.

Histologically, the visual cortex is of a granular type, with only a few pyramidal cells being present. Although the cortex is thinner (1.5 mm) than other cortical regions, the cell population is greater, the intercellular spaces being reduced. The general structure of the visual cortex resembles the primary sensory cortex in having six layers (this is summarized in Fig. 13-11). The cells in laminae II and III project to the secondary visual area (areas 18 and 19). The cells of lamina V project to the superior colliculus; those of lamina VI, to the lateral geniculate body.

The primary visual cortex receives afferent fibers from the lateral geniculate body via the optic radiation (Fig. 13-12). The cortex receives fibers from the temporal half of the ipsilateral retina and the nasal half of the contralateral retina. The right half of the field of vision, therefore, is represented in the visual cortex of the left cerebral hemisphere, and vice versa. It is important to note that the superior retinal quadrants (inferior field of vision) pass to the superior wall of the calcarine sulcus, while the inferior retinal quadrants (superior field of vision)

Figure 13-10

Diagrams showing the primary and secondary areas of the visual cortex. Note the position of the frontal eye field.

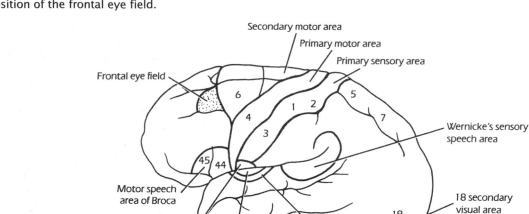

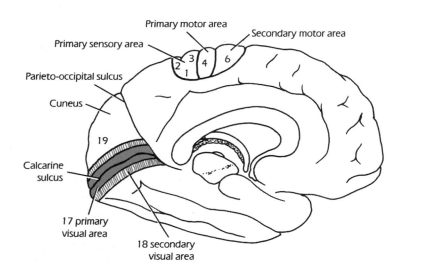

pass to the inferior wall of the calcarine sulcus. The macula lutea, which is the central area of the retina and the area for most perfect vision, is represented on the cortex in the posterior part of area 17 and accounts for one-third of the visual cortex. The peripheral parts of the retina are represented more anteriorly.

Secondary Visual Area (Areas 18 and 19)

The secondary visual areas surround the primary visual area on the medial and lateral surfaces of the hemisphere (Fig. 13-10). These areas are nonstriate and

Figure 13-11

Diagrams showing the structure of the primary motor cortex, the primary visual cortex (area 17), and the secondary visual cortex (area 18).

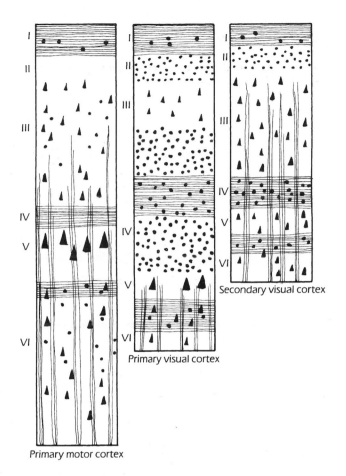

Secondary visual cortex

Primary visual cortex

Primary motor cortex

histologically show the usual six layers. The secondary association areas receive afferent fibers from the primary visual area (area 17) and other cortical areas, as well as from the thalamus. The function of the secondary visual areas is to relate the visual information received by the primary visual area to past visual experiences, thus enabling the individual to recognize and appreciate what he or she is seeing.

Area 18 also integrates the two halves of the visual fields by means of commissural fibers that cross the midline in the splenium of the corpus callosum. It is possible that area 18 is involved in sensory-motor eye coordination and is linked to the frontal eye field. Area 18 may also be linked by descending pathways to the cranial nerve nuclei controlling the extraocular muscles and be involved with smooth pursuit of visual targets.

Blood Supply

The visual cortex is supplied by the posterior cerebral artery. At the anterior end of the calcarine sulcus the middle cerebral artery may assist (Fig. 13-7). A further anastomosis between the posterior and middle cerebral arteries may exist on the lateral surface near the posterior pole.

Figure 13-12

The visual pathway viewed from below. Note that the inserts show the left and right primary cortices on the medial surface of the cerebral hemispheres.

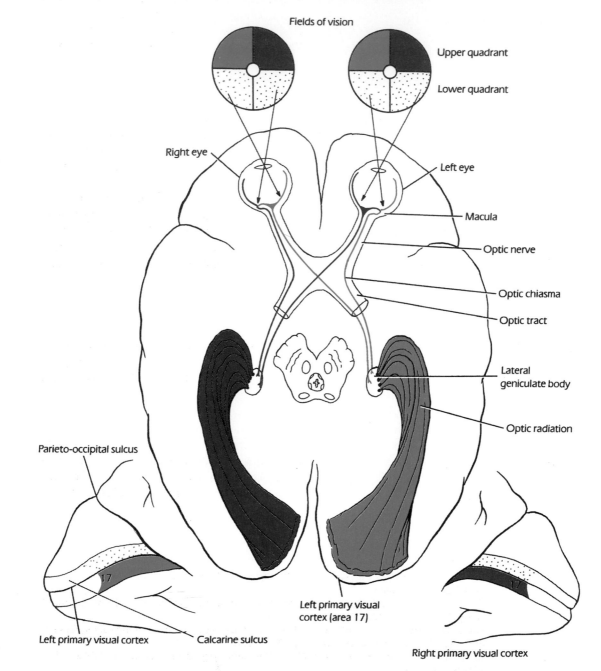

Fields of vision

Upper quadrant

Lower quadrant

Right eye

Left eye

Macula

Optic nerve

Optic chiasma

Optic tract

Lateral geniculate body

Optic radiation

Parieto-occipital sulcus

Left primary visual cortex (area 17)

Left primary visual cortex

Calcarine sulcus

Right primary visual cortex

Overview of the Retinotopic Organization of the Visual Pathway · · · · · · · · · · ·

This section is intended to be read only by those seeking a detailed knowledge of the visual pathways. The pathway taken by visual stimuli from the retina to the visual cortex has been ascertained as the result of a vast amount of research carried out on both animals and humans. Readers who are interested in pursuing this information in depth should consult the works of Polyak (1957), Graybiel (1975), and Hubel, Wiesel, and LeVay (1977). Extensive accounts are also given by Crosby et al. (1962), and Miller (1985).* A brief overview will be given here.

Retina

The visual fields are represented on the retina in a direct point-to-point relationship (Fig. 13-13). Because of the physics of the optical system of the eye, the temporal field is projected on the nasal retina and the nasal field on the temporal retina. In the same way, the superior field is projected on the inferior retina and the inferior field on the superior retina.

The nerve fibers from the ganglion cells converge toward the optic disc from all parts of the retina. On the nasal half of the retina, the fibers are arranged in a simple radial pattern. On the temporal half, the small fibers from the macula forming the papillomacular bundle pass directly to the disc, causing the remaining temporal fibers to pass above and below the macula on their way to the disc.

Optic Nerve

Distal Optic Nerve

The fibers are arranged exactly as in the retina. The most medial fibers are the nasal retinal fibers, and lateral to them are the temporal fibers (Fig. 13-13). The macular fibers, which form about one-third of the optic nerve fibers, are laterally placed in the nerve.

Proximal Optic Nerve

The small macular fibers have now moved medially and have come to occupy the center of the optic nerve (Fig. 13-13). The large nasal retinal fibers remain medial, and the large temporal fibers take up their lateral position. Fibers that originate in the inferior and superior retina remain, respectively, inferior and superior in the nerve.

*Crosby, E. C., Humphrey, T., and Lauer, E. W. *Correlative Anatomy of the Nervous System*. New York: Macmillan, 1962.

Graybiel, A. M. Anatomical organization of retinotectal afferents in the cat: An autoradiographic study. *Brain Res.* (96), 1975, 1–23.

Hubel, D. H., Wiesel, T. N., and LeVay, S. Plasticity of ocular dominance columns in monkey striate cortex. *Philos. Trans. R. Soc. Lond. B.* (278), 1977, 131.

Miller, N. R. *Walsh and Hoyt's Clinical Neuro-Ophthalmology* (4th ed.). Baltimore: Williams & Wilkins, 1985. Vol. 1.

Polyak, S. *The Vertebrate Visual System*. Chicago: University of Chicago Press, 1957.

Figure 13-13

The visual pathways, showing the detailed arrangement of the nerve fibers in relation to the visual fields and the quadrants of the retinae and the visual cortices.

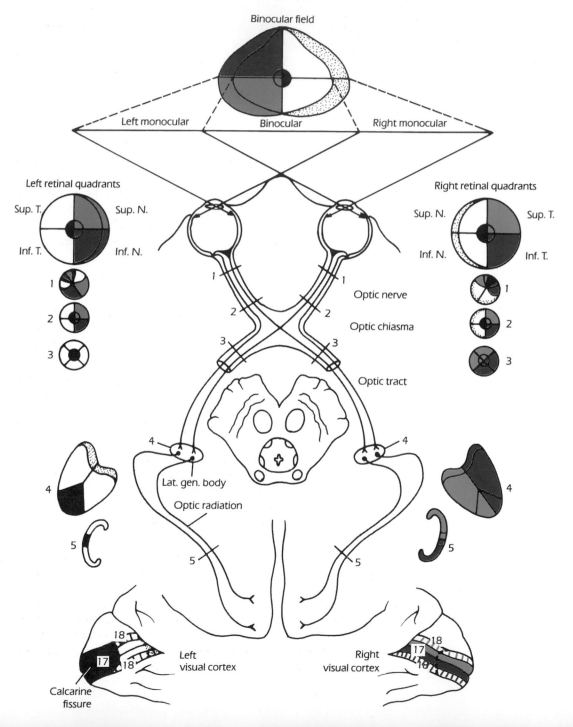

Optic Chiasma

At the optic chiasma the nasal retinal fibers, including those from the nasal half of the macula, cross the midline and enter the contralateral optic tract. The temporal retinal fibers enter the ipsilateral tract (Fig. 13-13). The crossed fibers tend to loop for a short distance into the ipsilateral optic tract before crossing in the chiasma or they go into the contralateral optic nerve for a short distance after they cross in the chiasma.

The macular retinal fibers that cross the midline do so posteriorly in the chiasma. In fact, the macular fibers and those from the perimacular region occupy the greater part of the central region of the chiasma.

Optic Tract

As the optic tract proceeds posteriorly, it undergoes a 90-degree inward twist, so that the fibers from the upper retinal quadrants pass to its medial side and those from the lower retinal quadrants pass to its lateral side (Fig. 13-13). It is in the optic tracts that nerve fibers from corresponding functional parts of each retina become associated. The nerve fibers from the superior nasal retina on one side become associated with uncrossed superior temporal retinal fibers of the other side, and inferior nasal retinal fibers become related to uncrossed inferior temporal retinal fibers.

Lateral Geniculate Body

In the lateral geniculate body the peripheral retinal fibers end in the anterior part, the upper retinal quadrants ending medially, the lower ones laterally (Fig. 13-13). The macular fibers end in the center and posterior part of the nucleus (Fig. 13-9). The temporal uncrossed retinal fibers synapse in layers 2, 3, and 5, while the nasal crossed retinal fibers synapse in layers 1, 4, and 6. It is thus seen that the uncrossed and crossed retinal fibers do not end by synapsing with neurons in the same laminae. However, fibers from corresponding functional parts of the two retinal parts end in neurons situated in neighboring parts of adjacent laminae.

Each retinal ganglion cell fiber, on entering its lamina in the lateral geniculate body, divides into five or six terminal branches. Each branch then synapses with a single geniculate neuron in that lamina. One geniculate neuron may, however, synapse with more than one incoming retinal fiber. Multiple connector neurons have been shown to unite genicular cells in a single lamina, and others have been shown to unite cells in different laminae. It should be emphasized that a single geniculate neuron does not receive afferent retinal fibers from both eyes. However, the connector neurons might bring about connections between bilateral retinal afferents.

The lateral geniculate body should not be regarded as a simple relay center. Evidence is accumulating that the incoming retinal pathway, although the main pathway, is probably influenced by corticofugal fibers that arise from the visual cortex. The presence of the many connector neurons mentioned above suggests that the lateral geniculate body may have an integrative function.

Optic Radiation and the Visual Cortex

The optic radiation is made up of nerve fibers that arise from nerve cells in the lateral and medial portions of the lateral geniculate body (Fig. 13-13). The lateral fibers are the projection of the homonymous inferior retinal quadrants and terminate on the inferior wall of the calcarine sulcus and the adjacent surface cortex of the primary visual area. The medial fibers are the projection of the homonymous superior retinal quadrants and terminate on the superior wall of the calcarine sulcus and the adjacent surface cortex of the primary visual area.

Other Areas of the Cerebral Cortex Associated with Sight · · · · · · · · · · · · · · ·

Occipital Eye Field

The occipital eye field is thought to exist in the secondary visual area in humans (Fig. 13-10). Stimulation produces conjugate deviation of the eyes, especially to the opposite side. The function of the eye field is believed to be reflex and associated with smooth movements of the eye when it is following an object (pursuit movement). The occipital eye fields of both hemispheres are connected through the corpus callosum by nervous pathways, and are also thought to be connected to the superior colliculus. By contrast, the frontal eye field controls voluntary fast eye movements (saccades) and is independent of visual stimuli.

Frontal Eye Field

The frontal eye field (Fig. 13-10) extends forward from the facial area of the precentral gyrus into the middle frontal gyrus (parts of Brodmann's areas 6, 8, and 9). Electrical stimulation of this region causes conjugate movements of the eyes, usually toward the opposite side. The exact pathway taken by nerve fibers from this area is not known, but they are thought to pass to the superior colliculus of the midbrain (Fig. 13-14). The superior colliculus is connected to the nuclei of the extraocular muscles by the tectobulbar tract and the reticular formation. As stated previously, the frontal eye field is considered to control voluntary saccades and is independent of visual stimuli.

Sensory Speech Area of Wernicke

This speech area is localized in the left dominant hemisphere, mainly in the superior temporal gyrus, with extensions around the posterior end of the lateral sulcus into the parietal region (Fig. 13-15). Wernicke's area is connected to Broca's area by a bundle of nerve fibers called the *arcuate fasciculus*. It receives fibers from the visual cortex in the occipital lobe and the auditory cortex in the superior temporal gyrus. Wernicke's area permits the understanding of written and spoken language and enables a person to read a sentence, understand it, and say it out loud (Fig. 13-15).

Figure 13-14

Diagram showing the nervous pathways involved in the visual body reflex.

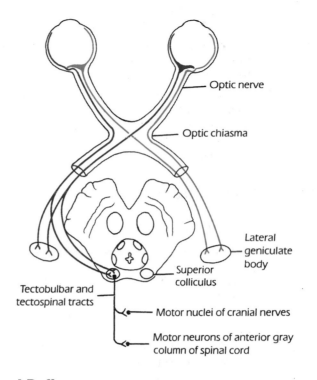

Optic nerve

Optic chiasma

Lateral geniculate body

Superior colliculus

Tectobulbar and tectospinal tracts

Motor nuclei of cranial nerves

Motor neurons of anterior gray column of spinal cord

The Visual Pathway and Visual Reflexes

Direct and Consensual Light Reflexes

These reflexes have been fully discussed in Chapter 12 (see p. 370). It should be noted that the afferent impulses travel through the optic nerve, optic chiasma, and optic tract (Fig. 13-16). Here a small number of fibers leave the optic tract and travel in the superior brachium to synapse on nerve cells in the pretectal nucleus, which lies close to the superior colliculus. The impulses are passed by axons of the pretectal nerve cells to the parasympathetic nuclei (Edinger-Westphal nuclei) of the third cranial nerve on both sides. The further course of this reflex arc to the constrictor pupillae is described on page 370.

Accommodation Reflex

This reflex is described in some detail in Chapter 12, page 370. The afferent impulses travel through the optic nerve, the optic chiasma, the optic tract, the lateral geniculate body, and the optic radiation to the visual cortex. Here it is believed that stereoscopic analysis of the object takes place in the visual association cortex (secondary visual area) (Fig. 13-16). The visual cortex is thought to be connected to the eye field of the frontal cortex. From here, cortical fibers are believed to descend through the internal capsule to the oculomotor nuclei in the midbrain. The further course of the reflex through the oculomotor nuclei to the medial rectus muscles, the ciliary muscle, and the constrictor pupillae muscle is described on page 370.

Figure 13-15

Diagram showing the probable nervous pathways involved in reading a sentence and repeating it aloud.

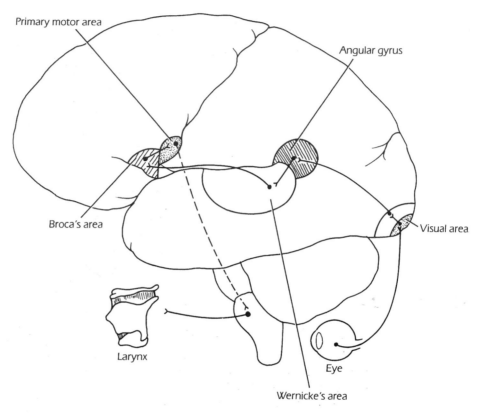

Primary motor area

Angular gyrus

Broca's area

Visual area

Larynx

Eye

Wernicke's area

Visual Body Reflexes

The automatic scanning movements of the eyes and head made when one is reading, the automatic movement of the eyes, head, and neck toward the source of a visual stimulus, and the protective closing of the eyes and even the raising of the arm for protection are reflex actions that involve the following reflex arcs (Fig. 13-14). The visual impulses follow the optic nerves, optic chiasma, and optic tracts to the superior colliculi. Here the impulses are relayed to the tectobulbar and tectospinal tracts to the cranial nerve motor nuclei and the neurons of the anterior gray columns of the spinal cord.

 Clinical Notes

General Observations

Vision begins with the formation of a focused image on the retina. The light patterns are absorbed by the photoreceptor cells, which activate complex connections between the horizontal cells, the amacrine cells, and the bipolar cells. The information converges on the final common pathway, the ganglion cells and

Figure 13-16

The optic pathway and the visual reflexes.

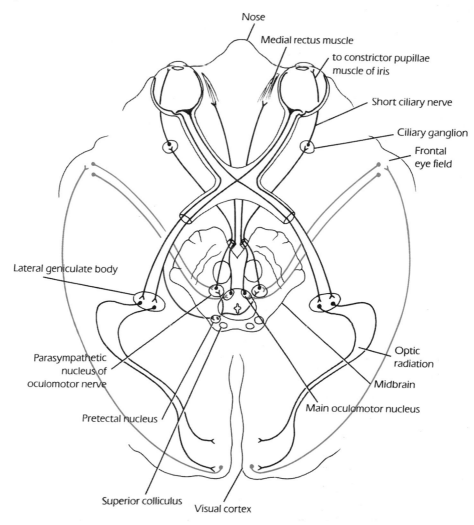

their axons that leave the eye. The retina is in fact a peripheral transducer that converts patterns of light energy into electrical nerve signals that are conducted via the visual pathway to the cerebral cortex for analysis.

Again it should be emphasized that the visual pathway is part of the central nervous system, and that the optic nerves, optic chiasma, and optic tracts are extensions of the white matter. In the central nervous system the simplest form of sensory pathway, from the sensory nerve ending to the cerebral cortex, involves three neurons (Fig. 13-17). For example, in discriminating touch, vibratory sense, and conscious muscle joint sense, the first-order neuron is in the posterior root ganglion, the second-order neuron is in the cuneate and gracile nuclei, and

Figure 13-17

Diagrams illustrating (A) the three-neuron sensory pathway for discriminative touch, vibratory sense, and conscious muscle joint sense, compared with (B) the three-neuron optic pathway. Note the similarities in the two pathways.

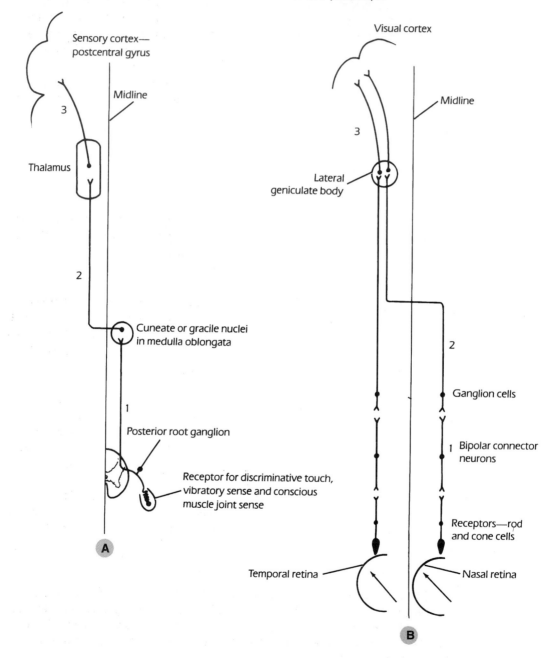

the third-order neuron is in the ventral posterolateral nucleus of the thalamus of the opposite side. The third-order neuron projects to the postcentral gyrus of the opposite side.

In the optic pathway, the first-order neuron is the bipolar connected neuron in the retina, the second-order neuron is the ganglion cell of the retina, and the third-order neuron is in the lateral geniculate body. These neurons project to the calcarine visual cortex. As in the other sensory pathways, the cortex of the cerebral hemisphere is concerned with the afferent information reaching the body from the opposite side, that is, in this case the opposite field of vision.

Because the optic nerve, optic chiasma, and optic radiation are identical to white matter, it follows that, like white matter, they have no powers of regeneration. The only part of the optic pathway that is equivalent to a peripheral nerve is the bipolar neuron in the retina. It would be interesting to know whether these neurons have regenerative powers similar to those of a peripheral nerve.

Optic Disc and Nerve Head

Epipapillary Membranes

Remnants of the hyaloid artery, including its supporting sheath, may persist as semitransparent, veil-like flat membranes overlying the surface of the optic disc. The diagnosis can be made with the ophthalmoscope.

Anomalies in Shape and Excavation of the Optic Disc

Small variations in shape, such as oval rather than round, are common and are of no clinical significance. A slight depression in the center of the disc is normal when it does not extend to the edge of the disc. A pathologic excavation due to glaucoma may extend to the disc edge. In a normal individual, the depression (cup)-to-disc ratio is about 0.2 : 0.5.

Myelination Anterior to the Lamina Cribrosa

Myelination of the anterior part of the optic pathway begins during fetal life, starting at the lateral geniculate body and progressing forward through the optic tracts, the optic chiasma, and finally the optic nerves. Myelination reaches the posterior aspect of the lamina cribrosa shortly after birth. Myelination does not occur anterior to the lamina cribrosa.

Very occasionally, oligodendrocytes extend forward into the retina during development and bring about abnormal myelination in the axons of the ganglion cells around the optic disc. Because myelin is opaque to light, this area of the retina is nonfunctional and the individual has an enlarged blind spot.

Cilioretinal Arteries

The presence of cilioretinal arteries arising from the short ciliary arteries and coursing over the temporal border of the disc to supply the papillomacular bundle has already been noted (see p. 189). If a patient possesses these arteries, they may provide an adequate blood supply to the macular region in occlusion of the central retinal artery.

Papilledema

Bilateral papilledema due to raised intracranial pressure has been fully discussed elsewhere. The raised pressure extends along the outside of the optic nerve in the tubular extension of the subarachnoid space. This causes the lamina cribrosa to bulge forward. In addition, the central vein of the retina, which crosses the subarachnoid space to enter the optic nerve, is compressed, causing congestion of the retinal veins and edema of the optic nerve head. Normally, the intraocular pressure on the optic nerve head is much greater than the cerebrospinal fluid pressure behind the lamina cribrosa. A rise in cerebrospinal fluid pressure can impede axoplasmic flow in the retrobulbar portion of the optic nerve. Persistent papilledema leads to optic atrophy.

Unilateral papilledema results from a large number of diseases, including inflammation and vascular and degenerative conditions.

Optic Nerve

Central Retinal Artery Occlusion

Complete or partial central artery occlusions most commonly occur at the level of the lamina cribrosa just before the artery enters the retina. Here, the central artery has the structure of a medium-sized artery and is subject to atherosclerosis (see also p. 192).

Blood Supply of the Optic Nerve

The major blood supply to the head of the optic nerve at the lamina cribrosa and the retrolaminar region is via the short posterior ciliary arteries to the pial plexus and the formation of the incomplete circle of Zinn (see also p. 282).

Trauma to the Optic Nerve

Although the meninges around the optic nerve are attached to the periosteal layer of dura within the optic canal at the apex of the orbital cavity, the fixed nerve is rarely damaged. This is probably due to the fact that the nerve is slightly S-curved and is not taut as it lies within the orbital fat. Injuries to the orbital walls, excessive movements during trauma to the eye or during orbital operations, and extreme exophthalmos rarely cause nerve injury.

Retrobulbar Neuritis and Sinus Infection

Only a thin plate of bone separates the optic nerve and its meningeal sheaths from the sphenoidal and posterior ethmoidal air sinuses as they pass through the optic canal. A spread of infection at this site could cause optic neuritis.

Optic Nerve Tumors

Gliomas of the optic nerve usually occur during the first decade of life and are often associated with von Recklinghausen's disease. Meningiomas of the meningeal sheaths covering the optic nerve also occur.

The removal of optic nerve tumors is commonly performed from the medial side via *medial orbitotomy*. This avoids the ciliary ganglion that is very small and located on the lateral side of the optic nerve.

Optic Chiasma

The close relationship of the optic chiasma with the diaphragma sellae and the hypophysis cerebri has been emphasized. Pituitary enlargement may exert pressure on the inferior part of the chiasma, causing damage to the nerve fibers from the inferior nasal portion of the retinae. The first signs and symptoms may be a superior bitemporal hemianopia. Later with the involvement of the nerve fibers from the superior nasal portion of the retinae which cross in the superior part of the chiasma, a superior and inferior bitemporal hemianopia would occur.

Lesions of the Visual Pathway

Lesions of the optic pathway may have many pathologic causes. Expanding tumors of the brain and neighboring structures, such as the pituitary and meninges, and cerebrovascular accidents are commonly responsible (Fig. 13-18). The

Figure 13-18

(A) Axial (horizontal) PET scan of a 62-year-old man with a malignant glioma in the left parietal lobe, following the injection of 18-fluorodeoxyglucose. A high concentration of the compound (circular yellow area) is seen in the region of the tumor. (B) Coronal PET scan of the same patient. The large size of the expanding tumor exerted pressure on the visual pathway. (Courtesy of Dr. Holley Dey.)

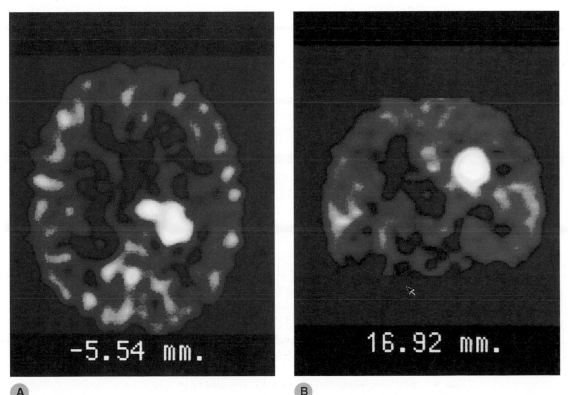

A   B

most widespread effects on vision occur where the nerve fibers of the visual pathway are tightly packed together, such as in the optic nerve or the optic tract.

Optic Nerve

Complete section of one optic nerve produces total blindness of that eye (Fig. 13-19). The pupil will not react to light directly but does so consensually. (The pretectal nucleus of the other side sends axons to parasympathetic nuclei of both oculomotor nerves.) The sight of the other eye is normal; the pupil reacts to light directly, but not consensually. The pupil on the injured side will constrict on accommodation.

If the optic nerve is sectioned close to its entrance to the optic chiasma, the fibers from the opposite optic nerve that loop forward within the optic nerve will also be sectioned. Thus, a section at this site will affect both optic fields.

Optic Chiasma

Sagittal section of the optic chiasma will produce bitemporal hemianopia (Fig. 13-19). The reason for this is that the fibers originating in the nasal halves of both retinae are sectioned. The pupils react normally to the direct light reflex, the consensual light reflex, and the accommodation reflex, provided that the light falls on the temporal retinae.

Lateral section of the optic chiasma on one side divides the fibers originating from the temporal retina on that side, producing nasal hemianopia. Of course lateral section on both sides divides the fibers originating from both temporal retinae, producing binasal hemianopia.

Optic Tracts

Division of the optic tract on one side will result in contralateral homonymous hemianopia (Fig. 13-19). If the right optic tract is divided, for example, a left temporal hemianopia and right nasal hemianopia will occur. The pupils react normally to the direct light reflex, the consensual light reflex, and the accommodation reflex, provided that the light falls on the seeing part of the retina.

Lateral Geniculate Body

Destruction of the lateral geniculate body produces contralateral homonymous hemianopia. The pupils react normally to the direct light reflex, the consensual light reflex, and the accommodation reflex, as stated above.

Optic Radiation

Destruction of the optic radiation produces contralateral homonymous hemianopia (Fig. 13-19). Here, again, the pupils react normally to reflex stimulation.

Nerve fibers arising from the lateral portions of the lateral geniculate body, receiving impulses from the inferior retinal quadrants (superior visual field) that fan out forward and laterally around the temporal horn of the lateral ventricle, if sectioned produce a superior quadrantic hemianopia. Lesions in the nerve fibers passing more directly posterior to the cortex cause an inferior quadrantic hemianopia.

Figure 13-19

Visual field defects associated with lesions of the optic pathways.
1. Right-sided circumferential blindness due to retrobulbar neuritis
2. Total blindness of right eye due to division of right optic nerve
3. Right nasal hemianopia due to partial lesion of right side of optic chiasma
4. Bitemporal hemianopia due to complete lesion of optic chiasma
5. Left temporal hemianopia and right nasal hemianopia due to lesion of right optic tract
6. Left temporal and right nasal hemianopia due to lesion of right optic radiation
7. Left temporal and right nasal hemianopia due to lesion of right visual cortex

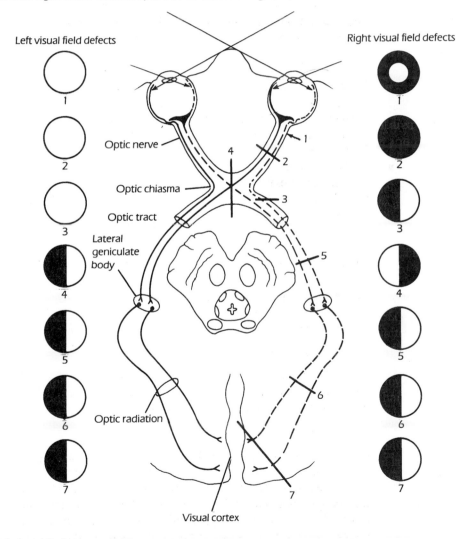

Lesions of the visual pathway, as it is coursing posteriorly in the posterior limb of the internal capsule, may also be associated with lesions of the general sensory and motor pathways lying within the capsule. The contralateral homonymous hemianopia is also accompanied by contralateral hemianesthesia and contralateral hemiplegia.

Visual Cortex

Destruction of the primary visual cortex (Fig. 13-19) produces contralateral homonymous hemianopia and the pupils react normally to reflex stimulation. In this condition the macula is often spared if the posterior cerebral artery is blocked by thrombosis. The possible anastomosis between the posterior cerebral and middle cerebral arteries at this site may explain the sparing of the macula.

CHAPTER 13
Clinical Problems

Answers on Page 411.

1 A 33-year-old man entered the Neurology Clinic with a history of eye problems and muscular weakness. Six months previously the patient had complained of a sudden onset of pain with extraocular movements in the right eye associated with a loss of vision in that eye. Examination by an ophthalmologist at that time revealed a central scotoma of the right eye with a loss of color vision; the peripheral fields of vision were normal. Ophthalmoscopic examination of the right eye showed a normal optic disc. The left eye was also normal.

Eight weeks later the patient noted a marked recovery of function. Reexamination by the ophthalmologist showed a residual central scotoma of the right eye, a persistent loss of color vision, and impaired visual acuity. The right optic disc appeared paler than normal, especially on the temporal side.

An extensive neurologic examination during this second visit to the clinic revealed that the patient's right arm and leg were weaker than normal, the weakness being worse in the extensors of the arm and the flexors of the leg. The deep tendon reflexes were hyperactive on the right side and the patient had a positive Babinski sign on that side. There was no evidence of weakness on the left side of his body. The patient experienced no numbness or paresthesia. What is your diagnosis? Why is the right central scotoma associated with color blindness? Why did the right optic disc show indistinct margins and then later paleness on the temporal side?

2 A 45-year-old woman was admitted to the neurosurgery unit with a tumor of the occipital lobe of the right cerebral hemisphere. On examination it was found that

her sight in both eyes was normal. However, when asked to follow a slowly moving object with both eyes, she experienced great difficulty in doing so to the right. When she was asked to look at a fixed object in a particular location, she had pursuit difficulty only to the ipsilateral side. Using your knowledge of neuroanatomy, explain this phenomenon.

3 When examining a patient with increased intracranial pressure, an ophthalmologist asked a fourth-year medical student to explain why the patient had enlargement of the blind spot in both eyes. How would you have answered that question?

4 A 40-year-old woman was operated on for a meningioma involving the lesser wing of the sphenoid bone and the optic canal on the right side. Ophthalmologic examination had revealed a right-sided visual loss and optic atrophy. Just before the operation it was noted that the patient had contralateral papilledema. Explain these signs and symptoms.

5 A 30-year-old man with a cerebral tumor involving both occipital lobes was found on examination to have a visual object agnosia, agnosia for colors, and an inability to remember the name of familiar household objects. Which part of the brain is not functioning in this patient?

6 A 68-year-old woman complained of sudden blindness in her left eye. She said she could see normally with her right eye. On examination it was found that she had left homonymous hemianopia. Was this patient in fact totally blind in her left eye, and was her right eye completely normal?

7 Lesions have to occur at two sites on the visual pathway to produce bilateral whole field loss. The lesions may involve both retinae, both optic nerves, both optic tracts, both radiations, or both visual cortices. Can you give the site of a single vascular lesion that could produce the same defect?

8 A 54-year-old man examined by an ophthalmologist was found to have a bitemporal hemianopia. Radiologic and biochemical examinations showed the pituitary gland to be of normal size and function. Can you name any other anatomic structure that, if enlarged, might press on the optic chiasma?

9 An 80-year-old woman was admitted to a hospital with a left posterior cerebral artery infarction. An MRI revealed that the artery was blocked near its distal end. On admission it was found that the patient had a right-sided homonymous hemianopia and receptive dysphasia and memory loss. After careful testing of the visual fields, it was found that the macula was spared. Explain the homonymous hemianopia and the sparing of the macula. What is responsible for the receptive dysphasia?

10 A 65-year-old man with hypertension was admitted to a hospital with a left middle cerebral artery infarction. The patient's eyes were deviated to the left and there was spastic hemiparesis on the right side, especially his right arm. He had a lower right quadrant facial weakness. On his recovering consciousness, the patient was found to have a right-sided homonymous hemianopia. Explain why the patient deviated his eyes to the left. Which part of the visual pathway was probably involved to produce a right-sided homonymous hemianopia? Would the patient have normal pupillary reflexes?

11 A 45-year-old man presented with the classic signs of acromegaly—enlarged, broad, spade-like hands, large feet, and protruding jaws. The patient complained of bitemporal headache that was associated with boring pain behind the eyes. Three days previously, he had noticed an impairment in vision. On attempting to cross the road he was nearly knocked down by a cyclist. A CT scan revealed a large tumor occupying the sella turcica and extending superiorly toward the third ventricle. Explain the boring pain behind his eyes. What might be responsible for his impairment in vision and the near accident involving the cyclist?

12 Bilateral infarction of both visual cortices produces cortical blindness in which the pupillary reflexes are normal. Some patients, although totally blind, may deny that they are blind. Explain this phenomenon.

13 An 8-year-old girl with von Recklinghausen's disease was noted to have subnormal vision in her right eye during a routine screening examination by her school nurse. An ophthalmic examination revealed severe loss of vision in the right eye, reduced color vision, moderate proptosis of the right eye, and papilledema of the right optic nerve. Suggest the location of this child's lesion.

14 A 28-year-old man suffered severe head and neck injuries during a motor vehicle accident. When he regained consciousness in the emergency department, he complained of blindness in his right eye. A CT scan demonstrated a fracture of the lesser wing of the sphenoid involving the optic canal. Explain the blindness that followed this injury.

CHAPTER 13
Answers to Clinical Problems

1 This patient has multiple sclerosis. The symptoms and signs related to the right eye were caused by retrobulbar neuritis. CT scans of the orbits revealed demyelination of the right optic nerve. Color vision is a cone function. The acquired loss of color sense affecting one eye occurs in diseases producing central retinal degeneration or optic nerve disease affecting central retinal function, as in this case.

The optic nerve head appeared normal initially because the optic neuritis was retrobulbar. Later, with glial scarring, the disc became paler than normal. In this patient the paleness was most marked on the temporal side, because the cone fibers leave the eye predominantly on the lateral side to take up their position later in the axial zone of the optic nerve. In this patient the axial zone of the optic nerve was most affected by the myelin degeneration.

2 With a tumor of the right occipital lobe, this patient had difficulty following a slow-moving object because the neoplasm had invaded the area of the cortex known as the occipital eye field. Eye movements on command are interfered with by lesions in the frontal eye field, especially in the dominant hemisphere. This patient had normal eye movements on command.

3 An increase in intracranial cerebrospinal fluid pressure causes bilateral papilledema, the severity of the papilledema usually being proportional to the rise in pressure. The blind spot, which is the area of the retina occupied by the optic disc and devoid of rods and cones, becomes enlarged by edema.

4 In this patient the meningioma had invaded the right optic canal, compressing the optic nerve on that side and producing the right-sided blindness. In addition, the tumor had obliterated the forward extension of the subarachnoid space around the right optic nerve. The tumor had also encroached on the intracranial cavity, raising the cerebrospinal fluid pressure; hence, the papilledema on the left side. This condition exemplifies Foster Kennedy syndrome.

5 Recognition of the names of objects, colors, and household objects requires normal function of the visual association cortex, areas 18 and 19. It is here that past visual experiences are stored.

6 Patients are often confused about loss of sight in one or the other eye. For this reason it is very important to test the fields of vision in both eyes. This patient was found to have left homonymous hemianopia, which meant that the right temporal retina and the left nasal retina were not functioning. The right nasal retina and the left temporal retina were normal. Subsequently she was found to have a lesion of the right optic tract.

7 A basilar artery occlusion produces bilateral whole field loss. The basilar artery gives origin to the posterior cerebral artery on each side. The posterior cerebral artery supplies the lateral geniculate body, the optic radiation, and the visual cortex.

8 In addition to the pituitary, the optic chiasma is closely related to the anterior communicating artery, the terminal portion of the internal carotid artery, and the dura and arachnoid. Aneurysms of these arteries and meningiomas may press on the chiasma, producing visual defects.

9 The homonymous hemianopia was right-sided because of a lesion in the left visual cortex. This meant the left temporal retina and the right nasal retina were not functioning. The macular area of the visual cortex is situated at the posterior pole of the occipital lobe, a site where the posterior cerebral and middle cerebral arteries anastomose. In some patients the contribution from the middle cerebral artery is sufficient to spare the macula. The receptive dysphasia was caused by the infarction occurring in the left dominant hemisphere with disruption of the nerve fibers connecting the visual cortex with Wernicke's area.

10 The patient deviated his eyes to the side of the lesion. Electrical stimulation of the frontal eye field usually causes conjugate deviation of the eyes to the opposite side. However, destruction of this area of the frontal cortex causes the eyes to look toward the side of the lesion. The left middle cerebral artery supplies the left frontal eye field; thus, this patient deviated his eyes to the left side.

The left middle cerebral artery supplies the left optic radiation. An infarction of the left optic radiation produces a right-sided homonymous hemianopia. The patient has normal light and accommodation reflexes because the pathways do not involve the optic radiation (see p. 370).

11 Later, at operation, this patient was found to have a chromaphobe adenoma of the anterior lobe of the pituitary. The slow, insidious expansion of the tumor caused pressure on the neighboring bone,

producing the boring pain behind the eyes and the bitemporal headache. In this patient the tumor had been pressing on the optic chiasma, producing bitemporal hemianopia. The loss of the temporal fields of vision was responsible for the near accident with the cyclist.

12 Bilateral destruction of visual association areas 18 and 19 may produce anosognosia of blindness or denial of blindness. This is termed Anton's syndrome. The basic cause of this condition is not known.

13 Optic nerve gliomas occur often in children with von Recklinghausen's disease. The tumor is usually confined to the intraorbital portion of the optic nerve but may spread through the optic canal to the optic chiasma and the brain. Children do not notice the gradual loss of vision because they compensate with their other eye. As the tumor enlarges, it can push the globe forward, causing proptosis. In addition, the direct pressure on the optic nerve will initially manifest as papilledema and later as optic nerve atrophy.

14 Traumatic optic neuropathy is a diagnosis made by exclusion. Following blunt trauma, decreased vision and an afferent pupillary defect may occur. When other causes of visual loss such as retinal vascular infarction are ruled out, the diagnosis of optic neuropathy is made. The etiology may be that a bony spicule from the fractured wall of the optic canal impinges on the optic nerve or there may be contusion of the optic nerve and its delicate pial blood vessels. Treatment includes surgery to remove the bone pressure at the optic canal, the administration of corticosteroids to reduce the fibrous reaction in the meningeal sheaths of the optic nerve, or both.

Index

Note: Page numbers with an *f* indicate figures; those with a *t* indicate tables.